AN ALZHEIMER'S
LOVE STORY

Robert John McAllister, M.D., Ph.D.

authorHOUSE®

AuthorHouse™
1663 Liberty Drive
Bloomington, IN 47403
www.authorhouse.com
Phone: 1-800-839-8640

Published by AuthorHouse   06/06/2012

ISBN: 978-1-4685-8800-2 (sc)
ISBN: 978-1-4685-8798-2 (hc)
ISBN: 978-1-4685-8799-9 (e)

Library of Congress Control Number: 2012907207

Contents

To Jane

To All Alzheimer's Patients

To All Their caregivers

May They Find Peace

ACKNOWLEDGMENTS

My gratitude to Harriet Lerner for her encouragement, enthusiastic support and helpful suggestions.

I am indebted to Sara Rubloff LCSW-C and Dennis Mauro-Huse, my good friends and colleagues, for their diligent reading of the manuscript, for their valuable insights and their enthusiastic support for the work.

My heartfelt thanks to Laura, Kathie, and Paul, our children, for their ready availability and stablizing support during the time of this story.

My love and gratitude to Jane for her resolute spirit, her courage and determination, and her continuing concern and love for "Robbie."

Finally, I thank God every day for the gift of Jane in my life, for the day we met, for the day she departed and all the days in between.

PREFACE

This book is a detailed account of what transpired between my wife, as Alzheimer's patient, and myself, as caregiver over a period of five years, three months. Jane was first diagnosed as having Alzheimer's in 2004. She was 74 and I was 85.

It is now obvious there were signs of the illness going back at least two or three years before that time. The signs became more prominent when we moved from a fairly large three-bedroom house to a two-bedroom apartment in a retirement facility. Although the distance was only a few miles, it brought us into a strange world where uncertain pathways and unexpected events gradually surrounded us and clouded our view of life and threatened our retirement years.

Despite my being a psychiatrist, we essentially had no information about Alzheimer's when the diagnosis was made. It must have taken a year or two before we began to think seriously about the meaning of the diagnosis. I got a number of books on the subject and read them with doubt and apprehension. I didn't want to think my wife's illness would be as predetermined as my reading suggested. On the other hand, I developed a need to look more closely at what was going on and not dismiss it cavalierly.

The need to look *more closely* brought me in December of 2006 to begin to write a journal about what was happening in our life. I did this for Jane's sake and for my own. As you'll see in the following pages we remained committed to talking openly about the process of this disease no matter how devastating its consequences. And while experts can chart the general course of the illness, each person's experience is unique, as was the journey Jane and I travelled together.

Perhaps, too, writing gave me a small sense of control over a disease that reminded me everyday of what Jane and I could not control. Through writing I came to new understandings of how Jane's mind was working, which allowed me to help her separate out the disease process from the "essential Jane." This is the Jane I describe in the kinder, calmer times: gentle, bright, affectionate, creative, quick-witted, full of life and love. That Jane was always there but often unseen, unheard and unrecognizable, hidden in the darkness and the fury of Alzheimer's emotional storms.

I feel fortunate to have remained in good health long enough to be Jane's caregiver until the end. I was 92 at the time of her death. There might have come a day when I could not have kept my repeated pledge to take care of her for as long as she lived. The caregivers of the world must never be criticized for what they are unable to do. None of us knows what our limits are until we reach them, and when we reach them it is time to stop. Then guilt is inappropriate; forgiveness is unnecessary.

The strength and force of the love Jane and I shared, and the depth and vitality of our faith in God were the two pillars that kept us together and enabled us to maintain our life and our bond through the Alzheimer's years. I was blessed to be her caregiver until the end. It gave me the opportunity to love her more fully, more unselfishly, and to return to her the gift which she had been to me from the day we first met.

Jane and I had fifty years together, following unhappy first marriages for both of us. We believed our meeting was providential, our love was extraordinary, our life was wonderfully fulfilling.

Jane died on February 23rd, 2012. Our Alzheimer's life is over. The story is finished. The details of her death close the book as they have closed my eyes to her beauty, my lips to her kiss, my arms to her embrace, my life to her bodily presence.

AN ALZHEIMER'S LOVE STORY

The following pages contain notes written during the years my wife, Jane, had Alzheimer's. Signs of the illness began in the fall of 2003. At that time, we moved to a Continuous Care Retirement Community in Columbia, Maryland. It was a few miles from where we lived the ten prior years. Jane could not remember our new address or phone number. She failed to recognize familiar scenes in the surrounding area. She would focus on select issues with an unusual tenacity and belligerency. On occasion, she lost her way driving.

Jane and I met in 1961. We were both in difficult first marriages. Jane was divorced in 1965 from Tom and I was divorced in 1966 from Marguerite. We were married that same year. We initially lived in Reno, Nevada, where I was Superintendent of the Nevada State Hospital. I am a psychiatrist. Jane worked in retail for a short period and later worked as a model at Nordstrom in Spokane, Washington.

Laura is our only child, divorced mother of Casey and Tara, often referred to as "the girls." Phil, Kathie, and Bonnie are Jane's children by her first marriage. Frances, Bob, John, Paul, and Patricia are my children by my first marriage.

Pertinent and contemporaneous excerpts from letters and emails (mostly to the children) are included in modified text. Asterisks indicate withheld material. The majority of the emails are to Laura, our child, or to Kathie, Jane's daughter, or to Paul, my son. The recipients of other emails will be further identified.

Jane became fully aware of her diagnosis when it was made in June 2004. These pages begin in December 2006. They are divided into six month periods. There is no basis for chapter headings; there is only measured time. There are no summaries at the end of chapters because ever-changing material cannot be summarized. There is only the passage of time, the inexorable advance of the illness, and our continuing love story.

PART 1 (DEC 06—MAY 07)

12/18/06

We're going to Laura's for Christmas. Jane began wrapping packages for Casey and Tara this morning. She enjoyed the task in past years and did it easily and well. Today she wrapped two packages and then didn't remember what was in them. She was devastated.

She was completely disheartened by the incident. After lunch she decided to go to bed. She appeared exhausted. I pulled the shades and tucked her in. She said she wanted to get the wrapping perfect because "this might be the last time I'll be able to do it." She may be right. In desperation she asks, "What are we going to do?" I tell her we'll do the best we can. What else can I say? I offered to sit in the bedroom and read as I sometimes do but she declined. We both cried a little and I left to do other things.

Jane is anxious to see Laura and the girls. She talked about it for weeks and worries about having enough time there. We will go on Saturday, 12/23. Jane proposed an earlier day but Laura and I agreed if we went too early, Jane might not make it through Christmas. Laura and I know the need for time limits based on previous experience.

12/28/06

On arrival we expected to have a quiet evening at home with Laura, since the girls were with their father. But Laura had made a reservation for dinner and included her friend, Frank. Dinner went well. We all talked freely and Jane was responsive and cordial.

On Sunday (Christmas Eve) Jane and I went to noon Mass at Our Lady of Mount Carmel in Tenafly, NJ. It was a blessed experience for us both, a sacred time, reverent, and a fine homily highlighting the place of women in the introduction of the Redeemer. We had lunch at the Tenafly diner—Belgian waffles. We returned to the church at 4p.m. for the Christmas service. Laura and Frank and the two children were at their church.

When Jane confronts things these days, she can't manage the whole scene at one time. She described eating the waffle at the diner and how she focused not just on each quarter section but on each individual little square, each with its ration of syrup. For her, life is like the waffle. Even the simplest situation needs to be approached in small digestible parts, and in doing so she is likely to miss the larger picture.

As we went through the ritual of gifts Christmas morning, I could not enter into a festive mood. The children's enthusiasm, Laura and Frank's affection for each other, the Christmas music in the background seemed to intrude into the sanctum of our lives. I watched Jane focus on one portion of "the waffle" or another, trying to digest what she could. I knew much of it was distasteful and would "stick in her craw:" the focus on monetary value, the stores things came from, the lack of personal warmth.

Saving bows and boxes is usually not supervised by a guest. It is an irresistible temptation for Jane. It was a piece of the scene which Jane could neither assimilate nor navigate. Laura knitted Jane a beautiful scarf which pleased her very much, but her later comment was, "I would rather have had some time with Laura just to talk."

Laura spent most of the day in the kitchen preparing an elaborate dinner. It was not a good visiting time. The girls were involved with their electronic gadgets. Jane and I were just "hanging out" or more accurately "hanging on."

By bedtime I suggested to Jane we go home on Wednesday instead of Thursday. She opposed the idea but the next morning she volunteered that Wednesday would be fine. We were all relieved when the visit was over.

Will we go again? No doubt, although I do not look forward to another visit. They are too stressful for Jane. She feels Laura should show more awareness of her illness. She wants to talk about it with Laura "before it's too late." There was never an opportunity.

Jane wants to hold onto those who are dear and feel the strength and solace of their love, **now** not next week or next year. She cannot depend on next week or next year. At Laura's house, I found Jane in the basement "visiting" the dolls of Laura's childhood. She remembered the origin and history of the more significant dolls. It reminded me of how gentle and loving and tender hearted she truly is. Are her children able to see that?

Jane hides behind harsh statements at times and anger from years ago sullies current comments often enough. But she expresses her love openly, verbally, easily and often. She and I voice our love for one another frequently. Now she needs to say it and hear it even oftener. Do the children doubt her sincerity when they hear it said so often?

Jane sometimes voices concern I won't always be able to care for her, but more importantly that I won't always want to care for her. She doubts the permanence of my love when she is despondent. That's not surprising considering the adults and peers of her childhood and young adult years. How can she believe in my lasting love when she never had the experience before? And how can I convince her before the fact?

Something happened the other day that makes me uncomfortable. When we came home from Borders, Jane had an art pencil she said she bought there. She looked for the receipt but couldn't find it. There was no bag. The charge never showed up on our visa bill. I don't know what to think. Jane is an honest woman; but sometimes I think she acts from a part of her brain which I have never known before. Is it just a more primitive part that escapes the control of judgment from time to time? So where will this go? These thoughts come to me in the disturbing hours of wakeful dark.

(Email to Laura 12/30/06)
I have the impression you have very little appreciation for how seriously the Alzheimer's is affecting your mother's thinking and her interacting with others. When she is with someone for a few hours she may seem to be her regular self. She can talk and joke and laugh and enter into the conversation quite well. It is deceiving. She has a hard time tracking what others say, and even if she understands the words the meaning can escape her. When several things are going on, such as the unwrapping of

presents, she cannot follow the whole thing but picks up bits and pieces of it all. She focuses on a small piece and loses the rest.

She says things she doesn't remember saying or she repeats what she just said. She forgets what others say or doesn't remember it correctly. When she is aware of this, it is embarrassing and depressing for her. She lives in constant awareness that her memory, mental acuity, and ability to interact with others are becoming increasingly impaired.

The time for her to "make some changes" is past. Changes are occurring which cannot be stopped and they limit her intellectually and socially. But emotionally they bring anger and sadness and fear, which provoke words and actions that are impulsive and without sense even to her. Understanding, patience, and love are the only real gifts any of us can give her now.

I'm not sure why I wrote all this. It makes me sad to reflect on this lovely, kind, gentle woman who is gradually losing her ability to demonstrate all these qualities that have made her the star in my life. If everyone else loses the ability to recognize who she still is because they never knew who she really was, she will always be my star.

12/31/06

Yesterday I wrote a lengthy e-mail to Laura trying to describe more clearly her mother's condition and gently chiding her for her attitude. Jane read it and approved it. Jane is filled with concerns about Laura. She is convinced we will never hear from Laura again. I suggested we go to Savage Mills Antique Mall and look around. She tried to be cheerful, but I fear the venture was a disappointment to her. Laura was still in her thoughts.

We planned to attend the 4:30p.m. Saturday Mass. When we got home, she was tired. I suggested she lie down and I would go to Mass alone. She readily agreed and remarked about giving up on the church and wondering whether God hears her. I woke her about two hours later and brought her Communion. It was a tender loving moment and I thought God does hear her prayers.

Jane becomes utterly exhausted in stressful situations. Sometimes she is not rested after her usual 10 to 12 hours of sleep. I must acknowledge these periods of sleep provide us both some surcease, although I feel a bit guilty for thinking so. She objects to sleeping because, "I want to be with you and it's lonely when I sleep."

Laura is still on her mind. "We will never hear from her again." When we came back after lunch, there was a message from Laura—pleasant, routine things mentioned. I encouraged Jane to call her back. It went well and was obviously a relief to her.

Jane often hears music when she lies down to nap and at bedtime. She is annoyed when I say I don't hear it. She often asks, "How can this happen? How can I hear music when there isn't any there?" She is irritated when I can't explain it. I say, "It must be due to the medicine you're taking." The music has gradually become less annoying.

This illness is a roller-coaster ride for both of us. It's frightening for her because she doesn't want to be on the ride. I don't like the ride but I want to stay on it to the finish. I don't pray for God to make Jane well. I know God could and God knows I want her to be well. But I will not stake my faith on a miracle and at this point it would be a miracle. I do believe God hears me when I pray I will always be here and able to take care of Jane as long as she is alive. I believe Jane is special in God's eyes, and God wants me to care for her through this awful time.

1/4/07

It is difficult to see Jane struggle with things she did easily a few years ago and now are too much for her. There are unfinished projects around the house, minor ones I am happy she rarely notices . . . a picture she intends to frame, an article she intends to repair, a book she began to read, a shirt that needs a button, a blouse she is going to iron. Does she not notice them or does she just not mention them because she feels so defeated?

The other day she said she felt like she was viewing things outside the car in segments and not taking in the whole scene. That is such an apt description of her current observation and attention responses. I need to be aware of her limited perspective and not flood her with several ideas at the same time, which I tend to do.

We recently looked at book covers because my book will soon be ready for publication. She became interested in a particular cover. As often happens, focus turns to obsession easily and she became irritated that I was not giving her comments the respect and attention they deserved. Reason leaves the scene and emotion rules. Anger, sadness, fear, isolation, disappointment, guilt, abandonment . . . all expressed in turn, and I know not how to respond. It is frustrating and discouraging.

1/5/07

Yesterday was a good day. We spent two and a half hours at the Candlelight restaurant over dinner. Jane was as bright, responsive and wonderful as she has always been. We talked of many things. She philosophized about how people respond to someone who mentions a serious illness. Some say "not to worry, everything will be all right." Others respond with "a pat on the back and feigned cheerful words." I asked what response would help her. She replied, "It is important to acknowledge the sadness of the other person and let that person know it is something you recognize."

I asked if it helps her when I say, "I know you are feeling badly and I wish I could do something to help you." She said it is helpful but sometimes is not enough. Some physical response is needed at times, and I don't always provide it. Touch, physical contact makes her feel less alone. I must remember that and do it more freely.

The evening went wonderfully. We talked and laughed and reminisced. It was like old times. We talked about her attention to small segments of a situation. She remembered few Christmas events at Laura's because she focused on what was happening to the bows and boxes.

Is it a natural response of an Alzheimer's patient to focus on a part of the environment so it remains clear and understandable and in the process the main event is missed or assimilated in a jumbled and distorted way? Does Jane try to compensate for her memory loss by an intense focus on one piece of what she is seeing or hearing? Her poor memory encourages the narrow intensity and the rest is lost.

It was a wonderful evening, overshadowed by the knowledge that this too may be a fleeting moment.

1/15/07
She slept until 11a.m. today. After breakfast she decided to go back to bed. As I was tucking her in, she said the book cover remains on her mind and we need to settle it. I carefully reminded her of our discussion yesterday and said we had agreed on it. She recalled it as I mentioned the details. She seemed reassured.

Jane's fatigue must be discouraging for her. I don't think it is the result of depression primarily, because it comes on suddenly and seems directly related to stress. It is difficult to define "stress" because different things may be involved. We have been going over my book galley. Jane read five chapters on Saturday and completed the last two chapters yesterday She points out word errors and raises excellent questions about content. She is usually correct and I make the changes. I wonder if the mental exertion of attending so carefully to something for so long is exhausting for her.

For two weeks I have marveled at how well she is doing and how easy and enjoyable it is to be with her. At other times I feel I am pulling her along. I must take care not to pull too soon or too quickly or too hard or too obviously. I have to learn her pace of walking, of talking, of thinking, of living. It is hard to remember this when she is doing well.

1/19/07
It was a good day. It was a bad day. It was an every day. How can days be measured when life is separated from the realities we used to know? When times are good, the old reality is closer but never certain. When times are bad, that reality is a memory and one Jane will remember less and less. I want my old Jane back.

The last few days had a sharper edge, an easy loss of patience over an insignificant exchange with me or someone else. We had dinner here with two other couples last evening. Jane had difficulty keeping up with the conversation. Today she said her hearing aids did not work well last night. I said maybe she doesn't hear things as easily when she is tense. She acknowledged the possibility and accepted the explanation.

1/20/07

I woke Jane a little before ten. She was in good spirits. After breakfast I suggested more sleep which she readily accepted. She slept until one this afternoon when I woke her. After lunch she started packing to go to Rehoboth beach tomorrow. After two hours trying to pack she became frustrated and unable to distinguish one thing from another. She became increasingly frantic. I suggested resting for awhile. She agreed. We talked for a few minutes and then she slept. I sat and read for a long time before I left the room.

Before going to sleep she said she was confused and uncertain about herself yesterday when we were at Mass at the monastery. She thought of stepping out in an area between the choir stalls and "dying right there." She looked at the granite tile where she would die. "Everything would be over for me, and you would survive well." I wept and told her how much I needed her. She said her head was full of worries. "Getting ready for the trip brings back so many memories." She gets lost in memories and has a difficult time getting back. Before sleeping she said, "Do you hear the organ music?"

Today she said, "You shouldn't worry. Things will be good sometimes and they will be bad sometimes, and it will go on quite some time before it gets terrible. Then I won't know and won't care but it will be hard on you. I think I've come to terms with it." Has either of us come to terms with this slow deterioration of her magnificent brain?

1/31/07

My book was submitted to the printer yesterday. It is a relief to have it out of the way. We are both pleased with the cover and the format.

The days at the beach went well last week. We went to breakfast at the Boardwalk Plaza the morning of the 24th, Jane's birthday. They would not seat us at a window table because staff planned to work there. Jane was not happy with the arrangement nor was I. We agreed to leave. As we left she went to the front desk complaining rather loudly and strongly. She became angry at me for not being more sympathetic with her position and therefore "not agreeing with her."

This sort of thing happens often. She takes a strong and harsh position about something that happens, and if I do not verbally support her, she becomes angry. I think this occurs for two reasons. First, it makes her feel alone and that is frightening. Second, she often regrets her reaction and recognizes it is excessive. She wants to feel, at least for the moment, her behavior was correct, and my agreement would support that feeling.

She focuses on being "right" or "wrong." If our opinions differ, she sees herself as being "wrong" because I am "always right" or "think I am." It is a recurring issue. We spent most of her birthday resolving our morning conflict. By evening it was over and we enjoyed a "birthday dinner" at the Boardwalk. For the next few days Jane often referred to the incident and expressed regret for how she handled it and "spoiled things" for us.

Since returning home Jane requires more sleep and is more tired. Are these symptoms due to neurological changes or are they simply reactions to getting through the day with cognitive limitations, decreased coping skills, and constant apprehension about the future? To face another day must take a great deal of courage and emotional resilience. And how does one maintain those when cells of the brain are attacked indiscriminately? Is it any wonder Alzheimer's patients undergo mood changes, personality changes?

Yesterday Jane was sad. She worries about who will get her things when she dies. She worries about not recognizing her things or remembering where they came from. She wonders about next Christmas. Will she be here? Will she know others? Will we be able to go to Laura's? She wonders about all kinds of things.

Sometimes I feel guilty about writing these pages and not telling her. We always shared everything and I feel uncomfortable keeping things from her. But reading this would not help her, although we discuss many of these topics and thoughts.

I wonder how to support Jane these days. What can I do to relieve the distress that is so obvious? How should I respond when she talks about her decline? It is hard to find the words, much less the thoughts to express. I have lots of feelings but they only bring me tears and wanting to hold her. She wants to know what is going to happen. "Why can't someone tell me what it will be like? Someone must know. There must be case studies. No one ever knows what to say. Why don't they tell me about it?"

I answer by saying cases vary a great deal and one can have Alzheimer's 2 years or 20 years. We both know that doesn't tell her anything. I point out she has bad periods and good periods and it is unpredictable. I don't mention the one predictable—it will get worse and she will either die of it or with it. She knows that. We don't speak of it directly. She sometimes refers to her death and when she is angry wishes for it soon. I wonder if she has the same wish even when she seems happy.

Today I see her despondency. She struggles to respond, to comment. This can go on for days and then recede, and she will be her usual bright self. Today the cloud envelops her. She was reluctant to get dressed. I never know what to do to brighten her day. Attempts at humor fall short or are taken as serious and become irritating. She commented, "I don't know what the matter is. I don't feel like doing anything except going back to bed." It is a safe haven for her but today the housekeeper comes so she must wait.

I suspect we are both dreading tomorrow . . . especially if she is not feeling better. She is going with her friend, Mary, to a birthday lunch of the pool group. She and Ellen have January birthdays. Then my son, Bob, and Wendy come for dinner, if their plane from Seattle is on time. It will be a long day, an unfortunate arrangement.

Jane just came to the door, completely dressed, and said, "Is it too late to go to church?" I was surprised. It was 11:30 but there was enough time since she was ready. We are going to Mass at the Franciscan Monastery. Mass there is a peaceful and pious experience for us, especially so this morning. The homilist reminded us of how ordinary people in our lives sometimes bring God to us. I thought of how much Jane has helped me become a better person and bridge me to the hereafter.

During lunch I asked Jane to tell me how she got from where she was earlier this morning to where she was in asking to go to Mass. She spoke about it in a studied manner. When I woke her at 10a.m. she felt "down" and did not want to get up. During breakfast she thought of going back to bed. She felt overwhelmed and had a difficult time recognizing objects as she prepared for the day. She couldn't distinguish individual items as she applied her make-up. She felt she was losing ground and feared the future.

I came in to see her and told her we have lots of good times still ahead. I embraced her and said how much I love her. As she was getting ready for the day, the thought came into her mind "it might be a good day to go to church." She began feeling better and could not explain why, other than to say the negative things in her head just went away.

Both of us believe miracles occur but probably not often. We have not lived with expectations of miracles in our lives, and we don't think there have been any. We do believe in divine providence. We often speak of certain events in our lives as special, unusual, providential. I think my deceased mother somehow brought Jane into my life at a time when I was at a crossroad. Do families or friends who have left this world have such influence on the deity? I would not try to convince others it is so, but I believe it is. Jane and I spoke of the morning as a "graced time." Which is what? A time or an event that stands out from ordinary happenings of life and says in a whisper there is a dimension we feel but cannot quite see or quite explain.

02/07/07

We went to my daughter's (Frances) 60th birthday party. Unbeknownst to me, the family chose to give Fran an album of pictures. Jane was sitting by Fran when she opened the gift. Everyone became interested in the pictures and began "family" comments. There were pictures of me with Fran's mother, Marguerite. Jane left the room and went in the kitchen where she began washing pots and pans in the sink. I got up and joined her once I realized she left.

Soon some guests were leaving and I suggested we go. Michael (Fran's son) told me he thought of calling about the album but he was unsure what to do. Too bad he didn't call. Jane was angry about the experience, and I support her criticism of the couple for not calling us or telling us privately about the gift.

Our days and nights have been very difficult. Jane brings up the incident every time we are together. She has "lost a whole family." She wants never to see any of them again. She expects one of them to call and apologize for what happened. I suspect the incident only registered mildly for any of them or not at all.

At the party Jane gave Fran a ceramic shard which we found in Virginia City, Nevada, many years ago. Fran had mentioned it when she visited us. Jane felt they have been closer lately and wanted to give Fran something special. Now she wants the shard returned.

The first copy of my book arrived today. Jane was as happy as I was. Later Jane came to me with something in her hand, "a gift in celebration of the book." It was this note: "My darling, what can I give you as a celebration of your wonderful book and the beautiful man you are? Unusual gift but . . . I know it will please you. I will never mention to anyone in the family we love and that loves us my days of sorrow. Forgive me for bringing you pain. I do and will love you always, Jane."

This is the sweet, sensitive, loving woman with whom I have shared so many years. I never lose awareness of that inner person, although it is difficult at times to keep it clear in my mind when she is angry and agitated. The sun shines again and life is good.

2/10/07

The respite ended the next morning. The birthday party remains the principal focus of Jane's thoughts and our conversation. Like the Christmas experience, this is now the center of Jane's thinking. All mental energy is focused here. It is painful to watch her struggle with an issue that is in reality quite insignificant in our lives. It is of central importance for her and it does tax my patience. I encouraged Jane to write to Fran about the shard and ask for its return. It is tragic this token of affection and bonding she extended to Fran has resulted in grief.

Jane lost ground cognitively this past week. Memory is increasingly impaired. Will her prior levity and responsiveness return? This was a harsh price to pay for attending a family gathering. It seems clear we will never attend a gathering of my children again.

2/13/07

The past week was difficult. On Sunday Jane continued angry, depressed and unreasonable. She wrote a letter to Fran asking her to return the shard. She read the final letter to me. I said I saw no errors in it. She sealed it, stamped it and left it to mail.

Later she said, "I decided not to mail the letter." I said, "It would be hard to undo it if you sent it." She was angry and said she thought I would respond differently. She said people do things that are not meant to hurt others but do them without thinking.

The next morning Jane tore up the letter and said the matter was over. She said the week must have been difficult for me. She knew how unreasonable she had been and how she repeated things over and over about the party. She was grateful how I responded to it all, letting her say whatever she wanted and not trying to tell her what to do.

This is the Jane I lived with all these years. She could get angry and unreasonable about an event or an offense but she would calm down and attain a much better perspective. Now her brain seems to get stuck in the initial process and she is unable to move on.

Today Jane is depressed. "Alzheimer's is a punishment. None of my kids cares about me; I do not want to speak to any of them if they call." She refers to the "thoughtlessness" at the party. I told her she is brave the way she carries her illness. We agree we have had many wonderful years together, and we expect to have many more good years. Although things are not the same we will stay close and keep going.

Jane does some writing these days. I will type it out so it will be available for "the book" she often talks about writing. I try to hold that prospect up to her so it will give both of us something to carry into our continuing struggle.

3/12/2007

The following letter brought the shard home to Jane. Fran's husband dropped it off with the concierge downstairs soon after it was written.

Dear Fran,   March 2, 2007

I have a request that may seem unusual to you, and I must admit it is unusual. It relates to the shard Jane gave you at your birthday party. The shard is something we dug up at Virginia City when we were digging up old bricks from the ruins of the Chinese settlement there. (We used the bricks in a ground level patio we made at our house in Reno.) To get to the crux of it, the shard has a great deal of sentimental and historical value to both of us.

The second thing I need to mention is that Jane sometimes gets on a track and loses perspective on the whole picture. She makes a decision impulsively and without consideration of its full meaning for herself. When you and Tom visited us, she was quite taken by the fact that you noticed the shard and commented about it. Afterwards she talked about giving it to you. I didn't comment, thinking she might forget about it. But when we were getting ready to go to the birthday celebration she got it and told me she planned on giving it to you. I had misgivings because I knew how much it meant to her but it was too late to intervene.

Now since she gave it to you, she continues to think about it and, of course, it becomes increasingly precious to her and occupies more of her thinking than it should. Because of this I suggested to her I write to you and ask if you would be good enough to return it. You could mail it (please, wrap carefully) or you could ask Tom to drop it off some day when he goes by the area. I would greatly appreciate this because it would do a great deal to help Jane obtain some peace of mind at least in this area.

Love, Dad.

3/19/07

It has been over a month since I last wrote. I haven't felt like writing though a great deal has happened. Am I too depressed to write, too frightened, too weary? I know the illness continues to move forward. There are signs!

Recently a friend said very seriously to Jane, "Someone who knows we often eat with you asked me the other day if I think you have Alzheimer's. To be honest, I don't see any evidence of it." Jane took the question to mean that people doubt she has the disease. She insists they assume she is lying.

Last Sunday Kathie visited and took Jane out for a walk. Later Jane told me they talked about the birthday affair, and now she can see how different it was from what she was thinking. She recognizes this battle was only in her mind and did not actually involve any of them. Kathie told her that others would not see the incident as she did.

Jane asked me to talk to her as Kathie did in the situation. I questioned whether she would accept that kind of statement from me. That was a mistake! She became angry because "I scoffed at her idea" and put the burden on her if it failed; and if it failed, "You would be finished with me and leave me." Things do escalate very quickly!

She became distraught and finally took her coat and left. I feared trying to detain her because it would only cause escalation. I sat and worried. If I went looking for her and she returned while I was out, she would either be frightened or more angry and desperate. She returned after about thirty minutes.

It is difficult to know how to deal with these episodes of anger and verbal attack. If I don't respond, I am "abandoning" her. If I respond in a calm and clear manner, then "you are treating me like one of your patients." I get exasperated at times. She becomes frightened and rather hysterical. If I try to embrace her, she is stiff and unresponsive. Her anger is vicious and unrelenting.

Later she acknowledges the extent of her anger and wonders how I put up with it. On rare occasions I become angry and say something hurtful or simply repeat some of the hurtful things she said to me. This is never acceptable. She focuses on what I said and reminds me of it for days, never seeing it as a response to her behavior.

These days I am careful about what I say and how it is said, and it puts a strain on our interaction. I am cautious about joking because she might see it not as intended. If she compliments me and I do not say thank you, she is irritated. If she makes a comment and I make no response (though it seems to me none is needed), she is annoyed and feels I am ignoring her. My comments must agree with hers or I am "taking the other side."

I write all this because I hope putting it in words may help me come to terms with it. When I tell someone Jane has Alzheimer's and they respond sympathetically, I end up in tears. It seems the tears are just waiting to be released and sympathy brings them out.

3/13/07

The past four days have been remarkably good ones. Laura came to visit last Saturday and left on Sunday. We gave Laura details about her role as executor of our estate.

Since Laura's visit, Jane has rarely mentioned Fran's birthday party. Her mind seems free of the hold the incident had on her. What a relief for me and I presume for her. Her mind has returned to the channel of every day life. The antipathy, the accusations, the interpretation of behaviors, all now seems to have disappeared.

The last four days were happy ones. We were out each day to Mass, to lunch, to stores, or to doctor visits. All went well. I left Jane at the Columbia Mall at 1:30p.m. on Thursday when I went to Loyola to teach. I met her as agreed at 4:15p.m. She enjoyed the time and bought some incidentals. She said the Mall felt unfamiliar.

We had dinner at the Candlelight last evening with two friends from church. Jane was talkative, laughed and joked. One would find it hard to believe she has Alzheimer's.

4/6/07

Good Friday. Last night we went to the monastery for Holy Thursday Mass. It was a solemn evening. Jane and I look for solemnity and piety in our lives. Not superficial piety, but a true sense of the sacred. The homily was about serving God and serving others. It seemed to inspire some new thoughts for me.

It became a meditation on our situation. God is present in my life in many ways, through many avenues. God is present for me in Jane. God lives in Jane in my life. Going to the monastery, Jane mentioned how beautiful the sky was. A dark cloud covered the setting sun, and the sun's light trimmed the cloud's edge with the white lace of its evening rays, as if to get attention before the light was gone. Jane is attentive to the beauty of nature in clouds and trees and shapes of living things. I said, "I'm sure God must love you very much because you appreciate all the beauty God has woven into the fabric of the world." Perhaps it was the earlier exchange that sparked my meditation during the homily.

If God lives in Jane, then I serve God in my care of her. It seemed so simple, so clear. It is something I must remember. If I am gentle with Jane, aware of her sadness and anger, attentive to what is going on within her, I may come to know God better. Her mind does not understand some things the way most of us do. She picks out pieces of information that, for some mysterious reason, are of marked importance and sometimes even comprise the whole of the event or scene for her. It may be a comment, a gesture, an action—but it becomes the core of a judgment or a decision she makes. And the judgment may live on in spite of evidence to the contrary.

I wonder if God is aware of little things we so easily slip by others . . . a caustic comment, an uncharitable look, a sly denigrating gesture. We felt it. We meant it. But we didn't want anyone to notice or to judge us negatively. Is it possible Jane picks up what others don't see or don't want us to see? Will God on judgment day say to me, "You are forgiven for this or that minor slip, but it seemed unworthy of the person you were trying to appear to be to others and to Me."

My voice sounds harsh, trying to explain or clarify something for her. I focus on someone else or something else distracts me from her presence or her immediate needs. I feel a need to hurry and I find her movements or her thinking slow. I show irritation and impatience. Does my good Jane think, "You are forgiven, but these times warn me that you may not always be as gentle with me as you say you want to be."

Perhaps I can translate this into my relationship with God. I try to explain my behavior to God, as if He doesn't understand already. I am distracted from my good intentions when my own needs or interests get in the way. And God knows I'm a clock watcher and try to keep the world running on my schedule. I must remember that things go along on God's time. The important thing is to be headed in the right direction. It doesn't matter how fast or slow we are going. We don't even need to know when we get there.

At Easter I celebrate the God of the Easter eggs. God has hidden all kinds of wonderful possibilities in our lives, marvelous surprises, happy events, secret treasures. All we have to do is find them. Jane is the Easter egg treasure of my life. Together we have found happy times that have been rewarding and fulfilling.

The God of the Easter eggs has hidden all kinds of fantastic surprises in the world that need only be revealed by those men and women who make remarkable discoveries and inventions, and sometimes act as if they created them. Children hunting for Easter eggs don't make the eggs; they only find them. God hides surprises in life whether in a spouse, a friend, a stranger or a discovery that brings health or happiness to others.

4/13/07

Laura, Frank and the girls came Saturday and left on Easter Sunday about 3p.m. I could hardly believe how relaxed Jane was. She was flexible with schedules, accepting plans and minor changes, at ease with the children, non-intrusive with Laura and Frank and their plans. She was ready to accept their leaving when they went.

Recently Jane wondered about charges on her credit card. I collected the receipts, added them up, and gave her an explanation of the charges. She became angry and very unreasonable. "You brought up the whole thing to discourage my spending and to check my expenses, going though the receipts in the middle of the night." She went on and on about trying to economize and worrying about not having enough money. "I will never use my charge card again." I calmly tried to explain why I gave her the accounting.

Later on Jane suddenly said, "I feel like I'm just getting out of the ring." It was a clear statement of an abrupt change of attitude. It ended her belligerence and her focus on money and the credit cards, as if something not working in her brain connected again.

Sometimes I feel Jane doesn't see me in the same way, almost doesn't recognize me. Not only am I unable to reason with her, she does not want me to embrace her, and when I do she is stiff. Her eyes lack the sparkle, the life, the love I normally see there.

She apologized several times and said how difficult it must be for me and wondered how a person can stay with someone who behaves this way for no reason at all. I said it is much harder for her than for me. I said this is not the kind of person she is, and this "happens" and is not willful or under her control. She recovered quickly, and it was not one of the 24 to 48 hour conflicts we have had in the past. They fill Jane with fear of abandonment and a feeling of isolation characteristic of her childhood.

Jane is writing a book and I am her recorder and scribe. These notes may serve as a separate section of her book to provide some view of what we were going through during her "writing period." A second reason for my writing is to have some outlet for things that go on that I cannot openly discuss with Jane. It helps me remain more objective. Thirdly, it is something to do with my time and my mind. I like writing, always have.

PART 2 (JUN 07—NOV 07)

5/26/07

It has been a long time since I sat down to these commentaries on our life. Sometimes I felt too tired or too distracted to write. Or was it too depressed?

The roller coaster ride continues. There have been wonderful times when we talked and laughed and remembered the past and planned the future, times full of closeness and expressions of affection, warmth and light, a sense of God and quiet peace. There have been Alzheimer's storms, angry words, paranoid accusations, misunderstandings, demands for clarification impossible to satisfy, tears, sleepless nights, threats of suicide interspersed with attempts to revisit our strong affection, rekindle our expressions of love, and realign ourselves with reason, peace, and faith.

To go from the good times to the bad is a grueling experience for both of us. When Jane is "apologizing" for her behaviors, I tell her they create much more pain for her than for me. She is merciless in her self-condemnation. She often says she has always been this way—argumentative, caustic, accusatory, angry, and demanding. Not so!

Jane is a passionate woman with strong feelings, easily and quickly expressed, likes and dislikes. She can fall in love with the shape of a tree, the texture of a leaf, or a heart shaped rock. She can be strongly attracted to a painting and want to get up close to it "where the painter stood when he painted it."

Her strong emotions have become more volatile, more invasive, and more overwhelming since the onset of her illness. They toss her about heedlessly when they dominate her being, as they sometimes do. It is especially painful for me when she develops an inappropriate anger or paranoid attitude toward one of our children, and I must take some middle ground until the storm passes.

When she is feeling less threatened, less vulnerable, less isolated, times are good . . . very good . . . like old times. She is funny, loving, observing everything, interested in everything, curious, responsive. She is not offended by her inability to remember something but gracefully accepts my prompt. We work together so smoothly the deficit almost goes unnoticed. Her sense of humor is as brilliant at these times as it normally was. She is loving in every way and unstinting in her affection.

I wonder, "Is her illness improving, going away?" I can deceive myself for a moment but not for long. When the storm comes, the world changes, and I am left to hold onto our past and try to find her in the tempest. In the midst of the storm I see someone else when I look at her. Her face changes, her eyes are unseeing, empty. They frighten me.

I'm doing better at coping with the torrent. I don't feel angry during recent episodes. I don't try to change her mind about a position she has taken. I don't disagree or try to explain. I focus on our love for one another, the safety of our present situation, my everlasting love for her, my determination to be with her "all ways and always." I tell her I don't want her to feel lonely, I am here beside her and always will be, and it is okay for her to feel angry and sad because the illness brings frightening feelings.

A different kind of episode occurred several weeks ago. We were talking about my years in medical school and I mentioned a nurse at Providence Hospital who once invited me to dinner at her house. Because of the distance I stayed the night. I was clear that the relationship was in no way romantic. Jane said she was glad I had such a friend.

The next morning it was a "cause célèbre." "Why didn't you tell me before about staying overnight with her? Why did you tell me now? Don't you know this will haunt me the rest of my life; it will be in my mind when I'm sitting in my wheel chair staring into space and unable to communicate? Don't you know how you have ruined everything?"

This situation brought on an Alzheimer's storm of considerable strength and length. It subsided and returned repeatedly for at least three weeks. By nightfall Jane would often acknowledge how wrong she was to pursue it; and by morning it would be back in full force. We spent hours on it. She did not believe I was honest but believed the woman and I were involved sexually. Finally she seemed to accept what I said was the truth. The subject has not resurfaced in the last three weeks. And this was all over a friendship I had with a nurse six years before I met Jane.

Jane becomes preoccupied with thoughts about her illness and the anticipation of an inability to communicate, to understand, to care for herself. Our plan is to remain in this apartment and get whatever assistance we need. She expresses fear that something might happen to me. I exercise daily and take care of my health. It is my hope and prayer I will be able to care for her. If I were not here, she could not maintain her current level of functioning. Alzheimer's patients must sink quickly into advanced forms of their illness if there is no one to help them battle the demons.

Jane sinks into an overwhelming sadness. She gets irritable trying to cope with simple situations that are now complex. As a child, Jane told her sorrows to her cat or her favorite doll. The cat died and her mother made her give the dolls away. It is hard for her to trust another, easy for her to close me out. She tumbles deeper and deeper into the grasp of her own despair. It happens before I am aware of it. She cannot respond to my attempts to catch her.

Caught in this descent into the hell of Alzheimer's, she thinks, "This is it. It is here. This is what happens." Each time she expects a sudden complete change with a rapid descent into oblivion. I remind her she said these things before, but then returned to our beautiful, active life together. I tell her, "We have lots to do, places to go, and years ahead to do it." I tell her Alzheimer's progresses slowly. But sometimes I wonder. When we awaken some morning will the Jane I have known for 46 years be gone?

6/07/07

Last week was stormy with two or three angry outbursts some days. We get through them more readily but not without emotional bruises. One evening Jane was having difficulty with her contact lenses. I came to the door to help her clarify the mix-up and hoping to bring some calm. She turned on me. "If you had only stepped toward me and held me in your arms and comforted me, everything would have been all right. But you failed me; you are no help; I can't depend on you or expect anything from you; you only stand in the doorway and offer nothing." She went on. I felt like someone else was speaking to me, someone who hated me, who had contempt for me.

I have not retaliated angrily to these onslaughts for some time now, but they wear on me. Jane apologized later and the next morning was totally remorseful. These episodes are harder for her than for me because she feels so badly afterwards. She said she felt she was talking to someone else, that it wasn't me standing in front of her. It was how I sensed the encounter, and it was deeply disturbing. How can I deal with this?

Initially Jane wanted to know about the illness but she gave me back an Alzheimer's book when she read "currently there is no cure for Alzheimer's." "If there is no cure, why read about it?" Now she shows an interest again. I ordered two books about Alzheimer's.

The last two days were wonderful. We enjoyed our time together and talked a great deal. She is more at ease about her memory failures. She is warm toward other people and engages them in conversation.

7/15/07

Some things have changed the past few weeks. Then I ask, "Have they changed or do they just seem different?" A few weeks ago Jane asked me about some of my studies. I mentioned my interest in philosophy. She asked what it is about. I talked superficially about the ideas of existence and essence, substance and accidents. Jane was interested.

I obtained a "Companion to the Summa" by Walter Farrell, who presents profound principles in a beautiful style. I read a few pages to her and she encouraged me to continue. I have read over 100 pages of the first volume to her, sometimes for an hour at a time. She is attentive and focused. She grasps the meaning well because occasionally we refer to it later and discuss something. I am fascinated by her response to this. While the words are simple, the concepts are complex, but she is "right with it." I have always believed Jane is very intelligent. This response verifies it, but not for her.

When Jane is feeling isolated, angry, desolate, frightened, I hear her talking out loud, condemning herself, her family of origin, and God. She gets angry at God and really tells God off. During a recent episode of this kind, she worked her way out of it in about 30 minutes. She said she asked God to help her, and it was "like a little voice inside telling me to come and tell you I was sorry."

Last week Jane had cataract surgery on her right eye. It went well. She gets anxious over new experiences. Her anxiety can take two forms. One is to become irritated by the imperfect behavior of others who are in any way involved. Her other coping method is to be solicitous for those who are involved in her care. She engages in pleasant exchanges with them and reassures them they are "doing a good job," "nothing is hurting," and she is "doing well." That's how she was during and after the surgery on Tuesday. She must be viewed by the caretakers as a very cooperative patient. She is!

When we got home, she was tense and brought up issues as far back as February, items which were resolved weeks if not months ago. In the evening she became confused and irritable. She noted she was "mixed up" and was concerned. I said it might be an effect of earlier sedation. In reality I think the stress of a day depleted her resources.

We go less often to the dining room. Having our dinner in the apartment avoids the stress of sitting at dinner with others for an hour or more. Jane is friendly and cares about other people, but extended social situations have become a strain for her.

(Email to Paul 8/28/07)
As you know Jane and I both designated you with power of attorney, guardian, and executor secondary to Laura. I am getting together a packet of information for Laura pertaining to our eventual death and I would like to give you a copy of the information I give her. It will have the copies of the necessary legal documents as well as names and addresses of various persons including CPA, broker, and attorney. The whole thing seems a bit macabre but it is obviously an appropriate thing to do. I know this is a difficult subject for you, but I also know we can have confidence in you and that you will be helpful to Laura in the event of our deaths. The distance makes her handling of these matters more problematic especially if quick response is necessary.

The past few weeks have been rather rocky, since our trip to Laura's. Jane's memory is clearly worse, and it disturbs her greatly. It brings her back to face the facts of Alzheimer's again. She had become more reconciled to the illness a few months ago and clearly had a more positive and accepting attitude. Now she focuses on the illness with its entire morbid story. As a result she is more depressed, more angry, and more unpredictable. I feel pretty helpless sometimes.

8/29/07

We went to Laura's in early August for three nights. It was a good visit. Jane spent several hours with the girls, all three of them drawing. It is the first time in years for Jane to sit and draw. She enjoyed it and, as always, showed genuine skill in her work. I encouraged her to continue it. But the door has closed again. She says, "I'm going to paint something next week" or "I think I'll do some sketching" but nothing happens.

Toward the end of our visit the strain was showing. Jane acted like a robot, moving very slowly and deliberately, watching others and participating minimally. She was more irritable with me the last two days and quite guarded with Laura.

The trip home started out well. We were talking and I said something which she found offensive. I have no recollection of the statement, but it couldn't have been a criticism. Things quickly went from bad to worse. Jane became rather hysterical and climbed over the seat to get in the back of the car. All of this at 65 miles per hour!

I stopped at the first available rest stop and persuaded her to come back in the front. We talked for 20 or 30 minutes to reestablish calm and peace. I drove on to Columbia. In our apartment things fell apart again over something insignificant and now long forgotten, but it was "the worst thing you ever said to me in our whole life."

Things have been on edge since we returned home. After a few days, disaster came again over some word I used or some comment of hers to which I did not respond or did not respond suitably. It is a "no win" situation.

I dread the march of Alzheimer's as it drives a wedge between me and my wonderful life partner. Something changed this past month. We both know it. She appears depressed, although she responds enthusiastically when we are out shopping. She is overly responsive and overly solicitous toward other residents and staff.

Jane spends hours in her bathroom "straightening things out." She comes to breakfast saying, "I can't find anything I need to get ready, and it's driving me crazy." If I suggest helping her sort through things, she is defensive. When I say "sorting through," to her the words mean "getting rid of."

She expresses resentment over our move here and our need to downsize drastically. We rented a storage facility before we moved. We had an argument every time we went there. I believe we were facing Alzheimer's at the time but did not recognize it. Although she is pleased to be living here, she is angry about the move. Jane says she got rid of things because I refused to get adequate rental space. The space had room to spare.

There was much to do when we moved and it was hurried. Decisions were difficult for Jane. They were sometimes erratic, almost reckless and at other times painfully slow. A friendly antique dealer bought most things we sold. Jane liked her and gave her much of her costume jewelry and other items she probably would never part with now.

For the past two or three weeks the distance between us grows. Jane is irritable and seems to wait for me to say something so I can be attacked. Her sense of levity, her keen curiosity, her gentle spirit are fading. I feel bewildered, lost, alone. Will her humor, her graciousness, her spirit return? Or is this the downhill path?

9/2/07
We've had a horrible week. We fought every day. What are we doing to ourselves and to our love for one another? Jane has threatened suicide, asked me the other day if I would help her do it, talked to Laura on the phone about her wish to die. Yesterday it all resolved without our clearly knowing why. I pulled her onto my lap during one of our go-rounds, and she was responsive this time.

I think a lot about the situation. I'm not fair to Jane if I don't take into account the devastation Alzheimer's is causing. She does not think clearly at times. Memory is severely impaired. The deficits are more noticeable to both of us.

I went to Sunday Mass at 8a.m. The sermon was about humility. It applied to me and fills my reflections. My responses to Jane are prideful, especially if she is critical or uses a harsh tone. "How can she speak to me like that after all I do for her?" or "I don't deserve that tone" or "I need to stop this behavior of hers." Now, I'm thinking, "Who do I think I am to be critical of anything she does or doesn't do, says or doesn't say?" How can I sit in judgment on her? Good God, what a frightening existence she has! A bright, beautiful woman, an amazing observer of all around her–now a person who cannot grasp a conversation, who is uncertain whether she observed something or dreamed it, and who finds the behavior of others hurtful without knowing why.

I have no right to be angry or retaliate for anything she might say or do to me. She feels conflict more painfully than I. But that is not the way I act when it happens! I am hurt and want her to know her angry words are hurtful. How can I hurt this sweet, caring woman who is the best part of my world, the focus of my life and my love?

She is very slow getting ready to go out. I try to be patient. I recently got some inkling of what it is like for her to get dressed in the morning or to get ready for bed at night. To go out, there are choices to be made, choices that were never easy for a woman of discriminating taste. Now, no choices come easily. It is a complex world she faces. Which skirt? Or pants? Which shirt or blouse? Do they go together? There are many options even in a limited wardrobe. Then there is make-up and depressed thoughts about how old she looks, and she sees herself as no longer beautiful.

After deciding, finding what she wants is the next task. She loses clothing she just took off. She can become hysterical, crying, throwing things, making critical comments about being crazy and stupid, looking everywhere and **seeing** nothing. Lost items are often in a place where she already looked. I usually find them before she does.

How frightening it must be to know that anything you have may be lost when you lay it down, and the image of it may get lost in the dark tunnels that are daily growing larger and darker in your brain! Tunnels that used to carry living messages full of faces and facts and creative ideas and even some dreams that never came true!

9/5/07

I have the misfortune of running a timetable in my head. I set time limits for doing things, important or not. When we go out, I set a time in my head when we should go. When we're out, I set a time in my head when we should get home. No particular reason why it is **that** time! I rarely just let things flow. I set my time to go to bed, to get up, to eat, to read the paper, and on and on it goes. It doesn't have to be the same time every day. It just has to be the time I decide it should be. The decision is entirely arbitrary.

I need to change that, not just for Jane but to give my head a rest. I need to be more available for her needs. Recently, when the evening show was over, it was **my time** for bed. It was postponed because Jane just remembered an actor's name. We talked for 30 minutes about her memory and how different it is at times. She was relaxed and content as we got in bed.

If Jane spends time looking at something or doing some little thing, it infringes on my schedule for bedtime, and I resent it. In reality, there may be something she needs to talk about or just wants to talk about. I need to be open to the "grace of the moment" and not be so concerned with "my time schedule." What can be more important in my life than to have Jane talk to me about anything that comes to her mind?

Jane's fear of being alone is apparent. She is afraid I will abandon her, because I get "so angry" and because she is "so mean" to me. She must feel the world is leaving her as her contact with others becomes more tenuous, more uncertain, more sporadic, more chaotic. She drifts away in her thoughts. She begins something and gets lost in countless distractions that take her to places she can't remember. It is a "land of lonely" where the web of faulty memories hides the past and confuses the present.

The "goodness" or "badness" of people and things and experiences are colored by emotional paint from unknown sources, of unknown shades, in meaningless symbols. The end result is to be a wanderer in a strange world where others act and talk and think in ways she no longer understands. How strange! How frightening! How alone! I must not let her be there without at least my hand, my voice, my love.

Jane's emptiness is magnified by the lack of order and accomplishment that engulf her. She plans; she purchases; she intends; she decides; she talks about it. But little happens and then only with painstaking struggles. She buys cards to send the kids. They sit on her desk for weeks and get put in with other cards not sent. She gets out thread to sew the hem of a skirt or the button on a shirt, but it never happens.

She buys books about art, but never looks at them. She buys drawing pencils, but they are set aside and eventually lost. She buys material to make pillows for the girls, but never makes them. I watch her "spin her wheels" and know she is helpless to move forward, and I am helpless to help her. My heart breaks for her loss in unproductive days. Each day she is "going to tidy" her desk, and each day it accumulates new items she cannot discard or give away. I try to convince her she should not be critical of herself for things undone, any more than she should be critical of herself for memory loss.

I write these things to read them later and remind myself of her world. I need to keep her world as clear as I can in my mind and refresh my memory of it as often as needed.

Email to Paul 9/5/07)
I should let you know that Jane has developed strong negative feelings about both Fran and John. These are based on small issues which have become magnified over the ensuing months. We will not go to any family gatherings and when John is in town I will probably meet him somewhere. This is more extreme than I wish, but I need to deal with Jane's feelings. I tell you so you will be aware of it when we get together. I make no effort to change her mind about these things because experience tells me that creates conflict.

9/21/07
We had a great trip to the beach Monday morning to Thursday evening. We walked and talked and shopped every day. Saw Phil and Eileen for lunch on Tuesday and again on the way home Thursday. Jane was relaxed. She got

frustrated one morning getting ready for breakfast. I held her and told her there was no rush. She became calm.

I suggested we go to Rehoboth for a month in the winter. Jane is enthusiastic about the possibility. We rented a one bedroom condo at Edgewater House from November 10 to December 10. The monthly rate is so reasonable we can afford to come home a few days if the time seems too long at the beach.

I have removed some of the time pressures I previously created for us. I don't challenge comments she makes, and if I inadvertently seem to challenge something, I apologize for the way I said it and try to right the situation. I work harder at keeping communication going between us. I am quickly reassuring if she seems confused or irritated.

I pray I can maintain this attitude. Each morning I dedicate my day to her and believe I serve God well caring for her well. My love for her increases each day, and I am aware I failed to recognize the needs this precious woman developed as a result of this illness.

(Letter sent to each of our children September 28, 2007)
We wish to provide all of you with some basic information about provisions we have made for our care during whatever years remain for us. We also want to provide some general information about funeral arrangements we have made. We hope this will not sound too grim or depressing. These are obviously important issues for us to have settled, and we thought it would be wise to pass some of our thinking on to you. We will sign this letter rather formally and place a copy among our other papers. Although it may sound official, it is sent with our love for each of you.

PLAN FOR THE FUTURE
* * * * * *

We plan on staying in our present apartment as long as we are able to do so and hire whatever help we need to continue to do that. We are both in good physical health with regular physical examinations and appropriate laboratory tests. We have every reason to believe we may both live a good many more years. We are not aware of any severe or chronic illnesses other than for Jane's Alzheimer's. We both appear to have full remission from former cancer.

It is my hope and prayer I will live as long as Jane is alive. I am careful to exercise regularly and do all I can to preserve my health. If my hope is fulfilled and my health remains reasonably good, then I expect Jane and I will both be able to remain in our current apartment. If we reach a point where I am truly unable to care for Jane here, she would go to the assisted living unit where I could spend most of my time with her. We both have strong beliefs such a move will not be necessary, but we know life is unpredictable. Separation would be very difficult for both of us.

We believe at this time most of our affairs are in order. Our funerals are prearranged and paid for. Laura is the trustee of our estate, has guardianship and power of attorney, and is the health care agent for the one of us who dies last or in the event of incompetence of the remaining person. Paul has agreed to serve in any or all of these capacities in the event Laura is unavailable. We recognize the burden this assignment places on Laura and potentially on Paul, so we request each of you assist them as much as possible in this difficult time for all of you. Laura and Paul both have instructions regarding our health care advance directives as well as matters after our death, including information regarding our physician, our attorney, our CPA, our investment counselor, and our funeral director.

FUNERAL PLANS:
* * * * * *

We both wish to be cremated. When one of us dies, the remaining spouse can then sign permission for cremation. When the remaining spouse dies, it is our understanding that the children must then sign permission for the cremation. It is our wish to be cremated, and we request that each of you respect that wish.

10/05/07

I had a frightening and thought provoking dream last night. I dreamed I was with Jane at a convention in a big city. Then I was no longer with Jane but with several persons whom I knew casually. In the crowd of people milling about, I suddenly found I had wandered off from the others. People were going in all directions. They all looked alike. I felt isolated and looked for someone to help me. A man handed me a cell phone to make a call but I didn't know how to use it. I wandered around becoming increasingly frantic. I felt lonely, completely isolated in the midst of all the people. They were walking faster now, and they didn't seem to see me. It dawned on me I didn't know where I was staying, and I wouldn't be able to tell anyone where I wanted to go because I had lost my memory.

I told Jane about the dream. I cried because of the feelings that came over me. I knew she has this experience: feeling totally alone in the midst of others, unable to communicate with those around her, unseen by them, desperate for help, unable to operate a simple cell phone, unable to know what to ask if someone was there. Jane thought my dream was not surprising, considering how close we are. The dream took me to the isle of Alzheimer's for a brief but chilling period.

10/27/07

A movie we recently watched mentioned a concentration camp in Austria where I was stationed as the war ended. I said I had been there. Jane began asking questions about it. My thought was, "it's time for bed." My answers were short and probably dismissive. More questions came. What did I do after the war? Where was I? What was it like? Where else was I stationed?

My clock said it was bed time, and the world should run on my schedule. Recently I have tried to avoid this kind of thinking. It is important to take the time Jane needs to talk about something or to do something. But I was working on my schedule. The result was horrendous.

I was annoyed we were not going to bed. I finally said, "I would rather not talk about all of this." That lit the anger fire. "In all our years together you never spoke to me in such a manner. Who do I have to talk to if I can't talk to you? I will never again refer to any of these subjects, and we will never speak about them again. What is going on with you that you don't want to talk about these things? Are you afraid to talk about them? Is there some big secret you don't want to share with me? What did you do? What have you been hiding all these years?"

I tried to calm her, to reason with her. No go! I tried to hold her. She was unresponsive. After we were in bed 20 minutes, Jane got up quietly and left the bedroom. After a while I got up to try to talk with her. The apartment was dark and cold. She was in the living room standing behind a chair looking out at the trees blowing in the wind. It was a rainy, windy night. I held her when we got back in bed, and eventually we both went to sleep.

The next morning she apologized for the night before. I got up three hours earlier, and I had time to think about it. I had failed her. She had questions! I did not take the time; I did not have the patience to answer them properly. I felt badly about what I did, and I told her so. Her questions deserved full answers. She faces an unknown world she does not understand. She was alone, isolated, frightened. She felt I deserted her, and I had.

Jane has new needs now. To spend time looking at little "treasures" we accumulated over the years. To ask questions or introduce ideas to be addressed and responded to. To repeat something she talked about just the other day and to develop the subject as fully as she wants. To spend more time with her make-up or getting ready because it is more difficult to achieve the result she desires. To stop and study the "faces" she finds in the bark of a tree or to linger in front of a building and admire the windows and count the panes of glass. These things help her stay in contact with the world she knew and now fears losing. If I fail these needs, I fail her.

As a psychiatrist, I spent over 50 years trying to know what the lives of my patients were like for them, to acquire as closely as possible a view of their personal world. In order to withstand the impact of that awareness on myself, it was essential to separate my knowledge of their world from my world and, in a sense, to insulate myself from the pain and tragedies of their lives.

It is ironic now to find myself searching to know the world that is becoming so misshapen and mysterious for "my love," as the tangles and twists of her brain cells begin to impose their "distorted view" of life as she sees it, hears it, judges it, and lives it. Now there is no way to insulate or isolate myself from what I learn, but only to try to live life with her as courageously and as cheerfully as she does.

PART 3 (DEC 07—MAY 08)

12/15/07

We rented a one bedroom condo on the boardwalk at Rehoboth Beach from 11/05 to 12/05. We stayed in that building a few summers in the 80's and a month one winter in the 90's. We were on the 6th floor with a marvelous view of the ocean. We talked every day about the beauty and solemnity of our view. We walked the boardwalk, the beach, the streets, three or four miles every day. I admire her stamina and her spirit.

Several large pictures of ocean scenes dominated the condo living room. Jane expressed doubt she could tolerate them for a month. "Why put up pictures of the ocean when you can look out and see it?" One day while I prepared lunch, she took the pictures down and stored them in a closet. The room looked much better. This behavior has been typical of Jane through the years. Her irritation with decorations or furniture that displeases her has become more pronounced since the Alzheimer's.

At the book store Jane bought three or four art books with a comment about "never having my own money." She brought several of her drawing books to the beach along with two boxes of graphite and colored pencils. They were never opened. I am not critical of her buying the books or the art supplies. I am saddened by it, by the loss it represents in her life, a loss which cannot be replaced by a book on a shelf or a pencil in a box. She made every place we ever lived a gallery of pictures and furnishings that pleased us and was admired by everyone who visited us. Each day I grieve her loss of the ability to create beautiful things. I know she grieves it too.

One day Jane seemed unusually enthusiastic about everything. The store was "magnificent." Many objects were "very unusual" and "excellent finds." I was uneasy about possible unwise purchases. The following day she described her attitude of the previous day as "feeling high." I was surprised she was aware of it. She said, "I was pretty crazy. You need to keep an eye on me when I'm feeling like that."

Adjustment to returning home was difficult. Unpacking and finding places to put things overwhelms her. Her bathroom is always a challenge with an excess of odds and ends. Going down to dinner for the first time was difficult for Jane. Everyone seemed older and more incapacitated. There were four deaths while we were away. It was a dreary, dark day—not a cheery homecoming!

At dinner someone mentioned the trees that were cut down. We had pine trees outside our windows and some of their branches could be touched from our balcony. We loved them. We lived in the tree tops. They were gone! Jane was devastated! "Those were our trees. No one had a right to cut them down without our permission, without telling us." She cried and threatened for hours. She was up during the night looking at the empty spaces.

The following day I asked about the trees. Everyone was notified before they were cut down. It was done because the trees were diseased and were impacting the building. This news was mildly placating for Jane. I'm glad we didn't know before going to the beach. It would have ruined our vacation.

We planed on going to Mass yesterday morning. She became hysterical because she could not find two black stockings that matched. I suggested she lie down. She reluctantly agreed. I massaged her feet until she slept. She was refreshed when she woke three hours later.

We plan to visit Laura and the girls at Christmas. Laura's boyfriend will probably be there. Five people for three or four days create a great deal of stress, no matter how well behaved everyone is. Jane is concerned this Christmas will be her last. She is losing ground these days. Is it the dreary weather, the disability and death at Vantage House, the loss of the trees? Or is it the advancing devastation of her unrelenting illness?

1/5/08
We were at Laura's five days at Christmas. Frank, Laura's friend, dampened the event. He was intrusive, pouting, attention seeking, in and out of the house as if he owned it. It was stressful for everyone and particularly for Jane.

We departed in good spirits on 12/29. The trip home initially went well. When we passed the Ripken stadium on 95, Jane said, "That reminds me of Paul." I asked, "Why?" She said, "Isn't that the stadium we pass when we go to Paul's?" I said, "No, we don't come this way when we go to Paul's." (He lives in the opposite direction.)

Jane's comment, "I'm never right. I'm so stupid." To lessen her self-recriminations, I said the stadium probably looks like something on the way to Paul's. Within no time she reached a point of bitter hostility! "Why do you always have to put me down? Why do you always have to win? Why didn't you just let it go and let me believe I was right?"

The rest of the trip was painful. Jane said she tried to talk with me and "look what happened. You made me out to be a fool. So there'll be no more conversation." Traffic was heavy. We had light rain and evening darkness. I devoted my attention to driving.

As I drove into the parking lot at Vantage House, Jane took her seat belt off, opened the door and started to get out. "I'm getting out of here. I don't want to be with you." I had no choice but to stop as she got out. I went the next 10 yards to our parking spot. By the time I stopped and got out of the car, she was gone in the darkness.

I could not look for her because there were several directions she might go or she might return to the apartment by several routes. I took the luggage in. If I went to look for her, I would have to lock the door. If she came home, a locked door would make her furious.

After 40 minutes I had a phone call from "Safe Return," the Alzheimer's program. Jane was at the Nordstrom store in the Mall, a mile or more from where we live. She had walked there in the dark and in the rain with rush hour traffic pouring through the area. I went over to get her.

She came home reluctant, angry, accusatory, paranoid. We tried to have a peaceful dinner, but she remained edgy, hostile, and argumentative. I was accused of not talking to her. I had little to say that might be useful. My words were more likely to incite her.

About 10p.m. she announced she was "going out." I told her, "If you go out, I will call the police. The police will look for you, and when they find you they will take you to Howard County Hospital, and the hospital will call me to come and bring you home, unless the doctors feel you need to stay." My words got her attention and quieted her. But she continued to dress to leave. I put a chair in front of the door, got a pillow and blanket, and planned on reading and sleeping there. She consented to go to bed.

The next morning she pleaded with me never to leave her and to take care of her. I told her the only thing that would prevent me from taking care of her would be her running away. For three days we tried to find the harmony we had before. It wasn't the same. We both knew it. She would pick on words I used or things I did and suddenly there was a chasm between us. We were separated and unable to reestablish the contact we had for over 45 years. She slept until about noon for several days.

Then one morning she "was back." I knew it in her eyes, in her smile, in her words, in her embrace. The episode was over. She was remorseful, full of apologies. She remembered most of what happened, walking to the Mall in the rain, the attention at Nordstrom's, the threats I made about the police. I didn't encourage her to dwell on it.

1/23/08
Jane will be 78 tomorrow. We'll lunch with a friend and then go to a movie and dinner.

Jane frequently brings up the lost trees, Fran's birthday party and her disappointment regarding Mary, her friend from the pool. Two days ago she had a difficult time focusing on anything. She was horribly depressed. She knew this is "how it is always going to be—it's happening fast—nothing will ever get better—the good days are over." She was irritable, with short answers, confusing things, accusing me of controlling her.

(For several years Jane went to the YMCA pool. She became part of a small group of women there who went places together and had monthly birthday parties for the group. Her friend, Mary from the group, was at the hairdresser's in October when Jane had a hostile parting with her hairdresser.) With Jane's permission I called Mary and told her Jane was upset because Mary had not called. Mary called the next day. Jane was dissatisfied with the call and insists the relationship is over. Jane decided Mary chose her loyalty to the hairdresser over Jane's friendship. The facts seem to support that idea.

Today we went out for lunch, some laboratory tests and minor shopping. Jane seemed so wise, so "with it," so warm. It was like we were back somewhere several years ago. And I kept thinking, "How can this be? What does this mean? How long can this last?"

I suggested to Jane some of the "little gray cells" (of Hercule Poirot) in her brain have been damaged or destroyed by Alzheimer's. If 40 or 50% of working cells are full of "the trees," "the birthday party," and "Mary," then she only has 50 or 60% available to cope with the world, so it becomes shrouded in a haze and is unintelligible. That is how Jane describes it. "Everything looks different. I seem not to recognize what I see. I seem unable to hear what people say, and if I hear it, I can't understand what they mean." When "trees" and "birthday party" and "Mary" no longer possess a major share of her brain, we can talk about other issues.

2/2/08
Yesterday we went to see the Matisse exhibit at the Baltimore Art Museum. It was a terrible experience. On arrival we went to the restaurant for lunch. The earliest reservation was for 2p.m.

Jane was angry and interpreted the exchange to mean that only members could eat there. I said I made a reservation for 2p.m. She kept returning to the issue and the special treatment for "the members," adding we could not eat there until after four o'clock. I repeated my comments and mentioned I told her before. "Don't ever again say to me you told me something before. It only reminds me of my illness and how stupid I am."

She became disoriented and frightened in the exhibit room. We left and sat on a bench on the landing and talked. She said she was always left out in life and never felt she belonged. She was certain those feelings would never go away. She felt like jumping over the balcony to the floor below and "ending it all, having it over."

She became calm so we wandered about the museum, and at her suggestion returned to the Matisse exhibit and went through it hurriedly. We agreed the sculpture was not worth seeing. We had lunch at 2p.m. Jane finally realized we could not get in earlier because we had not made reservations in advance.

At home Jane became increasingly angry because, "You don't talk to me." She began hearing loud sounds in her head "like motors running." I said, "I don't hear them." "I'm going crazy then." We sat on the sofa. I held her and she became calmer. She used to hear music sometimes in the evening. Now it is usually loud motors, more likely in the evening when she is tired. She accepts the idea it is "due to her medicine."

2/6/08

Yesterday Jane asked me to come to the window and look at the trees, how beautiful they are and how fortunate for us they are there. She said, "I'm okay with the cut trees now. I settled it in my mind. I know they are gone and I can accept it. I just wanted you to know." She said God would be pleased with her if she accepted what happened to the trees. I told her I think God must be very pleased with her endless appreciation of His trees and His skies and His sunsets, all of which she constantly admires and comments on. I love her love of all the natural beauty we find together. She said how much she appreciated my letting her make up her own mind about the trees. I didn't tell her what to think or what to do, but I gave her the freedom to work it out for herself.

2/6/08

God is good. A second writing today! One about the trees and there is more good news.

Today is Ash Wednesday. We went to the Monastery for Mass. We sat in the choir stalls on one side of the church. Suddenly Jane's son, Phil, was standing in front of us. He was waiting and hoping we would come. They embraced and spoke for a few moments. We sat together during the service. After Mass we had lunch together. It was cordial and a good visit. As usual Phil talked randomly about lots of things. He doesn't seem comfortable when something is said about his mother's Alzheimer's.

When we got home Jane took a nap. She said, "Emotional things tire me out, whether they are good emotions or bad ones. I'm just realizing that." It is certainly true. She was asleep in ten seconds as I massaged her feet.

When Jane is in the midst of an emotional storm, I ask God to help me deal with it and to help me know what to do. As a result I believe I have been more able not only to cope with these episodes but to help bring them to a speedier conclusion.

2/20/08

Last week was wonderful. Jane was vibrant, bright, engaged, and engaging, a bit over-talkative at times especially with others, but very appropriate. She told me she talked to God and felt God does not want her to be as angry as she is sometimes. She decided to make peace with a resident she has been angry at for the past two years over a minor issue.

Jane talked about how difficult she makes it for me when she "picks on me" and then is critical when I do not respond to "my silly and stupid and cruel accusations." She was seeing these episodes as an observer of self and more realistically.

A few days ago she mentioned our estate and said she dreaded talking about it because we did not agree. She had no memory of a recent conversation we had. I went over the plan I proposed a few weeks ago. She was fully aware and totally accepting.

When Jane is full of anger and memories of wrongs, she feels vindictive. But at some point her heart takes center stage, and she is moved by the kindness and love within her, and she cries out to touch and be touched by others. I pray she will have peace within herself and resolve or forget the recurring anger toward others—that the mountain will be made smooth and she will live in peace in the rich valley below.

Today the sun is darkened by clouds of bad memories, brought by the winds of loss and loneliness. After dinner I encouraged a nap. She agreed although an "unlikely time." She said how good the day together was. Just before she drifted off to sleep, she said, "Someday I won't even be able to tell you that." She slept. I wept.

2/21/08

Today we went to our accountant of 25 years. Jane sat beside me and was silent as he and I went through the details. I put my hand on her arm from time to time. When we finished, Jane asked, "How will I handle all of this if you are suddenly gone? I wouldn't know the first thing about it. It frightens me. You need to explain to me now what would happen if you weren't here and all this needed to be done." I said Laura and Paul and Kathie have all the information. The accountant tried to reassure her.

Jane seemed satisfied as we left the office, but in the hallway she began to cry. I held her and tried to comfort her. She told me what had been going on in her mind. She pictured me dead and knew she couldn't deal with anything if that happened.

We had lunch at the Mall and talked well over an hour. She told me her observations in the accountant's office, the pictures, one diploma with a ribbon and the other without, his use of an eraser, the color, size, condition of the eraser, his suit and tie, the one wrinkle in his suit jacket, the furniture, the size of the office, etc.

These perceptions went on as her mind was going through my death and her loss of ability to function. No wonder things get mixed up in her head. This is how she has always viewed the world, keenly and emotionally. Now she tries to cope with it as the tangles in her brain become more convoluted.

2/29/08

It was a stormy week. Although I had misgivings, one afternoon we went to a movie. During the movie she asked me something in a loud voice. I went "shush" because I thought someone else might do so and cause an angry reply from Jane. Well, "shush" was a mistake. After the movie she was hostile and refused to leave the theater. I tried to calm her. I get frightened of what she might do at times like this. She threatened to kill herself in the first opportunity. She was finished with life and dreaded her future. "It is obvious you will not be able to take care of me as I get worse and you will stop talking to me."

The evening did not go well. I tried to soothe her and achieve some peace and reconciliation. The following morning was better. Jane was full of remorse for "badgering" me the day before and expressed doubt I will stay with her.

She is convinced big changes are occurring. "I feel different about everything. I know I'm worse. You don't realize how different I feel. Everything has changed. I don't feel connected any more. I'm sure I will not get back to where I was two weeks ago." I let her know I fully accept what she is telling me and I don't know everything that goes on in her head, but I am trying to understand it and keep up with it as well as I can.

Today we went to Mass at the monastery and had lunch at the Mall where we talked for two hours. Jane was bright, connected, insightful. She brought up the area of moral responsibility for actions. I talked about emotions and how they limit or influence our freedom of action. She was attentive and absorbed it all. We talked about emotions influencing behavior and related them to actions in my life and in hers.

As a child Jane observed adult behaviors beyond her comprehension. She had no chance to explore or to express her resultant emotional turmoil because there was no one to listen. Her unexpressed feelings were paramount in her poor decision making of the past. When she is depressed she says Alzheimer's is a punishment from God. I tell her illnesses are not punishment.

Jane says she should do better and thinks she can. I tell her I admire how well she is doing because I see how frustrating and frightening and discouraging it is for her to forget so many things, lose so many things, be unable to follow so many comments by others, and feel helpless to do things that used to come so easily.

In church today I prayed for guidance in her care. I need to remain calmer when she attacks me. I know I bristle over a harsh remark she makes on a bad day because I feel her comment is not justified. It changes my attitude and she reads attitudes better than I can read my own name. I'm really not the victim in her hostile outbursts. I'm learning more about Alzheimer's and also more about myself!

3/22/08

Where are we with this illness? It is hard to tell. There are no bench marks. I finished reading "The Myth of Alzheimer's" by Whitehouse. Much of it I read to Jane, especially the positive, hope-filled passages.

There is increasing evidence that the emotional component and the memory component are quite separate. Memory continues to fail. Jane repeats things she just said. She fails at names and dates. Getting lost is obvious. I need to be careful not to leave her alone when we are out. These are the "stable signs" of her Alzheimer's cognitive decline.

On the emotional side, Alzheimer's has no constant signs. Recently Jane was in a calm mood at breakfast, but while preparing to go to an appointment, things changed markedly. She felt "out of it," "frightened," "strange," "different than I ever felt before." In the doctor's waiting room, "I don't want to go home to bed. I don't want to go to sleep. I don't want the doctor to give me medicine to put me to sleep." She behaved like a person in shock.

She was wary during the doctor visit. The doctor tied to reassure her with various suggestions. She asked, "Is this Alzheimer's?" He said, "No. I think you may have a secondary infection from your cold last week." "No" was the remedy. There was no secondary infection, but "No" relieved her concern.

After we left she said she was "coming back." We often talk about her "going somewhere" at times like this. At lunch we talked for two hours and by late afternoon she was bright and cheerful. I believe the episode of the morning was not directly attributable to Alzheimer's but to emotional stress. On the other hand, I believe Alzheimer's allows her emotional reactions to be exaggerated.

Jane recently lost one of the little books she writes in. When she was a child, her "things" were her security, her refuge, her private world. She shared a bed and a room with her grandmother until the day she was married. She had no private world apart from her possessions. They were not just dolls and boxes and scraps of paper and "junk." They knew her secrets, her sadness and any "badness" she felt. They gave structure to her world and meaning to her life. Eventually her mother made her give many of her treasures away and later her stepfather threw many of them away.

When the little book was lost, it contained "my thoughts," "my words," "my private mind." It was devastating. Her response was to become "numb," as a person who has experienced a tragic loss. The emotional episode was particularly meaningful because it connected to the losses of her childhood. Cognitive deficits of Alzheimer's keep her from evaluating current losses reasonably and modulating her emotional responses.

Each time Jane is angry with me, there seems to be some ingredient, no matter how minute, connected to the neglect she felt as a child. Something I say or do triggers a feeling in her portfolio of childhood offenses. She is not heard, not responded to, not seen, not part of a decision, not able to make a choice, not approved of, not accepted. Emotion takes over, and Alzheimer's prevents an appropriate response.

(Email to Laura 3/31/08)
I'm so glad you and mom had the long talk yesterday. It was great for her. It helped some of her thinking get back on track. She loves you a great deal and sometimes has such a hard time expressing it freely, especially when she gets so guarded and so afraid of being hurt. Thank you, thank you. Things seem to be a lot better this morning, and I'll try to keep them that way.

4/6/08
The world turned upside down a couple of times recently and I need to write about it. Laura and the girls came on 3/25 and left on 3/27. Laura and Jane seemed to be at odds most of the time. The visit was a strain on all of us and depleted Jane emotionally.

The day after they left, Jane wanted to go somewhere so we went to the Owings Mills Mall. Jane was irritable and critical of things I said. I became quiet. She went in the Dollar Store and told me not to come in with her. I waited outside for 30 minutes while she shopped. She was angry because I hadn't come into the store.

I tried to calm her during dinner. She refused to eat, was hostile and rebuffed my attempts to lessen the tension. As her rage increased, I became concerned and suggested we leave. She said emphatically she had no intention of going home with me. "I will call someone to come and get me. I will go to the police station if necessary." We were getting nowhere. It was close to 8p.m. What would happen when the Mall closed? Would she refuse to get in the car if we went to the parking lot? What would I do then?

A security guard walked by the table. I said to him, "My wife has Alzheimer's and is refusing to go home with me. What can we do when the Mall closes?" Jane jumped up, grabbed her shopping bags and ran from the eatery, screaming, "Don't come near me! Don't touch me! Stay away from me!" The guard and I followed at some distance. Another guard was waiting by the Mall balcony. Jane entered a jewelry store and was screaming at the clerk. The two guards escorted her from the store. She was cooperative.

One guard took me down the hallway and the other took Jane down another hallway. The guard with me went back and forth to talk to the other guard. Jane agreed to take a cab home. Then she agreed to go home with me. We were reunited under the watchful eyes of the guards. We left the store hand in hand. I drove home slowly on the right side of traffic, worried she might try to jump out.

She remained furious through the night and we both had little sleep. Saturday was a tumultuous day. Kathie called several times and wanted to come over. Jane insisted she not come. By Sunday afternoon things were a bit calmer. Kathie called and Jane agreed she could come. We had frozen pot pies for dinner and Kathie joined us.

After Kathie left, I suggested Jane call Laura. They talked for about 20 minutes. Apparently, Jane gave Laura and Kathie an accurate account of what happened at the Mall. She acknowledged she was out of control at the eatery and said she didn't know what she might have done.

The past week went reasonably well. Jane has been impatient, especially with herself, and insists her illness is much worse, expressing doubt she will ever get back to how good she felt a few weeks ago.

Then there is the other side of the world! Yesterday was the best day we had in a long time. How did things turn around? Who knows? But they did in spite of Jane's prediction that the good times were gone and in spite of the doubts that haunt me.

On Friday Jane slept until noon, and after a couple of hours, she decided to lie down again. As I massaged her feet she dosed off quickly and slept another two and a half hours. She was disappointed when she woke because she did not feel better. As often happens, she didn't improve until the next day.

Yesterday she was cheerful. The day went exceptionally well. After breakfast we went for a long walk in the woods. We talked over an hour at lunch. She recognized how much better she was feeling and admitted she thought it would never happen.

It was 3p.m. and we planned to go to 4:30 Mass. I asked what she would like to do with the time. She responded, "I have a wild idea!" I knew what her idea was and that we would never make it to 4:30 Mass. I decided that spending the time with her was more important and more sacred than preparing for church. Later I remembered there was also a 6:30 Mass on Saturdays, so we went to that. The best of both worlds!

After Mass one of those things happened that leaves its mark for years to come, so unexpected, so unusual, so touching, yet so simple. We said hello to Father Tillman, our pastor. He gave Jane a pastoral hug and said how happy he was to see her. Jane responded, "I've had a couple of good days and wanted to come this evening." He put his arm around her, pulled her close and said, "It's an honor to have you here. It's like standing in the presence of God."

It was so warm and so genuine! We were overwhelmed. Jane began telling him how good I am to her and all I do for her. I was teary-eyed and said, "I feel like I'm serving God in my own way." Tillman added, "You are." It was a graced moment!

4/17/08

Life is no longer a moving picture for Jane. It is a series of still shots which she grapples with as she tries to register them and make them into a whole. This is how she described things as we talked about them today. I think the still shots are hard to identify for what they are. I wonder if she can always "develop" them. She looks at missing objects and does not recognize them.

Today when Jane was looking for a sweater, I told her where she put it last night. She said it was a miracle I knew that. I said it was because I still have a memory that is working well and hers is not working well. I took her face in my hands and said, "I don't love you less because your memory isn't good. I don't love you because of all our memories of the past, many of which you may lose as time goes on. I love you not because of the past or because of what we did or had but because each day you bring a new vision to my life and a new inspiration to my heart."

I have new hope . . . not that Jane will improve . . . but that I may deal more effectively with the storm days. We have not had a horrible time since the time I called the security guards.

There were several days when Jane did poorly emotionally. If I set aside my irritation quickly and calmly, I achieve a much better attitude toward her with her anger and sadness and fear. I am better able to continue some verbal interaction with her. I do need God's help to see me through this opportunity to serve Him.

(Email to my daughter, Frances 4/17/08)
I thought it might be a good idea to drop you a note and try to give you some idea of my situation.
I don't know if you know much about Alzheimer's disease. I keep learning. I think it is safe to say most people with Alzheimer's have problems in relationships. They are often quite sensitive and easily misinterpret the behavior of others and even distort what may have occurred in certain situations. They often respond negatively to the actions of others and see those as hostile when they are not meant to be so. These reactions and responses may focus on particular individuals irrespective of the relationships that previously existed.

Jane has had some of these symptoms for some time now. Unfortunately, facts and reasoning are of no benefit in trying to change the direction of these attitudes because the thinking can become quite fixed and efforts to change it can only aggravate and exacerbate it. Over time these things are becoming an increasing problem for Jane.

All of this is the reason I have not kept in closer contact with you and others. I regret this is so, but my fidelity to Jane and my desire to keep her as undisturbed as possible cause certain limitations. That is also why

I resort more often to e-mail than to phone calls because the latter can be disturbing to her.

(Email to Laura 4/21/08)

I know Mom repeats stories she has told you before. After the call yesterday, she said she didn't know what month it was or if this was still the school year. She didn't want to let you know she didn't know that. I think it is difficult for her not to try to hide how much she has forgotten. That makes it difficult for her to fake her way through a conversation. I tell her it is important to let others know when she can't remember and not be embarrassed or feel guilty or stupid.

4/29/08

We went to Rehoboth for three days last week. Every day had its tension if not its crisis. Jane was angry daily over things that had no substance. We worked our way back to harmony each time as I tried desperately to calm the troubled waters.

The trip home was pleasant. Traffic was heavy because it was commuter time. When we neared home, I said I would get a cart to take our things upstairs. She thought it was a good idea. The plan worked well. In the apartment, she was suddenly angry because I walked by her and didn't embrace her and welcome her home. She went through a list: I didn't talk to her all the way home (not true), I bossed her around when we brought our things up (not true), and I ignored her after we got in our apartment (not true).

Later on she wanted to tell me something. She said she had no reason to be angry at me and she made up all the things she said and they were not true. She just felt angry, and the feeling pushed her into the accusations. It was so insightful on her part!

Why was Jane angry? Was there an external stimulus? Or is this similar to times when a person feels happy or light hearted but can't really explain why? Or someone feels "down" without an explanation. Is this anger of Alzheimer's just an empty shell, "a feeling?" Her comments addressed a real factor in this illness. Something in the brain makes a person angry. The anger reaches out to attach. The caregiver is the one most available. The "reasons" for the anger get filled in later by the "thinking brain."

Jane decided she didn't want to continue going to Mass at the monastery. One of the priests treated her coldly on an occasion, and she thought the priests showed preferential treatment toward certain attendees. Her sensitivity to these incidents is clearly related to "having to sit in the back of the church" during childhood years.

(From the letter I wrote to the Superior at the monastery 5/12/08)
When we began to come to the monastery Jane had become disenchanted with our parish. More accurately, she had acquired a good bit of hostility toward our parish, the priests, and the community. She had developed, over a few weeks time, four or five reasons why "I will never go there again." The "reasons" were, of course, not reasoned but were based on minor issues or actions of others that would have been insignificant, if it were not for the Alzheimer's. She was threatening to quit going to Mass.

This is what motivated us to come to you. It was renewing and refreshing for both of us. Jane's faith and religion is fundamentally based on emotion, not on reason. She was the only one in her household who went to Mass, taken and left there by her grandmother when Jane was very small. She had a few Sunday school classes taught by the parochial school sisters, who probably weren't too happy about the task and certainly not too welcoming to the kids who always had to sit in the back of the church. Through the years Jane has clung to that gift of her faith, and sometimes I wonder how she did it. Of course, she does fight with God regularly.

In any case, Jane offered to go to our Saturday evening parish Mass with me a few weeks ago. Father Tillman was as warm and welcoming to her as anyone could possibly be. One Mass led to another. We attended the 9a.m. Mass a couple of weeks ago, the one we went to for years. Many people embraced her like a long lost member. It was truly heart-warming. And all the reasons for never going back have faded away. We are home—for now.

I do not know what the future may bring. Jane's reasoning is very faulty at times, as her memory fails and her moods seem increasingly to be determined by cell matter and not by what matters. I work with her where she is and where she wants to go. I feel I can serve God by caring for her. So we may show up some day, and it may be for one time or for regular.

(From the letter I wrote to our pastor 5/12/08)
I very much appreciated your phone call of several months ago when you asked about Jane and very kindly offered to come over and see her. I mentioned paranoid thinking at the time. It does occur intermittently and with various foci. Certainly her hostility toward the parish was not based on anything of significance. It is almost like a torrent of anger springs from nowhere and paints someone or some event with a dark, frightening color. And the picture may last a few weeks or several months before fading away. Some of these "pictures" seem to endure and have affected our contact with some family and friends. Occasionally I get painted with the brush of anger, but I am learning to survive the splash and help Jane come back to "us."

Currently Jane is very pleased to be back at St. John's, and I am happy we are there. Your warm reception was of particular benefit in making her feel we are home. She has completely forgotten her grievances or, if she briefly remembers, will remark how unreasonable her feelings were.

Jane is being very courageous and for the most part often appears to be "her old self." Her memory increasingly fails and makes it difficult to attach today to yesterday, or even this afternoon to this morning. She is easily confused in simple conversations, especially when more than one other person is involved. She becomes disoriented quite readily and even gets lost in our building. Daily living is a genuine struggle for her and takes effort and concentration to cope with simple things. I believe all of this frustration is at the core of her anger and her depression and her fears.

May 15, 2008

The week is going quite well. Jane's emotional reactions are exaggerated. Whatever is lost is the most precious thing she ever owned. If I say anything critical, no matter how softly, it is the worst thing anyone ever said to her in her whole life. And when there is a frightening experience, it is the first time in her life she ever felt this. It seems she is exaggerating, but I have no doubt the experience is as she says it is . . . the worst experience, the cruelest comment, the most precious object. She has no memory of the prior incidents I so readily associate with the current one.

Recently we went to meet friends in a restaurant. Jane was tense and on the way said she knew she was much worse and she felt like Alzheimer's was taking over her life completely. She became irritated when I tried to reassure her by saying she has feelings like that from time to time.

The following day, she continued thinking about her fears of the prior evening. In the afternoon, we were active, making plans, talking about lots of things, past, present, and future. She was bright, focused, spontaneous, creative . . . . all those wonderful qualities we have enjoyed through the years. I took her face in my hands and looked in her eyes and said, "That's the same brain up there you had last night. See how wonderfully it works today. Alzheimer's doesn't suddenly get bad and then get better. What happened last night was not some sudden, permanent change in your condition or even some harbinger of what is to come. You need to try to remember that."

We have started something new. In the mornings when Jane does her hair and her make-up in her bathroom, her mind wanders to a long litany of negative thoughts . . . . all those sad stories of her mother, emotional abuse from her first husband, the disloyal relationship with the group from the pool, etc. These dark, destructive thoughts contaminate her mood, and their obsessive quality fills this time of routine. She finishes breakfast in a pleasant mood looking forward to the day. By the time she is ready for the day her spirit is deadened, her interest is dimmed, and her feelings are chaotic.

I started reading to her from the morning paper while she does her toilette. She follows articles well and refers to them later. She is pleased with the new arrangement. By the time she is ready, she is more likely to have a positive and pleasant attitude about the day.

She still collects a box here or there, a little piece of paper, a leaflet, a shop card, a toothpick from her sandwich, a bit of colored string. I suppose anyone who is an obsessive collector must have great difficulty parting with even the most insignificant treasure—because none are insignificant. Must be how God looks at people!

(Email to Kathie 5/20/08)
During your visit Mom rambled on as she does sometimes, especially when she is uneasy. This occasionally occurs with other people, and afterwards she seems to recognize it and feels embarrassed but also angry with herself and with them. After you left she became increasingly angry at you, at me, at Fran, at Mary (from the YMCA), etc. There was no reason for you to visit, you just felt an obligation, didn't I think you were different during this visit and the one last weekend, maybe you shouldn't visit, etc., etc.

There is never any value in trying to counter any of her comments when she is like that, but if I don't say anything that is even worse. I told her I thought you were tired Sunday evening, it had probably been a long day for you, you must have a lot on your mind these days, and we really have no idea how things are going in your life—but you are important to both of us and someone we both care about and who cares about us. * * * * * *

She thinks everyone in the family is leaving her, one by one. There will be nobody who will want to come to see her because they will all think she is crazy, and she won't be able to talk any more. * * * * * *

I have written this to try to give you some clear picture of how unreasonable and paranoid she can become at times. There is never any good cause and often not even a clear cause. I know you are aware of this sort of thing because you have learned a great deal about Alzheimer's and you are sensitive about it. It feels different when you are the object of it and not just an outsider to it. You know your mom has a great deal of affection for you and is bonded to you very firmly.

5/22/08

The vagaries of Alzheimer's! At lunch, we talked about recent Alzheimer's events. There were three days when Jane exhibited confusion, marked irritability, and despairing comments. She gets quite agitated, almost hysterical, when she is unable to find something. Sometimes the missing object is in front of her. Recently she is more willing to ask me calmly to help her search.

I reminded her forgetting things is like losing something. You had it and then it disappeared. I said she is going to continue to forget things and to lose things, and in either case she has no blame. This is her illness, and that is how her life is going to be.

A few days ago, we were robbed of $130, taken from our apartment by our housekeeper. We reported it to security, the police, and the housekeeping department. Jane feels violated, invaded, helpless. We want the housekeeper dismissed, but the facility cannot do that because there is no firm evidence she took the money, though there is little doubt. We will have a new housekeeper assigned.

Was Jane's reaction excessive? Alzheimer's is stealing things out of her head, and she has no idea what is going to be taken next time, and the time after that, and the time after that. Someday it may all be gone. There is nothing she can do about it! She remains vulnerable, defenseless, ready to be victimized again. The doors and windows are open. There are no locks, no barriers. What will be missing the next time she searches her memory? She won't even know if something is missing if she can't remember it.

Yesterday Jane had a philosophical attitude about her illness. "It is important to cherish the positive things in our life. We are physically well and enjoying the day. None of us knows how long we will live. Everything is great at the moment and that is the moment we are living." Her thoughts were solid, sane, coherent, and encouraging for both of us. I pointed out how well her brain works to develop and express this line of thinking.

Jane feels sad, tired, and hopeless today. She got up during the night and sat in the dark studio for a time. When she came back to bed, I was on "the far edge of the bed facing in the other direction." She felt lonely and abandoned. She told me about it this morning. I reminded her I want her to wake me if she is awake during the night because I don't want her to be alone. I suggested some additional sleep. She is sleeping now.

5/25/08

When we walk, Jane picks up little pieces of bark, small rocks, and twigs . . . . each in some way special to her. It is like walking with a small child. She stops to look at "faces" or "hearts" in the bark or the knot of a tree or in a rock too big to take home. Jane finds things all the time no one else sees, things that are objects of beauty to her. Her response to the trees and the clouds and the rocks seems primitive, like one might expect from a Native American. This is not a regressive phenomenon. She is in touch with things others do not see and do not understand. I know of it only through her, but it touches me deeply and affects my view of things.

Her sense of humor remains intact. The other day she was looking for something. I entered the hunt uninvited. When I found it and told her where it was, she said with a good deal of satisfaction, "That was just where I put it." We laughed together.

5/25/08

Occasionally we talk about our Estate Plan, which we agreed on quite some time ago. Jane and I are joined in a solid, loving, dedicated, permanent bond to one another. Our children cannot separate us by their behavior, so in a sense how one of them behaves toward either of us affects us both. Although I was the one who brought the check to the household, it was earned by both of us. We always made joint decisions about how to spend it, so we have made a joint decision about how to bequeath it.

There is the question of why money is given to anyone. Giving money to a young child is usually based on the giver's love for the child more than on the child's love for the giver. In the case of adult children, I'm not sure the same reasoning holds. I believe it is then appropriate and fair for a parent to consider the affection of the child.

In early 2007 I wrote a letter to the eight children telling them about Jane's current condition. They have known about the Alzheimer's since 2005. I wrote, "Understanding, patience, and love are the only real gifts any of us can give her now." Our children have responded with those gifts to varying degrees. A few have shown interest, concern, affection, understanding, appreciation. They give both of us courage and strength for the road ahead. Others have shown little interest, minimal evidence of affection, and no indication of understanding.

PART 4 (JUN 08—NOV 08)

(Email to Kathie 6/4/08)
I can't explain to your Mom why you said this or that or the other thing, or why this comment or that comment came up in her previous conversation with you. Every day she has been mulling over what was said or what she thought was said during your phone conversation, at the same time admitting she is not sure what either of you said. But she is full of statements about what you said and what you meant and how offended she was and is.

The whole thing seems to come and go each day. I think she is okay and then suddenly we're going over the whole thing again. It never makes any sense and never really reaches any understanding. Paranoia runs through it all. Then suddenly she is worrying that you will turn against her, etc., etc.

I'm not trying to unload this on you by any means. I'm sure she will settle down over time. I'm not suggesting there is anything you can do or should do except continue your affection for her and continue to be yourself. I just wanted to give you some idea of the lay of the land in case you call or come by.

(Email to Kathie 6/10/08)
First of all, I think Saturday went well as least from this end. Your Mom has not talked about any of it except to say she didn't know how she could be so wrong. It seemed to completely satisfy her. She was very pleased with the visit and I was very grateful. Hope it was not too trying for you. The whole thing was rather typical of how these things go from some blip in a conversation, to questions, to full blown accusations with frank paranoid thinking, and possible alienation.

(Email to Laura 6/14/08)

Mom is still disturbed if anyone here mentions the trees that were cut down. She doesn't want to even hear John or Fran's name. She is angry about my giving her car to Fran and thus to her daughter, Theresa. She is angry at Jim in Montana and doesn't like his wife. She still criticizes Don and our last two or three trips to Montana. None of this has any real basis in anything of substance. She blames me for things she gave away when we moved here, especially clothes she gave away. That comes up quite easily, although she rarely wears most of the clothes she has. But it always sounds like she had no choice in those decisions.

I am beginning to feel more alone because I cannot speak as freely with her as I have through all the years. We still have good times together. We go to the Mall and sometimes sit and talk for an hour or two, but I am always conscious of how precarious the situation is because something might set her off. Then there is an occasional day when she seems just like she always was.

I begin to doubt if we will ever come up to visit again. She doesn't mention it as much as she used to. She is very unpredictable and she can become almost uncontrollable at times. I love her as much as I ever have and I feel so sad to imagine how difficult and how painful it is for her to go through hours and days with big empty spaces in her life.

I doubt if Mom would survive more than a day or two in this apartment if something happened to me. She gets lost in the building. She would probably become hostile toward people here and not accept any help or comfort from them. She would be unable to take care of herself. She has a difficult time finding the usual things we use in the kitchen. I'm sure Kathie would be immediately available. I need to be well as long as Mom is alive and I pray most for that.

She was pleased with your phone call the other night. She told me you said you loved her and you were very understanding. She is often like a child needing to be told she is loved.

(Email to Laura 6/23/08)

Wanted to let you know that we had a wonderful week last week, probably the best we've had in a long time. Mom was a complete companion through the week. Had two or three problem points but she put some real effort into controlling her anger and keeping things on an even keel.

The past week makes me feel guilty for any criticisms I made . . . . and yet I can't help but be concerned that bad things will pop up again. Her mind gets focused on past items and they drag her down pretty quickly. This morning it was the women from the pool and how "they have all turned against me." It's too bad these aren't the things that are forgotten.

7/12/08

Except for emails to the kids and others, I haven't written anything for about two months. It has been a strange time with such variation it has been difficult to fathom and at times difficult to face.

For three straight weeks in June, life was hectic. There was some daily blow-up on Jane's part with anger, recriminations, accusations, long discourses that went nowhere, tears, despair, isolation, irrationality, arguments, charges, verbal attacks, and endless scenes. It was tiring, and I felt drained. When Laura and Paul and Bob called on Father's Day, I was feeling very alone, like I had lost my life's companion.

Jane and I talked about how wearing the days were and how they seemed to create a chasm between us. We wondered if the span would become too great for our love to bridge. We were both frightened! Jane is determined to handle things differently and not get angry the way she has been doing. I attribute the anger to Alzheimer's and wonder how much of it she can control.

There is a marked change the last three weeks. Jane is more relaxed. She is sleeping better and not having frightening dreams as often. We frequently talk for two or three hours at a time. She is alert, rational and engaging. Our exchanges are at the same broad intellectual level they were in the past. People ask me who supports me during this time. My honest answer is "Jane."

We talk about what we can do to try to maintain her level of functioning. I have tried to make some changes that I believe may help. 1) I bring in a chair and read a variety of articles to her while she does her hair and make-up. 2) If there is something on her mind, we talk in bed as long as she wants. I usually massage her back with a battery powered massager for a short time. 3) Jane can become tired any time of day. It is important to recognize when "her batteries are low" and encourage a nap. 4) We need to continue to monitor and curtail when necessary our social activities. We are going to stop going to the dining room for dinner. 5) I remind her more frequently of things we are going to do or places we are going to go. 6) I try to deal differently with her anger. I don't explain. I put my arms around her, tell her I love her, and say "Please, don't be angry."

Attending to these items has made a difference for Jane. Certainly our life has been more peaceful and happier these past several weeks. Will it continue? I think it can, and I believe Jane thinks it can. Her Alzheimer's seems not as threatening as it was. When we talk, it seems that memory loss is the only impairment Jane experiences from Alzheimer's. While that is reassuring, I know it is also deceiving.

(Email to Laura 7/28/08)
Mom has been much steadier emotionally for the past five or six weeks. There are brief flare-ups, but they are easily and quickly resolved. This seems to be a definite and I hope permanent change. It appears to be a fairly reliable new level of adjustment. At the same time, her memory has shown definite deterioration which indicates continuing loss of cells.

In view of all this, I think she would tolerate a visit to see you and the girls. I think she has some fear of losing track of you. She writes numerous notes to you on little pieces of paper when she is in the cafe or in the eatery at the Mall waiting for me to order for us. She buys cards to send the kids but rarely completes and sends them.

8/1/08
Two days ago Jane had a terrible dream relating to the hostility she feels between herself and Mary, the friend from the pool group. These ruminations return periodically and she becomes irritable, disheartened, and excessively focused on the negatives in her life. After breakfast, in an attempt to improve her mood, she suggested we walk the halls which we do two or three times

each week. We walk the 14 flights of stairs up and down, going from one stairway to the other on each hall.

We stopped at the café (second floor) for a cup of coffee. It was noisy. Jane didn't hear something I said. I repeated it, and again she didn't hear. I felt she didn't understand what I was saying, rather than not hearing it. I repeated it the third time. She was annoyed. We continued our walk. She was irritated, withdrawn and confused. In our apartment, I embraced her and tried to reduce the strain. She was angry because she asked me "What?" three times, and I still did not speak loudly enough for her to hear. I apologized and said I had been rude.

We talked about it during lunch at the Mall. I said it must be difficult for her to keep up with everything in her daily life and I admire her for the effort that is involved. What happened in the café was more than Jane not hearing me. It takes effort for her to stay connected and understand spoken words. As her constant companion, I am part of her immediate connection to the world. If the connection fails by my inattention, lack of response, or failure to speak loudly, it is threatening to her. If connections are lost, she is floating in a world she does not understand.

Back home we decided to play gin-rummy. I play so she wins most of the time. She enjoys winning and never becomes suspicious, no matter how frequently she wins. During our game, she brought up the episode at the café, and as we continued talking I knew she was getting increasingly irritated. I'm sure I sounded defensive. Her anger skyrocketed, and I was at a loss how to respond.

Then suddenly the playing field changed. She was the one in the café trying to explain something to me and I was the one saying "What." I couldn't believe it. I tried to tell her it was the opposite, and the fury mounted. "How can you try to get out of it by telling lies and pretending I don't know what happened? Do you think I'm an idiot? Are you trying to drive me crazy?" Now I really didn't know which way to go.

It was time for me to go get our dinners. I wondered about her being alone but I thought it might benefit both of us if I left for a few minutes. When I came back, she had changed clothes "to go out." She continued the same

61

hammering about our conflict in the café. I finally told her I couldn't continue talking about it because it was so muddled I no longer knew who said what. I thought this might move it to a "leave it alone" place. There is never a "leave it alone" place for Jane.

She decided I was losing my mind and I might leave her. I thought about it, prayed about it, and decided I had to confront this head on. I asked her to sit by me. I said, "I want you to listen to me. I have something to say." She was frightened and said, "Don't look at me like that!" I repeated "Just listen to me. Don't interrupt." I told her she was wrong, and I slowly went over the sequence of events in the café as they happened.

It was amazing! It was a change from dark to light, from confusion to clarity. She saw it all! It was something of a shock to her. She cried. We both did. She saw the significance of it, how wrong she could be in her judgment and thinking. She said she could not be trusted. She referred to it later in the evening and again the next day.

I thought about it for two days. It is a tactic to be used carefully. "Tactic"—an unpleasant choice of words. This is not a battle, a debate, a contest. It is a life relationship, a love relationship. I learned some important things these past few days. How fragile her connections! How vulnerable her psyche! How much more to learn about her! How many more ways to love her!

8/04/08

It is striking to watch two parts of Jane's brain working: the feeling brain and the thinking brain. There is the brain of emotional response and the brain of rational thought.

I see the emotional brain take over. I think of a half dozen things that quickly begin the tumult, things I try to avoid mentioning. These include: the trees, the stolen money, Mary, her first husband, and my daughter's birthday party. There are several others that send a red signal.

There are uncharted pitfalls in conversation. The other day we were discussing some bland insignificant thing. I said I was surprised she seemed "so concerned" about it. The storm came quickly. "How could you make such a stupid remark? How could you be so thoughtless? It was the cruelest thing you ever said to me. Don't you realize how strongly I feel about it? Don't you know how much it means to me? How could you abandon me? Go away and leave me alone. "Alone" is precisely what she does not want. I tried to hold her and said I was sorry. I tried to put the remark in a better context. That brought new charges that I was "defensive," "arguing" and "dishonest."

I was dumbfounded by her distorted view of what happened. I wondered if she really believed what she was saying, and yet I knew it was "her truth." I felt angry and betrayed that she could believe these things of me. I pray for help, for patience, for guidance.

Then it's like someone throws a switch. The thinking brain is back in charge. Jane is calm, apologetic, and aware of what she said and how foolish it was. She is embarrassed and asks me to forgive her. There is no need for forgiveness. It is obvious what occurred. I wish that ended it for her but the memory stays with her for a day or two.

After these episodes, Jane fears Alzheimer's will eventually bring her to similar behavior permanently. I tell her I have not seen or heard anything indicating this as the final stage of Alzheimer's patients. My remarks settle her mind for the moment.

Jane mentions her fears of late stage Alzheimer's: needing to be fed, unable to recognize family, unable to communicate, being empty inside. "What is going on in your brain when there are no memories there?" The overriding fear is she will be angry, volatile, and combative—"crazy."

8/9/08

When we were at CVS pharmacy, Jane looked at a hair clip and I encouraged her to buy it. She didn't want to spend three dollars for it because "we are saving money." I again encouraged her to get it. I asked her later if she was sure and she said she was.

At home Jane had a different view of the incident. She showed me the clip in the store. I said, "If you are sure you can use it, get it." "That is the kind of comment you always make when you don't want me to buy something." It was my idea to look for the clip. I showed it to her and I encouraged her to buy it. Her reply, "If I had taken my own money, I would have bought it." She often makes that statement and it irritates me. I told her it is "our" money, and if she wants to buy something, I put it on our charge.

We spent a few hours discussing it. She was hostile, tearful at times, threatening to harm herself some day, accusing me of lying, of being defensive, of attacking her, of abandoning her. When things like this happen, I feel helpless. I don't know what to say. I don't know what to do. Every response causes escalation.

We "made up" from time to time; but this never stops Jane from talking about it again and going over details that already caused our bickering. I keep trying to "clarify" things and, of course, to make my point. We both slept poorly.

The next morning I woke Jane with a hug and kiss, talked about the day, and opened the shades. I greeted her when she came in the kitchen and continued what I was doing. "So we're going to continue like it was yesterday! Every morning you hug and kiss me when I come into the kitchen, but I guess you don't want to do that this morning." My immediate thought was: "That is not true. I don't hug and kiss you when I am still working on the breakfast." I did hug and kiss her, but I was irritated.

During the day Jane had wild fluctuations of mood—angry, sad, remorseful, accusatory, threatening, pleading, crying. I can't adequately describe them—desperate enters into all of them. With some stability by 4p.m., we went to the Mall for dinner.

Friday when we were talking, Jane wondered if each of us could do something to avoid a 24 hour crisis like we just had. Two ideas came to mind. I said, "You always tell me when these things start that I could stop them if I wanted to. You are right. I need to hold you and comfort you and say I'm sorry and tell you things will be all right. Alzheimer's makes you unable to stop what you do, but I should react differently. The second thing I must do is not try to explain what happened and why I did what I did."

Jane and I witness the same event but each of us reports it differently. My conflict with Jane over an incident like the one in the pharmacy is utterly ridiculous. No wonder she speaks of those times as a contest. Are Alzheimer's patients "unreasonable?" Jane was being perfectly reasonable **based on what she believed to be true.**

During this discussion Jane realized her feelings and conflicts and comments about money are connected to her loss of independence. "I used to drive. I used to shop on my own. I could buy what I liked. Now I can't do any of that." She saw it all as a reaction to her feelings of loss as Alzheimer's tightens its grip.

It was an enlightening talk. Whether it stays with Jane remains to be seen. If it does not stay with me and influence my behavior, then I should be ashamed. Experts say I should not blame myself when things go badly between the two of us. There is truth in that, because this life can be burdensome. But it is also true if I want to be supportive of Jane, I need to understand all I can about what happens between us and put into practice what I learn.

(Email to Kathie 8-12-08)
I wrote an email to Phil and tried to explain what is going on with his mother. An email does help me get my thoughts together sometimes. Phil called yesterday and was quite upset. Unfortunately he seems to have little appreciation of what Alzheimer's can do to thought processes.

(Email to Kathie 8-22-08)
Your Mom was wondering yesterday why you never got back to her about seeing your dad. She said she would be ok to meet with him now, but "it better be in the next two weeks or so because I don't know how long this feeling will last." I don't think there's a big rush but perhaps the sooner the better. If we come up with a mutually suitable time, it needs to be with the provision it may have to be cancelled on rather short notice.

(Email to Laura 8/25/08)
I have for several days been struggling with whether or not I should write this email to you. Mom has been very much opposed to me saying anything about this, but somehow I think I owe it to you and perhaps to Mom to give you some idea of her feelings. I will not tell her that I wrote this email and it is better if you do not mention it.

You called last Friday and I passed the phone later to Mom. I am reluctant to go over this, and I want you to know it is in no way accusatory or critical. Mom's version of her call with you goes like this: "Mom was 'wound up' and told you about our trip to DC a day or two before and rattled on about the houses we went to see, the Shrine, etc., etc. She felt you were not interested and wanted to get her off the phone. Before long you said you had to get the kids ready for bed, so the conversation ended. Basically your part of the conversation was hello and goodbye." Mom accuses herself of being wound up and rattling on and taking up your time. (I know she gets into details and sometimes repeats things she just said.) She didn't believe it was time to put the kids to bed. (It was about 7p.m. I think.) She blamed herself for not asking about the wedding but also noted that you and I had already talked for half an hour.

I'm sure what I've written is not an accurate or complete picture of your conversation, but it gives some sense of how things can be interpreted. It is not unusual for her to get a "different message" in a phone call.

She feels you think she can't carry on a normal conversation and you see her as a person with Alzheimer's who needs to be handled differently somehow, to be pacified. She feels there is a wall between the two of you. Then she goes back over the years and finds little things to confirm her belief. Everything I say to remind her of the closeness the two of you had is to no avail.

We are three days from your call, but it remains prominent in her thinking and is one of those "recurring themes" we get into. Things like this drain her spirit and her energy. I've been wondering if some of the things I wrote to you have frightened you a bit in interacting with Mom. It probably gave you a negative picture of the illness. We talk and laugh and visit with people quite normally. Others often say they can't believe Jane has Alzheimer's. I am grateful for how well she is doing and much of it is due to her courage and her determination to cope as best she can. And 99% of the time she copes very well.

(Email to Laura 8/29/08)
Mom and I can be in a situation or see something happen and later when she tells someone else about it or talks to me about it, it sounds like she

is lying. But it is the way she perceived it at the time and is now only telling it as she believed it to be.

Her struggle with the phone call goes on. Some days she is just plain angry at you and vents it quite readily. She doesn't want to talk to you and doesn't want to visit. You have been—etc., etc. Other days she blames herself for her insensitivity, for not asking you about the wedding, for rattling on about what we had done the day before. Then she feels guilty and more understanding of your behavior. She talks then about visiting and about writing to you. All of this is difficult for me because I know how close the two of you have been, and I have no doubt of your love for each other.

At present she says she does not want to talk to you if you call, and that might be best. Phone calls are difficult for her. She gets mixed up as to what people say. It happens with Kathie sometimes. She doesn't like to make calls. Gadgets are stress producing for her. She doesn't like to work the TV remote, the camera, the cell phone, etc. Anxiety leads her to faulty perception and erroneous judgment about what was said, what happened, and others' intentions.

8/30/08

Events are definitely more overwhelming for Jane than they used to be. The latest was a phone call from Laura a week ago. I covered the incident in an exchange of emails with Laura. The event plagued Jane all week. She brings it up frequently, and when she is not talking about it I know she is thinking about it. Her thinking is unreasonable, unrelenting, unforgiving, unshakable. Then suddenly she is understanding, blaming herself, wanting to visit Laura and the girls again, writing a note to her.

Laura separated herself from us long ago as an adolescent and moved away from us emotionally. At that time Jane accepted what happened and acknowledged it was what teenagers do. The healthy separation that occurred during those years is now relived for Jane but with a lack of understanding.

This week Jane found old letters from Laura that were affectionate, informative, enthusiastic, and optimistic. Now they are no consolation to her because she judges them to be insincere and not a true example of Laura's feelings. If I

67

suggest anything supportive of Laura and her love for her mother, Jane is irritated and responds, "Laura was always closer to you than to me."

Laura was close to both of us. I perhaps got along with her a bit better. I was more circumspect in our exchanges, more careful in choice of words, and more able to recognize her developmental stages. Jane was prone to be overprotective and quicker to comment more critically on things Laura might say or do. Jane and I typically agreed on decisions about her, but I went about it more quietly. We each made our own mistakes.

Jane is conscious of diminishing cognitive ability. She looks at things as if they are strange. The tiniest evidence of memory loss is not tiny. It is gigantic! Someone breaks into the treasury of priceless memories and who knows how many will be stolen. The thief leaves his calling card every time.

Someday forgetting may be less troubling for her, when she is no longer as conscious of it. But that is a day she thinks about too, and it only increases her sense of despair. She fears the loss will separate us. If it does, then my priceless treasure, my jewel beyond value will be stolen from me by the same thief that haunts her now.

(Email to Laura 8/31/08)
Thanks for the emails with the pictures and especially the note you wrote. Mom was pleased but still insists you said you needed to get the kids ready for bed. I told her you may have mistakenly said it, but obviously you didn't mean that. She was pleased you addressed that and the time with me, etc. The note will mend things well. I appreciate your response to the need.

Mom shows signs of increasing confusion. We watched a news show today and during a short segment she understood the exact opposite of what the man said. I did not try to tell her what he said because that would only confuse her more. This continuing deterioration is hard for both of us. She is very aware of it and suffers as a result.

(Email to Laura 9/2/08)
Just wanted to let you know how wonderful it was to hear Mom talking and laughing with you over the phone. It was great for her and helped blot

out all the negative feelings she had before. That's how easily they all go away when the time is right and the connection is good. She had one or two times with Kathie that got shaky for a while. A phone call set one of them off. Anyway, thanks for coming through on this. It is much better for her because the angry states only make her miserable and detract from our time together.

9/3/08

Last week Jane "knew things have changed" inside her head. She made the usual statements: "I never felt this bad before," "This is the worst it has ever been," "I'll never get back to how I was feeling before," "This is definitely a new phase." These dire superlatives are standard at a time like this. The desperate attitudes and comments disappeared completely the day after Jane's restorative talk with Laura.

Two days later we went to IKEA. Jane was irritated by new displays in the store and nothing pleased her. The appearance, serviceability, and price of things became personal irritants to her. She never wanted to come to the store again. It became another loss in her life. She was irritated because I did not express the same feelings.

As we left the store she apologized for her attitude. Then she accused me of "not talking." I sympathized with her conflicts about the store. She acknowledged she feels "left alone" when I don't have feelings and opinions that correspond to hers. I told her I agree with her but often don't feel as strongly about things as she does.

The conflict continued well into the night. The following morning she wanted to talk about the previous day. This rarely helps because it is simply a recall of unresolved issues. I became angry and spoke harshly about her repeated complaints I don't talk. I said I don't talk because talking only makes things worse. I am being defensive if I state what I think happened. If I apologize or sympathize, I am just trying to placate her.

Whenever I speak in an angry tone, it is devastating for Jane. I should never do it! She is frightened, feels abandoned, and believes she is being attacked. "This is what the future holds for me if I stay alive with Alzheimer's." She wants to die and threatens she will one day kill herself. All the emotional neglect of her early life fills her with sobbing and self-criticism. It is a horrible scene and fills me with guilt and shame for my behavior.

I cannot, I must not cause this part of her tragic existence to reappear. She gets lost in emotional turmoil caused by simple events in her life, such as the IKEA displays. That is not her fault or her conscious doing. These emotional reactions drive her behavior. Reason and common sense are absent. Comments are misunderstood, misinterpreted, confusing. When I speak harshly or critically to her, I feel I have abused an ill person whom I cherish and admire. And I ask myself, "How could you do that?"

Negative situations remain in Jane's head for a long time. After a period of conflict, I can move ahead and leave it behind. Thoughts remain but the emotional impact is gone. Not so with Jane! The strength of her emotional responses embeds them in her most active cells. They are not lost in the tangled web of Alzheimer's.

9/9/08

We partially recovered from the IKEA episode after two days. Then Jane's mood took a downturn for no apparent reason. I asked if anything was wrong. She was thinking of the IKEA clashes. She distorted much of what occurred but had the essentials right.

She decided I attacked her with the desire to hurt her as deeply as I could, and she would never forgive me. "It was the worst thing you ever did to me, in fact the worst thing anyone ever did to me. You were very deliberate in how you talked to me and you had never been that angry in all our years. You must hate me. There must be something wrong with you. Maybe you should find someone to talk to. You must be keeping something from me now and probably all our married life." She grew silent. There wasn't much I could say except to try to reassure her. My statements only gave her fodder for her claim, "You don't accept what I say. You have to prove me wrong."

When we went to bed she lectured me about it for some time and said we had to talk about it the next day and I had to tell her why I was so cruel and hateful. I offered to talk about it then. That made her angrier. "You never listen to me. I said we could talk about it tomorrow. Why don't you pay attention to what I say?"

The next morning I went to 8a.m. Mass and brought her Communion. I prayed for guidance and strength and peace of mind for Jane. We talked for three hours. I tried to explain to her how I feel when she becomes irritable or angry. Her heightened irritability makes me anxious, even threatened, because I worry about what she might do, how far she might go in some impulsive gesture. I am less relaxed, less spontaneous, less natural. I don't withdraw from her (as she claims) but I focus more intently and more tensely on her. She misinterprets my feelings as anger and withdrawal.

She carefully followed what I said and responded with understanding and acceptance. She will not remember what I explained, but it was valuable for me to realize more clearly my feelings. We talked for another three hours during the rest of the day.

Our internist of the past four years is changing his practice to a "concierge" practice, taking a limited number of patients and charging each one an annual fee of $1,500 for the privilege of being his patient. The MDVIP plan which runs this scheme passes the abuse doctors' experience from Managed Care on to their patients. Jane has been smoldering since friends informed us of the doctor's plan.

I had a routine appointment with the doctor this morning and was informed of the plan. In the afternoon we spoke to our in-house nurses and got the name of a recommended internist. We have an appointment in a couple of days to interview him.

Toward evening Jane became irritable, angry, despondent, frightened. She talked about Alzheimer's and said it is a punishment. After her first thirty horrible years she doesn't deserve this. She can't face it, she doesn't want to live with it, and she wants to die. She became angry and verbally abusive several times. Each time I talked with her at length, apologizing, consoling, comforting as best I could. Each time she eventually relaxed saying she was sorry and how difficult it must be to live with her. "You should find some place to put me." I assured her it is my plan to live with her here until we die.

Jane knows I exercise every day at 6a.m. to preserve my health and my strength for precisely that reason. I am ten years older than she, so the odds of me outliving her are not great. But my health is good, and I sometimes say

I have a deal with God it will happen that way. I don't have it in writing but I have it in my heart.

9/11/08
We had a good trip to IKEA yesterday. During lunch Jane asked how one would use the word "indignant." We had quite a discussion as a result. She said she was indignant about our internist's change of practice and took it as a personal offense.

We talked about why she might easily have feelings of indignation. As a child her individuality was not recognized or acknowledged. Her mother dragged her around to serve her needs, and her grandmother tried to shape her into a kind of puppet. She had little to establish her basic human dignity. So when a situation seems threatening, she interprets it as an attack on her integrity, her dignity.

Jane can engage in this kind of discussion and contribute insights of her own. Her reasoning and thoughts are clear, and her intelligence and good judgment work well. She asked me to remind her of the word "indignant" so she can remember the conversation.

We talked about how thoughts of Alzheimer's have flooded her mind recently. Fear of the future is the horror story of the moment. She says, "I will be going crazy soon." I tell her persons with Alzheimer's don't go crazy; "crazy" is an entirely different disorder.

(Email to Laura 9-12-08)
It was so wonderful to hear you and Mom chatting like you used to, and it meant so much to her. She thrives on attention and expressions of love. They seem to pick her up out of the negative feelings she gets into at times. I think the worst thing about Alzheimer's is the fear generated by thinking about the future. From what I have read, the final stages are not as horrible for the patient as the patient anticipates, possibly because awareness is greatly diminished by then.

In any case, it has been a good week and Mom has been able to adopt a positive attitude again. We had a long talk a couple of days ago in which I described what the future may hold but with more positive aspects, and

I was able to emphasize how important it is for her not to see herself as stupid or crazy or wicked because of what she forgets or what she loses or what anger she expresses. I often reflect on how much courage and strength and control it takes for her to get through even a small piece of the day.

9/20/08

Today during lunch in the cafe, Jane described what sometimes goes on in her head. She is standing by a train track and knows the train is coming. She is not sure she wants to get on it but something compels her to do so. She already has her ticket. The other day when we had a tiff in the cafe, she could see a red train coming, and when it stopped, she got on even though she didn't want to. Once she gets on the train, all the doors are closed and soon there are no doors, so she can't get off. The train goes to a horrible place where she doesn't want to go. She can't understand why she gets on the train when she doesn't want to, but "I've done it all my life." The train separates her from me, and the longer she is on the train the farther away from me she goes. She knows when she goes to sleep she will be off the train when she wakes.

We talked about this for some time. It was a creative analogy for her unwanted trip into anger, an analogy I think most people who experience strong anger can relate to. It was remarkably insightful. It pointed out how unwitting and unwanted the trip is and how isolated and desperate she feels when there are no doors to get out. It is a trip she dreads, and it never has a good outcome. After an angry episode when she feels so separated from me, she often uses the phrase she needs to "get back."

She asked me how the trip usually ends. She did not remember her bitter verbal attacks and the lengthy sessions repeating the details of what caused her anger. I reminded her I hold her and talk to her, and that seems to help her get off the train. Sometimes when she uses a harsh tone, she quickly asks me to forgive her. I suggested this might be a way to get off the train before it starts.

9/28/08

We went to the beach last Monday and returned Thursday. It was mostly a disaster. We stayed at a motel where we stayed many times before. Jane felt lost there. The whole town was strange to her. She became confused several times and was generally uncomfortable. It was very windy so we had little time on the boardwalk. She reminded me I knew she didn't want to come. She was pleased with the idea when I made the reservation. Later she became concerned about going. We agreed we will not return.

Before leaving, we met briefly with Phil at our motel. His daughter had her first baby the previous morning. We talked a bit about the baby. Jane asked for his daughter's address so we could send a card. Phil seemed rather distracted during our visit, probably focused on his new granddaughter.

10/3/08

Casual relationships are easy for Jane, if the contact is not too lengthy. Jane is very friendly with staff here and with the people we know well and see occasionally. These encounters can become problematic if they extend over a period of time. In brief contacts, other people often think, "It's hard to believe Jane has Alzheimer's."

The situation is markedly different when it involves someone of significance in our life, e.g., our pastor, a friend, a physician, or especially one of our children. These contacts are loaded with emotional baggage, treacherous terrain, and high expectations. These relationships cannot survive on a "casual basis," even though that might be their true level. There is a new element in the equation. It requires a new level of response. That level of response is not sympathy, nor coddling, nor catering. It is caring, understanding!

Alzheimer's increases the value of some ingredients of life, and it lays waste others. Jane has no memory-box for names. She doesn't know the president's name or the name of anyone who lives or works here. But when someone significant offends her, the vivid memory is glued in an active part of her brain and remains there for weeks.

Parallel to all of this, there is a swell of tenderness for others who respond to her. She cherishes and is cheered by affection from others, and she is lavish in her expression of affection for them. The darkness of her illness makes the light of another's love a small miracle in her world. It is temporarily restorative. But everything is "temporarily."

We reflect on the responses of the important people in our life. When our pastor welcomed Jane on our return to the parish, his comments were caring and loving, clearly personal and heartfelt. The coldness of a priest in the parish brought Jane to want our previous departure. The aloof attitude of a priest at the monastery brought us back to our parish. The recent decision of our internist to set up a concierge practice was offensive to Jane. For her it was a personal abandonment. For me it was an example of the deterioration of professional medicine into corporate practice.

One might say, "Well, that is just the paranoia of the Alzheimer's patient." If one used the term "hyper-sensitivity," I might concede the point. In the examples above, I had the same "gut reaction" Jane had. But I saw the relationship with those people as a casual one. I did not need their understanding or their caring response. There is almost always a basis for these seemingly paranoid reactions Jane exhibits. When Jane's "I've had it" reaction sets in, almost every time I can honestly say, "I understand how you feel. I agree it was offensive."

Family and friends present examples of this complex issue. Some show concern and deep affection for both of us and sensitivity to Jane's feelings and behaviors. Their love and loyalty are comforting and reassuring. On occasion, something happens: a confusing phone call, a misunderstood comment or behavior, a general "doubting time." But questions can be answered and uncertainties cleared up, because Jane is aware of the strength of the bond and because the other person has the affection to do whatever is necessary to preserve the relationship. The validity of the bond is there.

Others show little response to the illness and its gravity or the havoc it brings to both of us. No cards, no notes, rare phone calls, uncomfortable visits, if any. At another time, all this might be disregarded or amenable to resolution. But this is not another time! This is not a time when relationships with significant persons can survive at the casual level where offensive behavior can be ignored. It is not that time!

Alzheimer's rules are different! For Jane! For me! For Jane, offenses do not easily go away, lack of affection is not ignored, and unpleasant interactions do not easily get resolved. For me, one does not minimize my wife or her illness, one does not offend "my love," one does not ignore the realities of her **new existence**. I support her position no matter how warped or distorted it may seem to be. What she loves I love. What she hates I hate. I maintain no ties with anyone with whom she has no ties. When she is wrong and something convinces her she is wrong, **then** I will change my position.

Why should I consider any other course? Our lives have been entwined for a long time. How else could I feel if someone offends her? Is her position often exaggerated or even wrong? Exaggerated? Yes, even grossly exaggerated at times. But a grain of truth, a piece of reality also catches my attention. Flat out wrong? Yes, occasionally. But if she is wrong and the relationship is insignificant, then it usually dissolves quite rapidly.

If she is wrong about an incident involving a person with whom she has a sound and caring relationship, it can be resolved with a little time and a little patience. If she feels (erroneously) someone offended her, and that person is clearly affectionate and expressive, I help her focus on our loving relationship with that individual. Jane is soon able to recognize the error of her thinking.

But if she feels (erroneously) someone offended her, and if that person maintains an emotional distance from her or has a casual relationship, there is no basis to try to effect a change for Jane. The immediate incident is not the problem; the ongoing relationship is the problem and prevents any genuine rapprochement. I invest little effort in trying to correct her view of things. There is little benefit in trying to repair a relationship that would be labeled "casual" when "caring" is required.

Some individuals are less capable than others of demonstrating affection. I am sorry for those whose lives are emotionally stunted. However, affection has become the coin of the realm in our life.

10/7/08

Jane sleeps more these days. It is often 11p.m. by the time we get to sleep. I get up at 6a.m. and exercise for 30 minutes. I do some spiritual reading, read the paper or a novel, and do some writing or editing. I look forward selfishly to the three or four hour period before Jane wakes, because it is the only time I have to myself.

Jane has extreme difficulty sorting things. Each object she picks up becomes an individual challenge. What is it? What's different about it? Where should it go? She doesn't think: "all pencils go here, all pens go there, paper clips go in a box." She can't hold onto an over-all plan. She tried to sort hair pins, cosmetics, safety pins, and pencils. Her circuitry couldn't handle it and basically shut down.

When we talked about it, Jane understood what happened and was relieved. Her calm and reasoning brain could recall and picture the details in a different light. I said when this happens, she should leave what she is doing and come and talk to me about it. When I mentioned coming to me, she understood why she should do that but wasn't sure she could because, "I don't think I'm thinking clearly enough to do that." When I said I saw her reach this state of "shut-down" on previous occasions, she said she never experienced anything like this. If a person remembers a dire event from the past and remembers recovering from it, a recurrence is not so threatening. Alzheimer's does not allow for this.

(Email to Laura 10/8/08)
Mom told me when she was talking to you she suddenly didn't know what to say and she couldn't think of the girls' names or anyone's name. She felt badly and thought maybe you were offended. I told her I would send you an email and explain. Actually she seemed quite confused and somewhat irritable after we finished dinner. Then she decided she wanted to give you a call "just to hear your voice." She dialed twice and got mixed up, so I dialed for her. It upsets her whenever she tries to dial and makes a mistake. Actually it wasn't a great time for her to talk. She felt embarrassed because she didn't know what to say. That's why she switched you to me.

10/20/08
There was a disastrous event last Thursday. Jane and I went to our café for lunch. There were 13 paintings on the café walls where the pleasant masterpieces previously hung. The paintings were done by a resident, who hung twice that number of paintings in the same area three years ago. After numerous resident complaints the administrator at that time made him take them down.

Jane was overwhelmed with grief and anger. She began to cry and became quite verbal, expressing anger and desolation. The Administrator was in the area. I approached her and told her I was angry and why. She defended the exhibit stating she saw it done in a similar facility. I said the pictures were ugly and we don't have a choice of places to eat.

Persons with dementia are very sensitive to the environment. The sound of our air conditioner can be extremely annoying to Jane, so disturbing I may turn it off for a while. Visual sensitivity is also sharpened. Mismatched clothing, misplaced furniture, poor lighting makes Jane emotionally uncomfortable. Visual stimuli are more striking for her because of her artistic abilities and her perceptive awareness. (She is a graduate of the Moore Art Institute in Philadelphia.)

Facilities for the elderly strive to provide soft lighting, gentle surroundings, calming furnishings, and soothing décor. To suddenly impose changes, particularly when they are harsh and unpleasant, is particularly disconcerting, especially if dementia is present.

I was so angry at this assault I wrote a memo to the administrator. I made over 200 copies and distributed them to all the residents, asking them to contact the administrator if they were in agreement with my thoughts. A copy of the memo follows.

Jane's anger fluctuates. As it mounts, she becomes verbally threatening. She got a hammer, some magazine pictures and nails and was going down to nail the pictures up in the café, the lobby and the hallways. At another time, she got a knife and was going to destroy the pictures. I was direct and forceful with her on these occasions. I said, "You must not do this! This is dangerous for you and for me! This will get you in trouble! The police will be called! You will be charged! We will have to pay for any damages!" Once I said, "If you do this, the administration may say they cannot take care of you and they will insist you go to a facility for Alzheimer's patients, and then we will be separated." She never left the apartment to carry out her threats.

Her sleep has been disturbed with horrible dreams. Her energy is drained. She is listless. Last night she referred to a fear she will wake up in the morning and "everything will be gone." She won't know me or her things and she doesn't want to live that way.

I am angry at the administrator. It is more than the obnoxious pictures. It is her total lack of appreciation for factors which contribute to the emotional well-being of elderly persons, most of whom are experiencing some cognitive decline, many of whom are living alone, and all of whom need to have an administrator whom they can trust and believe has their best interests at heart.

(From letter to Administrator 10/17/08)

A few years ago one of the residents put up some of his paintings in the café. Later he was told by the Administrator of Vantage House to take them down because there were numerous complaints by the residents. As I recall the Administrator said resident fees would not be used to pay for the staff time of changing them and repairing the walls.

Now we have a repeat of the same situation by the same "resident painter." The question of propriety and fairness returns. The café is not just a "common area." It should not be used for the personal aggrandizement and financial gain of one resident. It is an area where residents must go to purchase and eat food. There is no alternative to this venue. The food is good, the staff is wonderful, the service is great. It provides a pleasant, relaxed and social atmosphere for eating. Now it has become an exhibit room, an art gallery that contaminates the pervading tone.
* * * * * *

This is an area where our food is served, and I do not believe we should be subjected to any individual resident's choice of pictures no matter how pleasant or how disgusting. It is our taste for the food that is important here. Individual taste in art should not be a criterion for being comfortable in our café.

Professionals who work with the elderly are usually aware that the environment is an important factor in their well being. The art work at Vantage House is generally non-intrusive and non-offensive, though perhaps not liked by some residents. Professionals are well aware that sudden dramatic and drastic changes in the environment can be disturbing to

elderly patients, particularly those who may have one of the illnesses which cause dementia. Considering the age of the population here, I believe it is statistically sound to say that seven to ten percent of the residents must have some early signs of cognitive decline. A part of our small world is radically threatened.
* * * * * *

When I spoke to you about this you suggested that other residents will also be able to exhibit their work. No thank you! Not where we go to eat, socialize, and enjoy some time! Put it somewhere else where we aren't obliged to see it every day or any day if we would rather not, some place where the majority of us can avoid it if we prefer.

(Following note attached to each resident memo)
If you agree with the principle stated here that the café should not be used for the display of personal paintings or other objects of any resident, I urge you to contact the Vantage House Administrator.

(From a note to President of Board of Directors October 17, 2008)
A matter has come up that has greatly disturbed both of us. My wife has had Alzheimer's for the last four or five years. Generally she is doing quite well, but as with all patients who are elderly, and especially those with some form of dementia, changes in the environment or in routines can be very unsettling for them. Yesterday she had a very frightening, irritating, and discouraging episode during our visit to the café where we routinely go for lunch. The entire décor of the café had been changed because a resident hung over a dozen of his paintings on most of the available wall space. In my opinion most of the paintings are revolting. But the subject of them is beside the point. I think it is completely unjustified to change the environment in the café for the brash egotism of one resident, no matter who it is.

I have made my argument in the copy of the enclosed memorandum. I believe there has been a gross exercise in poor judgment on the part of the administrator who yesterday defended her action when I spoke to her.

I have a doctorate in psychology and in medicine, and I was a practicing psychiatrist for over fifty years. I am fully aware that stark changes in the environment of the elderly (especially without any basis) are an assault on their peace of mind and their emotional composure. On a more personal basis, this "administrative decision" caused a calamitous setback for my wife and has aggravated me beyond measure. The effect on my wife will continue for days and it will contaminate our stay here for months to come.

(Note to painter after I discovered the administrator asked him to display the pictures. 10/21/08))
I clearly owe you an apology for attributing motives to you that were in error, and I hope you can forgive my behavior and the precipitous position I took. I discussed the pictures with the administrator before I wrote the memorandum. While I cannot say she led me to believe you had asked to put them up, she said nothing to suggest otherwise. I made the assumption and she said nothing to dispel it. I offer that not as an excuse but as an accompanying circumstance.

Jane was terribly disturbed by the sudden and unannounced change in the café, a place that has become something of a haven for us where Jane can enjoy some socialization without the stress of sitting through a full meal in the dining room. Until a person has had some direct experience with Alzheimer's, it is impossible to imagine how devastating an unexpected disruption of routines or of the environment can be. We have just spent five days of fear, sadness, and anger, all wrapped together. My comments about your paintings were based on those days and not on any feeble ability I might have in art appreciation.

10/23/08

The pictures were taken down during the evening of 10/20. Almost 50 of the residents expressed appreciation for my memo. But it is not over for Jane. It has taken its toll and how soon she will recover remains to be seen. She has lost ground. She has been more irritable and focused on the inevitable future of her Alzheimer's.

We were in the Mall on 10/21 for lunch. Jane commented about the picture incident. I was trying to decide how I might redirect the conversation. She became angry because I did not respond immediately. She pushed her lunch away. "You dropped off, turned away, abandoned me. I can never trust you again. That is the meanest thing you ever did to me." I put my arm on her shoulder. "Don't touch me, don't look at me." I begged her to forgive me. I said I would never abandon her. She became loud and didn't seem to care who heard her. Several people looked at us.

This went on for over 30 minutes. I wondered if I could get her home without involving the police. It is rare she becomes this hostile in public. Finally, she said, "Let's make peace." We embraced; she finished her lunch. We walked to the car and came home.

At bedtime she recalled the issue of the afternoon. She said I completely shut down; I never said a word most of the time; I never apologized; I never reached out to her in any way to resolve the issue. It was clear she forgot much of what occurred.

We both slept poorly. The next morning it started again. There is no way I know to settle these things. If I mention something other than what she believes happened, I am defending myself, calling her a liar, or being out of my mind. If I say little about it, I'm shutting her out, isolating her, condemning her to loneliness. If I agree with her, she needs an explanation of why I did the horrible things I did. And I'm without an answer. Several times I asked her to make up. Suddenly she did. There were no magic words on my part—just a magic time. Why or from where I don't know.

Later I was going to pick up our dinner. Jane, out of nowhere, made a cutting remark. I said I thought it was unnecessary. She apologized. She said, "I heard it come out of my mouth. It seemed like another person said it. At first I couldn't believe it was my voice that said it." I believe it was exactly as she described. She said it is frightening to say words she never intended to say. Referring to the incident, she asked, "What happened in my brain?" a question she has genuine curiosity about. I suggested it was possibly a spontaneous reaction to a similar event long forgotten. A better answer: "Who knows?"

Apparently my memo to the administrator was a major force in the picture removal. Numerous residents told me how much they appreciate what I did. I am grateful for their comments, but I would not have acted if it were not for the effect on Jane. The administrator issued a letter to the residents on 10/20 about her plan for a "Resident Art Exhibit Program" to be held at some later date and in some as yet undecided place.

(From letter to President of Board of Directors 10/28, 2008)
I appreciate your reply to my letter of October 17. I believe the matter of the paintings was satisfactorily resolved as of October 21. I had about 50 residents who expressed appreciation for my memorandum to the administrator. They were clearly supportive of the objection to the placement of the pictures. I do not wish to imply they were critical of the pictures themselves.

I am enclosing a copy of a note I wrote to the man whose pictures were the subject of the memo. My criticism of the content of the pictures was clearly inappropriate. That was really not the issue.

11/02/08
Last evening after a good day, Jane began worrying, "Will I go down hill again? I know today was unreal and it cannot last. I wish I could stay like I am today." What can one say to quell the fears of a person with Alzheimer's? I talked about slow and gradual changes and said she experienced several good days. They had faded from her memory.

She slept twelve hours and woke with a positive attitude. Her comment on mood today was, "I won't name it. I'll just try to live it." Not a bad idea.

Jane "thinks in pictures," not in words. When she is interested in a subject, she gets pictures of it in her mind. The word "Alzheimer's" brings up a view of end stage disease. She **sees** herself bedridden or sitting listlessly in a chair wondering what is going on around her! It is so vivid that **she is there**! She is not only there but she is observing herself being there, and she reacts with overwhelming fear and anger and sadness.

The present becomes an annoyance rather than a comfort. I become an outsider rather than a participant. The environment becomes a threat rather than a distraction. The happy times of yesterday become part of a dark night that surrounds her. She is alone, helpless, abandoned, not unlike the "motherless child" of her own childhood. In her despair, she cries, "It's unfair! I did it before! I shouldn't have to do it again."

I wonder, as I stand helplessly by trying to sooth the agony of her loss, am I really trying to smother the persistent demons of her childhood memories—of being alone, helpless, emotionally abandoned?

11/15/08

Variation seems to be the theme of this illness. Ten days ago we had a difficult time. Jane was irritable and dragged conflicts out indefinitely. In reality I think she just can't end them. The issue drags her along more than she wants to continue it.

I can usually avoid negative reactions to her accusations or verbal attacks. I make some response but try not to contradict her view of things. I have a more patient and sympathetic attitude which helps decrease her feeling of isolation from me and the fear and loneliness that entails.

The past week was remarkably good. Jane puts more effort into maintaining a better mood. I don't believe she can control her mood, but her attitude about the illness helps.

We recently met a woman in the Mall who waved at me as she passed. It was a social worker I knew from work years ago. Jane asked questions. "Who was she? Where did I meet her? How did I remember her since I left the hospital six years ago?" I thought my answers settled the matter. At lunch I found the matter was definitely not settled. "She was an average looking woman. How could you remember her after all those years? Why didn't she stop and speak to us? How often did you see her at work?"

The whole thing was ridiculous. I never worked directly with the woman. I saw her occasionally at meetings. I did not treat the questioning as ridiculous or unimportant. I provided full answers. It seemed adequately settled after 30 minutes.

Before we left, Jane apologized and acknowledged jealousy has been a recurring problem in our marriage. She has never had reason to question my fidelity. She was embarrassed by the episode. She wondered what happened in her past that made her so vulnerable. The issue has not been mentioned again. What a relief to be able to work through something that could have continued for a long time.

My son, Bob, and his girlfriend arrived from Seattle and visited us yesterday. We had dinner downstairs and then a nice visit in our apartment. Bob and Jane have been very close for many years. Bob refers to her as his mother.

11-28-08
Thanksgiving Day
I woke Jane about 10:30a.m. After breakfast, she looked tired. She accepted my suggestion to lie down. I massaged her feet and she was soon fast asleep.

Before she slept she said, "I am often close to tears these days." I can guess she is thinking, "Will I be here next Thanksgiving? What will I be like if I am here?" Is that why she was content to go to bed? It isn't to retreat, to hide, to run away. It's to catch her breath, to get her strength back, to help her cope. She is not a quitter. She is fighting to remain "my companion" as her memories disappear.

When Jane is willing to sleep it gives me time to read, do some writing, or tidy up something in the apartment (noiselessly). It is similar to the time I have in the mornings from 6a.m. until Jane is awake. I selfishly welcome these alone times.

(Email to Laura 11-28-08)

I was so pleased Mom and you had the long conversation. From what I heard her say on the phone, she certainly responded with the love and tenderness and caring she has always felt for you. It was sort of miraculous it happened so smoothly. Your telling both of us how much we mean to you and how important we are to you was very touching and we are both grateful. Mom's response was remarkable.

In spite of the fact that Mom had been pretty sad and a bit edgy during the day, she rallied around very quickly once you started talking to her. She was, from what I heard her saying, being very understanding, very reasonable, and very caring. That is her real self, her old self, her true self. I think you may be more like Mom temperamentally than I realized. It may be difficult for others sometimes to understand you, especially when you expose some of the emotional edges. But when someone comes to appreciate you deeply and fully (as I have your mother), then they know how fortunate they are to know you.

11/29/08

Today Jane met with Tom, her first husband. He suggested this, and it was arranged through Kathie. We all met in the Mall. I had a nice visit with Kathie while Jane and Tom talked for about an hour.

Tom told her they were both very young when they married, perhaps his explanation of what went wrong. We all were grateful the meeting occurred. It may have brought some closure for Jane and, I presume, for Tom. Kathie joined the two of us for lunch so Jane had a further chance to "debrief."

When we got home, everything I said made Jane angry. She decided she wouldn't go to 6:30p.m. Mass as we planned. She was mad at God. "Why should I go to church when God repeatedly abandons me?" When it was time to go, she was ready and waiting. Jane said she couldn't be mad at me in church because God would strike her dead.

On the way home, she apologized for her "horrible behavior" and was sincerely remorseful. She berated herself for the things she said. "I'm a horrible demon." I told her that is not true and that Alzheimer's causes her reaction. I said we always got along well and she is still the same person she was then. This behavior is similar to forgetting things. She can't help it and is not responsible for it. She says, "No excuse."

She remarked how glad she was we went to Mass. I agreed. I prayed she would find greater calm and peace for the future. Perhaps both our prayers were heard.

PART 5 (DEC 08—MAY 09)

12/7/08

There are three items to write about. The first is especially difficult and very disconcerting. It occurred seven days ago. Jane was very hostile over nothing one evening and continued it late into the night and again the next morning. Finally, she calmed down and had the usual feelings of remorse and guilt, with profound apologies.

Later that day I felt I didn't love her anymore. It was shattering. I didn't feel angry or sad. I felt numb and nothing seemed to matter. It wasn't comfortable. I didn't feel guilty about it. It was there, sort of a fact of life. I wondered how I could hide the feeling from her. We are very close and expressive both verbally and physically. How could I maintain a facade to assure her of my love, when it was no longer there? How could I give her the care she needs and the consolation she deserves with my changed feelings?

I struggled with these thoughts for two days. I wasn't comfortable with my feelings or with her. She did not notice the change. I said I was feeling a little tired, hoping it would temporarily cover the change in me.

I didn't want to write about it at the time, the old idea, "if you don't put it into words, maybe it will go away." It has gone away as quietly as it came. Was it depression? Was it fatigue? Was I worn out by her assailing me time and time again? Could it return? If it does, it will not last. I know my love for her cannot change!

The second thing that happened was positive. Jane became angry over nothing. Her hostility escalated quickly, and as always I caught the brunt of it. However, in the height of her anger she said very clearly and forcefully, "I am not angry at you. I am not angry at you. You did not do anything! I am not angry at you." She said this in loud, angry tones. When she got in bed later, she was okay. We talked awhile and she soon slept.

The next night Jane referred to her anger of the previous night. She talked about "what happens in my head. It is hostility that is just suddenly there." She doesn't know why she feels hostile but she knows it isn't toward me. She said, "I take it out on you even though you don't deserve it and did nothing to cause it." She seemed comfortable, objective, and insightful as we talked about her "abrupt and uncontrolled hostility." I mentioned my feeble attempts to help at those times. She said there doesn't seem to be anything else to do but what I do.

At times there seems to be no Alzheimer's. But when there is too much happening, too many people, too much that destroys her focus and distracts her, she loses her connection, and everything goes bad. She is alone, hostage to her disease, and the world abandons her. She wanders in a wilderness of words and phrases and sights and sounds having no meaning, no coherence, no language she understands. Unleashed hostility is the result!

The third event of the past week occurred yesterday. Jane said her mind goes to negative thought patterns when she is in her bathroom or the bedroom "tidying up" or looking for something. That is why I began, some months ago, reading to her while she does her hair and her makeup. Previously the task took two or three hours. Now she finishes in thirty minutes. She admits the thought patterns are unhealthy and occur in that setting.

She will try to spend more time in the studio with me. I would love to see her there. She has a large desk and a comfortable chair. She could write, go through her art books, look at her magazines or do a little sketching. She agreed she likes to do all those things.

She was pleased with the conversation. As we drove to evening Mass she said she forgot what we talked about, but she knew it meant a great deal to her. Could we go over it again? I repeated the discussion later. Will she remember in the morning?

I think a healthy part of Jane's brain has walled itself off from less healthy parts. As long as her mind is within a certain perimeter, it functions extremely well, even with a memory deficit. When she slips outside that perimeter there is relative chaos, because that area does not contain reasoning power or common sense or self control. It does not contain considerateness or kindness. It is driven by forces she does not control or perhaps even know. It is dangerous; it is dark; it is more frightening to her than to others. It is desolate! It is hell!

I must keep in touch with her when she goes outside that perimeter. She must know I love her when she is **there**. I must never abandon her no matter how small the healthy brain, "my Jane brain," becomes. Can I do anything to prevent her ever going there?

12/15/08

Jane was edgy all day Saturday, ready to enlarge on everything. We ate dinner at the Mall before we went to 6:30 Mass. Everything at Mass made her angry: the music leader, the weak voiced reader, the African priest with an unintelligible accent. She said she would never attend that church again.

At bedtime she was unable to find her hair net in "the place where I always put it." "I'm a failure. I'm stupid. I'm crazy. It's a punishment. I can't live with this. I don't want to be here any more." This went on for an hour.

She was still awake after two hours. She took another sleeping pill I brought. I didn't say anything when I got back in bed. This "horrible neglect and rejection" on my part was "too much." She got up, put on her robe and left the room. She would not sleep with "someone so uncaring." I thought about going to her in the living room, but I feared it would only agitate her. After an hour she quietly returned to bed. I feigned sleep to avoid more wrath. Later when she returned from the bathroom, we hugged and kissed and spoke our love.

The next morning Jane was apologetic for the prior evening. After lunch some insignificant thing set her off again. She was furious, unreasonable, demanding I talk to her, and judging every comment I made to be hurtful, sarcastic, defensive, stupid or irrelevant. We finally achieved "peace" and ate dinner. She accused me of being angry at her. She "sees it in my face." Her behavior worries and frightens me. The change in my expression, she interprets as anger.

After a three hour visit with Kathie, Jane said she was happy because we made up and I wasn't mad any more. I agreed I was glad we made peace but stupidly added I had not been mad at her. That set off a new tirade. How could I make her suffer all afternoon by letting her think I was mad at her? I had told her several times I was not mad at her. She denied I ever said it.

Her anger continued to escalate. She screamed at me with a wild, frightened look. There was no way of calming her, no way of consoling her, no way of containing this horrible anger. She struck me in the chest and pushed me so I stumbled backwards. Then she burst out crying and was remorseful. She asked forgiveness saying her assault would ruin things forever between us, and she would never forget it.

Her accusations about my anger continued. Finally, I was angry. I said in a stern voice, "Now I am angry. If you want to see my anger, this is it, so pay attention to what my anger looks like. I'm getting tired of what's been going on today. I can't take much more of this shit. I've been trying to comfort you and to calm you. I'm not able to control you, so you're going to have to do something more to control yourself. If you can't achieve some better control, then I won't be able to continue to take care of you."

She fell into my arms and wept and pleaded. I held her until she was calm. She took the medicine she previously refused. She got in bed. I sat on the edge of the bed and talked to her. I turned off the lights and got in beside her. We hugged for a long time. I massaged her back. I waited until I knew she was asleep and then I slept.

(Email to Laura 12-22-08)
Don't think I mentioned before that Mom talks out loud to herself a lot of the time when she is alone, and sometimes she whispers to herself even when I'm around. She is pretty open about it, but I just don't mention it. She sometimes does.
(Note to Laura re Christmas—attached to above email)
Mom has difficulty making decisions and making choices. If I suggest two or three possibilities for the day, it may only complicate the day, because she has difficulty sorting through and understanding what the choices are. I try to keep the choices to two things, or I may just ask, "What would you like

to do this afternoon?" Or I just suggest one thing we might do that I think she would like.

When I explain something to her or tell her about something, I have the bad habit of "starting in the middle" or somewhere down the road. It's better for me and for her to make it clear what I'm talking about even before I talk about it. Perhaps the important thing is to start out slowly and try to make sure she is following. She can also get irritated sometimes if I speak in too simplistic terms. But she is usually good about picking up what the story is about and following it.

Mom makes radical statements about a lot of things. (She always did do some of that.) Politics, world affairs, news items, people—she can make rather harsh criticisms that sound awful sometimes. I never challenge them; just try to make some neutral remark. I would never comment to Mom that anything she said or did was inappropriate. On rare occasions when I have implied it, she was either completely devastated or severely irritated. It is not worth it to make such a comment to her. She makes harsh unjustified comments about people, what they wear, how they look, what they say. I don't dispute them.

She tells stories sometimes about something that happened and the stories are quite erroneous or exaggerated. I let them go the way she tells it.

Mom can't handle too much input from rapid changes in the environment or from numbers of people involved. She has lost some of her ability to follow what is going on. A TV show or a movie can become too complex for her to follow, and explaining it may not help. The news is too complex for her, but when I read an article from the paper to her she follows it well.

Displays of affection, both verbal and physical, have become very important to her. You and Kathie and Paul and Bob are the only ones who openly express real affection for her, and it makes all the difference in the world. Her feelings about the others are either flat or negative.

I'm sure during this visit Mom will be thinking it will be our last, and that will bring a good bit of sadness to both of us because it is probably accurate. We have agreed we will not go to Rehoboth again and an overnight trip anywhere else would be too stressful and too confusing.

On occasion, Mom gets overwhelmed by whatever is going on around her. She becomes confused and may even say I don't know what I'm doing. She sometimes acknowledges it would be good to lie down and get some rest. She will be reluctant to do that at your house because she will be "losing time."

Going out to a restaurant may be problematic, unless it's pretty informal and relaxed—sort of like we do at the eatery. Coffee and a cookie somewhere would probably work great.

Mom has difficulty with a time schedule because she can't remember it and because she gets lost in the process of getting ready. She gets distracted and may wander off to do something else when she is supposed to be getting ready. If we are going out, let us know pretty clearly the approximate time and I'll work closely with Mom. The same thing will happen with meal time.

Mom likes to help out because it makes her feel useful and in control. I sometimes think I do too much and cut her out of doing things. But it takes patience to let her do things because she can be slow and too meticulous.

Mom can be very sensitive when others are distracted during a conversation. I've upset her greatly on occasion by glancing at my watch when we are talking. Obviously you are going to have distractions when we are talking. I just wanted to make you aware of her sensitivity in the area so you can be alert to it and try to compensate in some way if it occurs.

I know you don't need a handbook about how to deal with your mother and I hope you won't feel "guided" by these remarks. There really are no "rights" or "wrongs." It is the attitudinal part that is important and you certainly have that. Just be your loving self, aware that Mom is different because of her illness, but knowing she always loves you dearly and deeply.

12/28/08

These notations began two years ago. There have been marked changes over this period of time, but I am grateful the changes have not been more devastating than they are.

We went to Laura's on 12/23 and returned on 12/26. Jane was under a great deal of stress for two or three weeks before we went. Yesterday she described it as "being a test." It was! We all wondered how she would do and would this be the last trip.

The days before we left were hectic. The gift wrapping became my job, with Jane in reluctant agreement. I did it while she took a couple of long naps, exhausted from the routine preparations to go. She often said, "Let's not go" or "I don't want to go."

The evening of arrival passed nicely with Laura and the girls. They planned the following day well. We made Christmas cookies.

Christmas morning after breakfast, we opened presents by the tree. Suddenly the wrapping paper became more important than the gifts, the same distortion that occurred the last two Christmases. Laura told me later it was the same every Christmas since she was born. The wrapping paper, bows and ribbon became Jane's major interest. All the Christmas spirit was gone. Jane was angry and ready to show it to the world. She was tired, exhausted. I suggested a nap. She described it as "being put to bed like a child who has spoiled the party." I massaged her feet until I thought she was asleep. Ten minutes later she was putting things together for our trip home the next day.

She became calmer and agreed to be courteous toward Frank, who is seeing Laura again and was joining us for Christmas dinner. We survived dinner in spite of the tension. Then the girls gave their presents to their mother, Frank, and both of us. It was pleasant enough with the children in charge. Laura and the girls gave us a violin concert.

The following morning Jane woke as furious as when she went to bed. She and Laura had a conversation in the kitchen which seemed to pacify Jane. The farewell with Laura was particularly touching. She was very affectionate toward her mother. I left thinking, "Laura has now seen the face of Alzheimer's, and she too is frightened."

To my surprise the trip home went well. We talked agreeably and Jane remained calm. She said, "The time there was not long enough." It never is—even when it's too long.

Our first day home was difficult. Jane was concerned about her behavior and how Laura felt about it. She said, "I've lost her. I know I've lost her." I said Laura is "our daughter" and it was good she had an opportunity to see how Alzheimer's affects her mother. Laura now knows Alzheimer's patients exhibit unusual behavior and may say things that are harsh or hostile or critical. Laura knows, as we all do, the person's behavior and comments do not mean the person is crazy or weird or cruel.

Jane worries the illness has radically advanced these last few days. "I woke up one morning about a week ago and I felt different. It has changed. Something new has happened in my head. This is a big change and will just get worse." She experienced increased anxiety the past few weeks. I encouraged her to wait a few days before she determines how much change has really occurred.

(Email to Laura 12-30-08)
Mom sometimes behaves like she is a different person. Even though some things are not new (e.g. saving paper) they reach a point of irrationality that can be frightening for me and for her. You have seen her Alzheimer's about at its worst, so far. After the episode is over it seems unreal to look back and know it did indeed happen. She is always filled with remorse once she is aware of the strange, sometimes foolish, sometimes hostile

things she has done. Then she worries about the future and what she "might do."

12/30/08

For two days after our return Jane was full of worry and tears and hostile defenses of her behavior at Laura's, commenting about how Frank is "bad" for Laura and about Laura's "hostility" over the wrapping paper.

Today she insists she has lost Laura. I reminded her she had a phone conversation with Laura several weeks ago and told Laura she would support any decision Laura made about Frank. She recalled how cold, if not rude, she was toward Frank. Now she is embarrassed by her behavior. She wants to talk to Laura, to go see her, to tell her she was wrong. She called Laura and was very comforted.

This trip was a striking example of how Alzheimer's changes Jane's attitude, emotional responses, and behavior. Jane felt Laura grabbed wrapping paper out of her hands to be mean. Jane was rude to Frank and saw nothing wrong with it. Now she can't understand any of that behavior and is embarrassed by it.

I've dealt with this kind of duality for months, but I am still shocked when it happens. Each time there is disbelief. This cannot be my sweet, loving, kind wife who appears vicious, vindictive, and unreachable. Briefly, Alzheimer's takes over our world.

1/3/09

Life is terribly sad. Jane asks the same question repeatedly. "What day is it?" "When was Kathie last here?" "Did the visit with Laura go well?" This morning she said, "How did we meet?" It felt like a final goodbye. It hurts when I think about it. We often talked about our first meeting. Is this a step away from her not knowing who I am?

Jane has been sad for several days. Yesterday was an angry day. She often complains about the TV sound. She is offended because I think the sound is good. After ranting about it yesterday, she promised never to refer to it again. She has promised that many times.

In the evening on return from the Mall, Jane mentioned she is afraid to be in the apartment when it gets dark. I've noticed she likes "lots of lights on."

1/4/09
Today is my mother's birthday. The thought of her prompted me to write a short note. She was a saintly woman, quiet, loving, sensitive, and caring of others. Her inspiration permeated my life and my work as a psychiatrist. She cared deeply about others. She influenced my life in later years as she did in my childhood and adolescence. I believe she played a part in my meeting Jane. We believe our meeting was providential. I ask my mother and father to intercede for Jane and me and help us in the life we now have.

I thought of my brother, Don, who took care of his wife, Helen, for several years on the ranch, as she deteriorated with a dementia from Parkinson's. Some days I think of how lonely and difficult it must have been for him.

Jane's demeanor and behavior today is more like her old self. She was pleasant and agreeable, reacting with humor and clarity. It was a good day. She had a 90 minute nap in the afternoon and awakened refreshed. We went to the Mall for dinner.

1/12/09
Jane struggles with overwhelming emotions. She is sad to the point of despair, thinking about the future. She is angry to the point of harsh self-criticism and hostile behavior toward me as she grapples with an increasingly complex world. She attempts to isolate herself but cannot stand the separation.

A couple of days ago we sat and talked for three hours at the Mall. After we got home I was clearly visible to her preparing our pill boxes for the coming week. Jane became angry at me for "going off on your own," "not telling me where you are going," and "ignoring me." She stormed about the apartment. "Leave me alone, stay away from me."

I embraced her and asked her to sit with me. She cried and said how sorry and how sad she was to hurt me again. Something new occurred to me. I was not "hurt" by her comments. They really didn't offend me. I realized what she was saying was not from Jane but from her Alzheimer's. I said I was sorry for my neglect and for offending her, but I was not hurt. She seemed relieved. I hope this perspective remains with me.

Jane said she would like to promise me she would never get angry and say mean things again. I said it would be like promising she would never forget anything again or would never lose anything again. She understood my point.

(Email to Laura 1-16-09)
Things are going pretty well. Some days are rather difficult. On those days it seems Mom can hardly remember anything. On good days she is alert, bright, and talks about things quite easily. We have recovered from the Christmas visit, but it still comes up at times. Last night she remembered again her talk with you about your seeing Frank, and she said she couldn't believe it when she remembered she had not spoken to him. Then she said, "Do you think Laura knows how bad the Alzheimer's is?" I assure her you know.

1/17/09
Jane loses segments of the past. She has no recollection of giving the girls and Laura gifts or of gifts from them. Last evening she said, "Did we ever go to Laura's for Christmas?" I told her we have gone every Christmas since Laura came back from London. She didn't comment, as if it didn't surprise her she forgot.

Definite changes are occurring. I can't help but wonder about next month, next summer, next Christmas. I get frightened about the future. And I feel lonely on a day like yesterday when she slept so long. I wonder, "Will I be able to manage whatever comes?" On good days, "together days," the future does not loom so dark. Yesterday Jane found no peace, no real calm, nothing positive. And so it was for me!

1/20/09
The night before last, Jane was despondent, wanting to die, inconsolable. She lost a slip of paper on which she had written her thoughts. It was loss, and loss is intolerable. I'm sure it represents the loss of memory, of contact, of life slowly but surely leaving.

We spent four hours at the Mall yesterday. We had lunch, talked, walked and watched the children in the play area. We met a young woman who manages Starbucks where we used to go. She was dressed well and looked attractive. I didn't recognize her but she told us who she was. We exchanged pleasantries. Jane told her she looked nice.

Later Jane asked how I knew that "attractive woman." I said we knew her from Starbucks and we had talked to her there on a few occasions. We continued walking and talking. I thought everything was fine. It had been a pleasant afternoon.

At home Jane attacked me for my "horrible, thoughtless behavior" in the Mall. She felt "completely left out" when we talked to that woman who "came onto you." "I saw how she looked at you and smiled as she was approaching." She denied ever seeing the woman before. "You didn't say a word to me all the way home." Not true. Trying to tell her the facts only increased her anger. I embraced her and tried to calm her.

Her hostile, tearful, desperate comments continued for almost an hour as we sat together. We went to the kitchen to prepare dinner. She turned and put her arms around me. She said, "I know why I get so angry and I'm sorry. I just remembered when I had these same feelings as a child." She cried as I held her and consoled her. She continued, "My mother went out in the evenings and left me. I wanted her to stay home. I knew someone else was more important to her than I was. She came home one night after someone had beaten her. I was frightened. I use to feel hurt and angry when she left but there was no one I could tell." I held her and said, "My poor sweet babe, sweet love."

After her discovery Jane was relieved. She said, "Maybe now I won't get so angry at you." I told her it might still occur because "sometimes emotions just show up and overwhelm you, so don't worry if it happens."

People with Alzheimer's have "emotional incontinence," so I doubt her "insight" will change her angry episodes. The connection she made to her childhood experience was interesting. During her angry episodes I often sense that something else is in play. Her comments are irrational and irrelevant but they are consistent and coherent—as if they are being addressed to someone who is guilty of what she is saying.

1/27/09

The woman we met in the Mall did not fade away. Jane brought it up several times in the next day or two. Finally I lost my patience in spite of all my promises to myself not to do so. I told Jane I was angry and tired of her accusations and innuendos.

It was hurtful to her. It was "the harshest things you ever said to me," and "I could not believe you could be so cruel and without understanding." I felt badly. I held her and apologized and said I was sorry we ever saw the woman. We made up.

Later in the day Jane told me she was awake the previous night creating scenes about my relationship with the woman. She decided the woman would keep track of us, and when Jane died she would return to my life. She realized how ridiculous it was. Perhaps the subject is ended.

Jane was irritable the next three days. She took afternoon naps without noticeable benefit. After my episode of anger I was more sensitive to her mood, and I weathered each storm by holding her and comforting her with loving words. The periods of anger were brief, and recovery was complete. She was then remorseful and self accusatory. I tell her these times are caused by her illness. The important thing is they go away.

The other day Jane said having Alzheimer's is like walking on a carpet with sharp nails sticking up. Wherever and whenever you take a step, you are reminded of the kind of carpet you will always have.

1/27/09

I finished writing a half hour ago but I have the impulse to write more.

Midmorning one of the staff knocked at our door to check something. I woke Jane before noon. I kiss her, hug her and make a few comments about the day. She said, "Why didn't you tell me who knocked on the door?" I said I intended to but was giving her time to wake up. She was angry. I told her about the staff person.

When she came in the kitchen, she was still ready for a fight over it. I took her in my arms, saying, "I'm sorry, my love. Please, forgive me. I love you.

I'm sorry." She started crying and said she is frightened about the Alzheimer's and she dreads losing contact with everyone. She said, "Let me go. Why can't I go and have it over? I don't want to be here any more. I'm afraid." I held her until she was calm.

After breakfast I put my arm around her and laid her head on my shoulder. I stroked her cheek and spoke softly to her. She relaxed. I asked if she wanted to lie down for a bit. She did. I closed the blinds, tucked her in and massaged her feet until she was asleep.

She slept two hours. She is rested and her mood is good. After lunch we talked. I told her I believe God sent me to take care of her, His waif. She believes it too. I told her now there are many new ways to love her and I'm happy about that.

1/30/09

It was a good week. There were brief episodes of irritability. She was irritated today, because "you left the room without saying anything to me." I held her in my arms, told her I loved her and I was sorry. And it was all over. If I reminded her that I told her I was going to shave, the fire would spread. I need to continue gentleness and humility.

We had a wonderful evening with my son, Paul, last night. He is loving, genuine, and gentle. He talks to Jane in a caring and insightful way. He is a remarkable human being, and I feel complimented when Jane says he and I are much alike. He has genuine insight into Jane's illness and is very supportive of us.

(Email to Kathie 2-2-09)
It was helpful to have you here yesterday, because I've been hoping for an opportunity to challenge your Mom's idea that she visited her grandmother and her mother in the same place and they had both been in cages. The story began to surface about six months ago and reappears quite often, especially when she is upset and thinks "someone is going to have to lock me up in a cage someday." I'm cautious about confronting things like that because it can lead to all kinds of difficulties. Your comments yesterday gave me the chance to confront it pretty directly. Your Mom and I continued

to talk about it and I believe she was convinced neither of those things happened. Of course, they may resurface any time.

2/5/09

The past week had some wonderful days for us. Minor episodes of anger were quickly dissipated by an embrace and soothing words. Last Monday we met my son, John, for lunch at the Mall. It was a good visit. Jane was warm and friendly toward him, like the old days. She said it was good to see him.

The next morning the atmosphere changed. Jane was irritated by minor things as soon as she came in the kitchen. Her irritability spread, and before long everything I said was wrong or defensive or ridiculous or critical or clever or psychiatric or self-serving. The other comment at such times is that I don't talk to her.

She said she slept poorly and spent time going over everything about Fran and the car we gave her and "everything else." She seems to have a list of wrongs she visits when one memory starts her off. Probably John's visit brought back the birthday party for Fran.

The day was miserable. Jane has bits and pieces she needs to settle before her anger and obsessive traits will let them go. By evening, she did not remember what started our conflict or much that was said during the day. But that didn't mean the conflict was over.

She said I told her earlier in the day I didn't love her any more, I was going to leave her, and I enumerated stupid things she did in the past. She acted like she believed all this to be true. I felt terrible and told her repeatedly I never thought such things and I could not possibly have said something so untrue. I repeated it many times, embraced her, and told her how much I love her and I would never leave her. It seemed to quiet her fears. She could not remember just what I said that caused her fears.

She told me several times how much she wanted to die. "Jumping off our balcony might not be high enough to kill me." Then she said she couldn't do that to me. I respond to these threats by saying how much I love her and how much I need her.

In bed she began talking about "the horrible, unforgivable things you said to me today." No specifics. It was like she couldn't stop the train. She got up and left the bedroom. I went to find her. She came back to bed reluctantly. We kissed and embraced. She slept within a short time. I slept eventually.

I felt drained the next morning. When I woke Jane about 10a.m., I tried to be cheerful and loving. She seemed okay when she came in the kitchen. Suddenly all hell broke loose! She had put on cosmetics and fixed her hair, and I didn't say she looked nice or say I loved her, or ask her if she slept well, or how she was feeling. I had embraced her and told her I loved her.

I told her we "made up" before we went to sleep and everything was settled. She didn't remember that, and there were still some things I said about not loving her and about leaving her that needed to be settled. She refused to say our morning prayer. "I will never pray with you until you apologize for how terrible you've been to me and for the horrible, mean things you said to me." I apologized for my behavior, for everything I said, for upsetting her, for making her sad and angry.

It is sad to see my loving wife go through this turmoil. Her anger is so ridiculous, so exaggerated, so unreasonable, so wild, so uncontrolled. Her sadness is so severe, so complete, so encompassing, so unreachable. Her fear is so palpable, so primitive, so devastating. I see it begin and watch it develop and I am helpless to stop it. It scares me, the uncontrollable recklessness of her mood shatters my confidence that I can take care of her.

There is an angry, bitter piece of Jane's mind in touch with the misery of her earlier life. Hostile comments about her mother and her first husband emerge frequently. Now the conflict with Fran returns to feed this strange "need" to be angry and have a foe. Does anger help her **keep a connection**? Does anger help her **feel** she has control? She exhibits pretty adept thinking during these periods and refers to winning or losing as if it is a contest of some kind. Is she compensating for loss by trying to beat me down in some imaginary contest?

I thought we were headed for another hurricane day. Jane was brighter and more cheerful when we returned to the apartment after lunch. We reminded each other of our love. All was well again after 36 hours of misery for us both. We returned to a crossword puzzle.

Jane said she was sorry for how horribly she had behaved and begged me to forgive her. I said there is nothing to forgive, it is not her fault. Her guilt will hound her for a short time. I ask her to forgive me too.

She enjoys crossword puzzles and is good at them. Numbers are a foreign tongue to her, but words are her forte. The puzzles are engaging. She is alert and focused on the immediate and responds well to it. I realize what happened earlier may already be gone.

When I contemplate these past few days and the drain they have been on us, I sometimes think "what's the use." But when Jane returns and her companionship is so fulfilling, so exhilarating and so comforting, I know those times of struggle are worth every painful moment. When I see her beautiful, relaxed smile and hear her laugh and watch her pleasure in eating a Subway wrap or watching the kids play at the Mall, I know it is important for both of us to keep her as active and as connected as possible.

My greatest fear is someday one of these episodes will not end. Will it be worth it then to see it through—when there is no "through?" That is her greatest fear too. She voices it often during and after an episode. "I will go crazy and stay there. They will have to lock me up somewhere." She fears it more than I do because she faces the unknown. I face the unknown, but I know my Jane. I know the warmth of her love. I know the depth and the breadth of her bravery. I know the strength of her faith and her closeness to God.

I know if I gave up and turned against her for her bad moods and bad behaviors, it would be the end of walking and talking, of sunshine and blue skies, of fairness and virtue, of love and of life. It would be the end of Jane, and it would be the end of me.

2/6/09

Today Jane said she wanted to tell me something. "My mind works strangely. You know how observant I am. Now I can't seem to stop sometimes. Sitting here talking, I look at the room, the pictures and the lamps. I study them and try to figure out if both corners of the room are exactly the same height, and if the three ceiling lights are exactly the same, and are the pictures aligned just the way they should be. It drives me crazy, but I can't stop it. It happens all the time. I always observed things but now I get obsessed with things. It is ridiculous. I get afraid when it happens because I don't understand it."

She gave several other examples. More things are leaving her memory bank daily. When we wake in the morning, our minds are probably filled with memories of the day before, thoughts of our current situation, and plans for today. But what if the screen was blank? Then we would try to remember information to orient ourselves. But what if nothing comes up readily about plans or activities or people? Then we might focus on our physical environment, a "where am I?" moment.

Maybe this happens often to Jane. If her mind has no available memories to orient her as to who she is or where she is, her mind may search the physical environment for some sense of place and of her own identity. An obsessive quality searches for answers in details.

She spoke of "a haunting feeling, difficult to describe. It may be of death but I'm not afraid to die. It's a little frightening and I don't know why. It's out there somewhere but it's also within me. It makes me feel strange."

I said it is difficult for me to remember how difficult it is for her to remember. When we have a conversation like this, she is as focused, as connected, as intelligent, as responsive as she has ever been. I think, "Where did the Alzheimer's go?"

2/10/09

If I tell Jane something and refer to it again later, she may have forgotten I told her. She asks, "Why didn't you tell me that before?" She can be irritated or suspicious about why I waited to tell her. If I say I did tell you before, she is disturbed because she forgot and says she is stupid. If I make up some excuse for not telling her sooner, she is annoyed because I failed to tell her the story earlier.

Jane brought up some losses for which I bear responsibility. In 1966 when she moved from Richmond, I suggested throwing away her year book from the Moore Art Institute. When we moved to Vantage House five years ago, I suggested throwing away our long play records because we sold the record player. Two years ago, I gave my daughter the car Jane drove, when it needed one thousand dollars in repairs. Jane was not driving so we had no need for a second car. These are recurring issues for Jane. I apologize repeatedly for these actions, acknowledging how wrong I was.

When one of these incidents comes up, Jane is sad about the loss and hostile toward me for my decision. I condemn my insensitivity and acknowledge her feelings in each case. I am ashamed of what I did, especially with the yearbook. I am annoyed when these things are brought up because I'm not comfortable with how I handled them.

Last night Jane brought up the records. I tried not to show my annoyance. In bed she started crying. She felt terrible for talking about the records. "I know it was unkind, and I don't know why I was so mean and hateful toward you when you are so good to me." She begged me to forgive her. I kissed her and told her I had been insensitive about the records and had not been fair to her. She slept well.

2/19/09

These are sad days. Jane has a marked decline in memory function. She mentions it often. "I'm telling you this because I don't think you know how bad it's getting." I know. I see it all the time. She no longer remembers where dishes go, where to turn lights off, what we did yesterday, where we keep things.

She has moments of marked sadness when these "reminders" strike her. She may cry or get irritable. I embrace her and ask her to sit with me so I can hold her. I tell her I see her memory failing, and it makes me sad too. She thinks of how much worse it will get. I say we will be together, and my memory is "our memory." I tell her I am grateful she is in my life, and it will always be wonderful to be with her. The other evening she got "a little lost." She began to cry and said, "I feel like I'm saying goodbye to things." That must be what it's like for her—saying goodbye to the world in bits and pieces.

Jane is child-like in many ways. When we go to the Mall she is interested in everything, fascinated by odd little things. She picks up free leaflets as if they were treasurers. Stray boxes are claimed as valuable possessions. The bag from our cookies, the paper our food comes in, the cup that held ice cream, may all find their way home with her. She hides them in different places so I won't see them. I do, when we look for other lost objects.

What will happen to all these possessions? Someday it will be my sad task or Kathie's or Laura's to transform these treasurers to trash. The goal now is to make life as comfortable and as full as it can be for my love!

(Email to Laura 2/20/09)
Mom frequently speaks of sending cards to the three of you. In fact, she has cards picked out. But like many things she talks about doing, she never quite gets to the doing. But I see the goal of each day to help her be as calm and peaceful as she can be and to do whatever we can to make that happen.

2/27/09
Jane had a difficult week. Memory is feeble. Sadness and anger are strong. It is so hard for her to control her anger and so difficult for me to respond in any helpful way.

Phil called three days ago and talked of coming Sunday to visit for a short while. He has not shown a great deal of sensitivity for Jane's condition. His deficiency regarding Alzheimer's is not his fault, but it does have a negative impact on Jane. She noted he is going to AA; he recently went to a retreat; and he is trying to make some important corrections in his life.

Jane was crying today and said how badly she wants it all to be over. That has been the theme this week. She is so aware of the losses in her mental abilities. She is embarrassed by her "stupidity" and unforgiving of her limitations. She says she achieves nothing, has no goals, and is incapable of doing anything useful.

She took a nap and I lay beside her for a while. I was overwhelmed by her sadness and the dark future that looms ahead. I said, "I will pray for a peaceful and early death for you, if that is what you want so badly." She said it is what she wants. She wondered what would happen to me. I told her she can watch over me from heaven.

3/3/09

I sometimes think about what I might do if Jane died. I think of visiting Montana again. I would move to a smaller apartment. I would go to more of the activities here. I'm not a very sociable person by nature. I was not unhappy being alone when I was young. It's not a bright picture, but on days when Jane is sad and irritable with me, it has an aspect of relief. On the other hand, Jane has been the only person in my life with whom I have felt genuine closeness. Her death would create such a black hole for me I'm not sure I could do much of anything without her.

3/6/09

Phil visited on Thursday. The visit went well. He brought a copy of Jane's high school year book which he found on eBay. Jane was delighted with it. Phil talked about himself and spoke about going to AA, making some positive comments about the program.

After Phil left, Jane refused to eat lunch. She kept badgering me, screaming, weeping, and threatening to kill herself. Nothing calmed her. She said I was not friendly toward Phil during the visit. I told her I would call him and apologize. I didn't feel it was necessary, but I had to appease her. Jane left the apartment and wandered in the building. She gets confused about where she is when she is by herself, but she left before I knew she was going. She returned in 20 minutes.

She was still angry. Before Phil came I said we could go to the Mall for lunch or dinner. She insisted we go for dinner. I said she was too distraught to go. This made her angrier. She said she would go alone. When I said I would not let her leave, she dropped the matter. She finally joined me for a chicken pot pie.

We made a fragile peace before we went to sleep. The next morning we were in the same battle. She went over and over all of it with the same questions, the same arguments, the same accusations. It didn't get anywhere. I lost my patience and walked out of the room and shut the door behind me. She came out screaming after me. When we reached the living room, I told her I had enough and could no longer stand her bitching at me.

She broke down and cried pitifully. I held her and told her I loved her and tried to calm her. Finally, she was calm and we talked a bit more rationally. As usual, she said it was "the worst thing you ever did to me and the worst thing you ever said to me." I hate to display that kind of anger and harshness toward Jane, but sometimes it seems to be the only thing that can bring her back to the real world.

For Jane these periods of conflict are "win or lose" situations. "You are smarter. You say things to put me down and to earn points. That is the goal of everything you do or say—to win." I told her there is nothing to win. We both lose. I say things only to respond to her anger so it will go away. She doesn't believe that. "You're out to win, to outsmart me, and that's so easy for you to do. Losing makes me feel stupid and a 'nobody.' Kids did that to each other and to me when I was young."

Jane referred to Alzheimer's as a source of her rage, and I agreed. I praised her for the effort she makes to combat the angry feelings. Peace today is such a blessed relief. I'm not feeling as strong as I was before these last few days. I called Phil yesterday and left an apology on his cell phone.

Jane took a nap again today. Before going to sleep she talked about dying. She doesn't want to leave me alone. I told her I am willing to let her go and I will join her soon. She said, "What if there isn't anything after death? What if we would never meet again?" I told her something in her heart and something in my heart tells us there is a life after death and we will see each other again. I massaged her feet until she slept.

(Email to Kathie 3-12-09)
I appreciate the generosity and love involved in your coming up yesterday. It was a hectic afternoon and a terrible experience for your mother. I dread these times because they are so traumatic for her and leave me with a feeling of helplessness. I woke up this morning with fear that the administration here might begin to think I can't adequately take care of your Mom and push me to transfer her to our health center or even to a facility for Alzheimer's. Both of us would have a tremendous problem with that. And sometimes I fear at some point I won't be able to care for her in the apartment.

Her distorted view of things I said or did are hard for me not to confront. But we found our way through it, and all is well this evening. She is lying down for a nap. She slept poorly last night.

03/13/09

The other morning Jane was out of sorts and having a difficult time focusing. Something insignificant set off her anger which grew and grew. I tried a new approach. I held her and said, "Please, don't be angry at me. It is important we stay close together. I would not do anything to offend you." Nothing helped. She wanted to call Kathie and ask her to come up. She took her phone book and abruptly left the apartment.

She apparently wandered about the building for a while and then went in and talked to staff in the clinic. They helped her reach Kathie by phone and kept her in the clinic area. Kathie came in 30 minutes. The social worker called and let me know Jane was there.

Jane and Kathie came to the apartment. Jane looked "wild" and frightened. The three of us tried to talk. Jane was accusatory toward me. It was all my fault because "You wouldn't talk to me." Kathie's attempts to put things in a different perspective only made her the recipient of Jane's anger.

Jane said she would leave the apartment after Kathie left. I said if she did that, the administration might decide I am unable to take care of her and want to place her in the health center. The comment made her furious. "You are threatening to put me away, to lock me up." Kathie tried to clarify what I said, but her comments were met with anger. Kathie left the room, and Jane and I reached enough harmony so Kathie could leave. There were no more threats from Jane. We ate dinner, watched TV, and went to bed.

Jane is remorseful about the episode. She is embarrassed by her behavior and worries "everyone will know about it." I tell her there is no reason to be embarrassed. She said the social worker told her if she "left the building," they would take her to the assisted living section of Vantage House. Jane now has reason to fear that could happen.

I assured her I am totally dedicated to caring for her and want her to stay with me as long as she lives, if I can give her the care she needs. The administration may impose security measures if Jane continues to leave the building in a fit of rage. If my health remains good and I outlive her, she can be with me until she dies. That is what we want and pray for. I fear she may become so belligerent she will be unwilling to stay in the apartment.

3/22/09

Laura came to visit four days last week. One could say the visit generally went well. One could also say it was a disaster.

The day she arrived I took her to Hagerstown to see my son, Paul, for some "after hours" dental work. Paul asked Sharlene, his wife, to assist him. After the work was completed, we all went to dinner together.

Jane has been irritated with Sharlene for several years, mostly because Sharlene and Paul do not get along well. Because of the hostility I debated whether I should tell Jane about Sharlene being with us at dinner. I decided to wait until the next morning because I anticipated she would be angry.

She was furious when I told her, although she regained her calm by the time Laura came for breakfast. In the afternoon when we were alone, Jane began again about "the dinner" and became increasingly disturbed, highly unreasonable, shouting, and threatening suicide.

The next two days passed without major incident, but because Jane was on edge, Laura had a difficult time dealing with her. Jane's over-solicitous behavior annoys Laura. Jane wants Laura to take things home from the apartment and is angry when Laura refuses.

Laura left Friday morning. We walked to her car, carrying three packages for her and the kids. We hugged and said goodbye and waited and waved as she drove away. Thirty minutes later Jane said, "I wish we had walked to the car with Laura when she left."

Jane has been sad and angry about the visit and about the dinner in Hagerstown. There is little I can say other than "I'm sorry it happened." Surprisingly the anger is not at me. It is focused on Laura and Paul and it grows with each recall of their "misbehavior." These two days have been sad for me, and they have been tiring, very tiring.

(Email to Laura 3-23-09)

I know mom makes comments that annoy you. She is critical of lots of things, always was, but it used to be in a light hearted or pleasant sort of way. Now it carries a feeling of anger and resentment sometimes. And I know she bugs you when she asks you to take things home. Since you left, I'm sure she has said at least ten times each day, "I can't understand why Laura wouldn't take the flowers home with her." I know it feels like she is trying to tell you what to do, and she senses your resentment. It's almost frightening to me how she picks up on some of my feelings that are not expressed. Thirty minutes after you left, mom said, "I wish we had gone to Laura's car to say goodbye to her." She has still not remembered doing that, but unfortunately other little things remain foremost in her mind.

3/25/09

Jane always had strong feelings about people and about things. As a child she was lonely. The adults in her life took care of her adequately, but no one seemed to care about her hates, her desires, her anger, her wants. She never had a close friend to talk with and learn more about her own feelings and those of others. Feelings remained a mystery to her, and thus they became, in a way, more powerful and more frightening.

Feelings have not controlled her life but they have often dominated it. Her religion is based almost solely on feelings. Her relationship with God is an emotional one, but it is genuine and strong. Her relationships with others are based more on emotion than on intellectual appreciation. Those feelings too are genuine and strong. Her response to other people is based partly on feelings they have toward her. It is difficult for her to move beyond her feelings to more valid reasoning. Feelings are the coin of life.

She gets angry at God when God seems not to respond to her weeping and pleading. She gets angry at her children when they seem not to respond to her emotional needs. All she wants is God's love and her children's love. Without it she feels desolate and irate.

As Alzheimer's progresses, Jane's interaction with others becomes even more an emotional one, and she is more expressive of her feelings. Unfortunately she expresses negative feelings as readily as positive ones. She is not just judgmental about people and things; she expresses her opinions in a harsh and sometimes caustic manner. There is no longer much "neutral" in her emotional engagement with the world.

Loss is the dominant feature in her current emotional landscape, and the darkness of depression colors it all. Alzheimer's has many streets for her to travel, most of them from the past. She readily talks to others about her childhood losses as if that might somehow provide restitution or at least solace. She tells others she has Alzheimer's, even people she hardly knows. It's not for sympathy. It's to know she is not alone with the terrible, frightening feelings she carries. It may help her avoid the sense of isolation and loneliness that pervaded her early life.

Jane was never afraid of pain. Surgeries, childbirth, injuries were faced with calm and courage because she was not alone in the experience. Friends, family, or medical personnel, expressed concern, affection, and kinship for her in these trials. The hurt was visible, and the response of others was ready and generous. How does one respond to a person who has loss of memory, mental confusion, waves of raging emotions? Without some knowledge of what is happening, **no one responds**. Jane feels angry, frightened and isolated when others have no idea of the pain and suffering she endures. No one appreciated her feelings when she was a child and could not express them. Now she can and she wants others to know what she feels.

I never really understood why she married her first husband. They had few, if any, emotional ties and apparently no strong physical attraction, at least on her part. It may have been an extension of her prior experience—someone to provide the essentials of existence with no connection to her emotional life.

Her feelings were meaningful to me. I connected with the reality of her inner world in a way no one else ever had. Our relationship began with those emotional ties, and they were genuine and strong. With time, a deep and lasting relationship developed—fidelity, integrity, communication, mutual interests, the richness of a loving, lasting bond.

Jane is an intelligent, sensitive, caring, and soundly good woman, and she always has been. But "feeling" is the fuel that keeps her alive and functioning.

When others do not or cannot respond to her "feeling," they lose the meaningful connection with her heart.

(Laura 3/30/09))
It has been a rather difficult week since you left. Mom goes over and over the same things, the same complaints. She gets angry quite easily over nothing and trying to explain what I said or why I said it only makes her more irritated. And then if I don't respond, she gets more upset. We've had these periods before and then they seem to go away. I wish this one would.

(Laura 4/2/09)
Mom still talks of a card to you. It startles me how the days slip by. Mom is up usually between nine and ten. We listen to the news during breakfast until 10:30 or 11. Then it takes Mom an hour or more to get ready with some help on my part. We have lunch then at the Mall or in our cafe and by the time that's finished it is three o'clock or later. There's not much left of the afternoon. If we work on a crossword puzzle, it's soon time for dinner.

Mom talks a lot about things she would like to do. Recently she talked of getting material to make a skirt. She got material to make a skirt soon after we moved here. I can't mention that material because she would decide I was trying to avoid buying more. I've encouraged her to shorten a couple of her skirts for summer before she starts to make a new one. Neither of those things is likely to happen. It is sad to hear all her great ideas and know she can't do them.

4/5/09
Isaiah: 50, 6: "I gave my back to those who beat me, my cheeks to those who plucked my beard. My face I did not shield from buffets and spitting."

The above quotation was read at today's Passion Sunday Mass. I must remember it and think about it. The homilist spoke about suffering in our lives and the incongruity, the mystery, the incomprehensibility of sickness and pain and destruction—all becoming meaningful with the knowledge of the Resurrection and our own rising to eternal life.

My thoughts brought me to evaluate the resentment I feel when Jane makes unfair, critical and harsh comments. "How can she say these things when I do so much for her? Why does she treat me this way?" The remarks are made in an angry mood—or is it just "in a needier mood?"

It is humiliating to acknowledge these remarks chill my attitude toward her. And she senses the chill! I try to hide the response because it disturbs her. She decides I am angry. I deny it. She insists, and I get increasingly irritated because she won't let go of it. My anger frightens her because she feels isolated and abandoned and she becomes increasingly dependent on me. This often leads to hysterical outbursts of sadness and anger, for which I deny any responsibility. But I have some responsibility and I need to do something about it!

The quotation from Isaiah is meaningful. I need humbly to accept the "assaults on my integrity" and see them in the light of this scripture passage. If Jane is "beating my back, plucking my beard, buffeting me," they are minor items which strike my foolish pride because of "all I do for her." I need the courage, humility and grace to look at my "suffering" in the light of Jesus' passion or perhaps in the light of Jane's cross. Pride would indeed destroy me, if the relationship with my love were irrevocably harmed. I need to accept the pain when she yanks my beard a bit!

4/22/09

Jane's memory continues to deteriorate. We had lunch here with Kathie on Monday. By evening Jane forgot the lunch and most of the morning.

At times these past two weeks, Jane has "yanked my beard" but I kept calm and helped her settle down quickly. Last evening we watched a movie about the Nazi occupation of Holland. I mentioned I was in Austria during the war. By the time the movie was over she was furious and screaming at me. "You could have turned the movie off for all I care. It wasn't my war; it was your war. Why did you bring that up? Why didn't you ever tell me you had been in Austria? Leave me alone. Don't come near me. Do you say those things to try to upset me? If you get angry now, I will never forgive you."

She initially rejected me but I held her and said, "You know I love you, sweetheart. I'm not angry at you. I love you. You are my wonderful companion, my love, my life. I'm sorry I upset you. I'm sorry I said that. Everything will be all right. We're together and we will always be together. I love you and I would never do anything to hurt you."

She became quieter and we talked calmly. She was apologetic and self accusatory. I told her, "Its okay. Don't worry about it. I love you and you love me. There is no harm done. Nothing is broken. There are no cuts or bruises, no damage. We are together and always will be." She replied, "I don't know why I do this. I would never hurt you. I hear the words coming out of my mouth and I can't believe I'm saying them. This is how I'm going to be someday and how will you live with me then? It will be hard for you."

I responded, "When this happens, I know it is just a storm going by and I know it is harder for you than for me. It must be horrible for you to feel the things you feel. This is what Alzheimer's does to people. And I don't believe this is how you are going to be. This is not you. You are a loving, caring, gentle, good woman. These storms come and go and they will come again. The important thing is not that they come but that we get over them as soon as possible." I pointed out this storm lasted only 30 minutes.

Today was wonderful. Her memory seems better and her attitude is remarkably improved of late. During lunch Jane acknowledged how much better her attitude is about Alzheimer's. She is not angry about it. She accepts the poor memory. She does not get as frustrated and "hysterical" when she misplaces something. The contrast with what happened last evening is striking and almost shocking.

4/26/09

My son, Bob, and his partner, Wendy, visited yesterday. Bob speaks softly and Jane had difficulty hearing him. After they left Jane was in a daze. She explained what it was like. When she can't hear what someone is saying, she can't understand what is being discussed. Then she pictures a time when she will be with others and not have any idea of what they are saying. Their lips will move but her ears will not hear the words or her mind will not register them. So there it is! The end stage of her Alzheimer's!

4/28/09

We are having some unusual days. Jane is more thoughtful and at the same time more forgetful. She appears more concerned about me than about herself. Even though we have always spoken intimately to one another, a deeper spiritual sense is present.

Yesterday Jane was a little paranoid about recent exchanges with a staff member. She was insightful and said she realizes she does that sort of thinking. She believes it is related to earlier relationships with peers. She said she knows the thinking isn't right.

Jane talked about eventual "deterioration" as she called it. She is concerned at some point she will not recognize me. She visualizes a time when she may be unable to speak. She joked about how talkative she is. Talking is how she maintains her connection with others. She always wonders what others think of her and she thinks that motivates her.

Jane is more attuned to the spoken word than the written word. When I read to her, it registers well. She pictures the scene in her mind. As a child she attended to things adults said to one another because they said little to her. She became the listener and the watcher trying to understand the world around her.

Jane's emotional storms show marked improvement. She puts effort into controlling her irritation and readily says she is sorry if she speaks harshly or critically. I think this is based on her desire not to hurt me or make me sad. Our love has always been a powerful force in our lives. It motivates her to put effort into being the kind of companion she has always been. It motivates me to be aware of the changes she is experiencing and to accommodate in every way I can.

Alzheimer's has not affected our love for one another, but our love has affected Alzheimer's. We converse at least two hours almost every day. We go to the Mall five or six times a week. It provides exercise and an occasion to talk. The store windows provide stimulation for Jane. She observes and comments on everything. Jane would be much farther into Alzheimer's if it were not for our love which is physical, intellectual, spiritual, sexual, emotional—uplifting, inspiring, undying. Each day we become more appreciative of each other and the love that exists between us.

(Bonnie, Jane's daughter 5/4/09)
Wanted to let you know how much we enjoyed your visit yesterday. Your Mom was especially pleased and thought you seemed to be doing very well. She said she would be writing to you, but I wanted to let you know she often talks of writing to people but it almost never happens. It is a real problem for her to get a letter put together even if she does remember she wanted to do it. I will try to remind her from time to time to call you. Even phone calls get to be a burden for her and she puts those off to "another time." Anyway I wanted you to know she thinks about you often and frequently brings up your name and wonders how you are doing.

5/6/09
Last Sunday Bonnie was in the area and visited us a couple of hours in late afternoon. Jane was relaxed and afterwards said she was determined to stay relaxed. She was pleased with the visit and felt comfortable with Bonnie.

Two days ago Jane was irritated with Paul because he continues to see Sharlene, the wife from whom he is separated. I said we knew that for some time, and I am confident it does not change his feeling of affection for us. Today Jane said how unreasonable her attitude was and how ridiculous her ideas are when she decides how someone else should behave.

Jane's memory continues to disappear. I mention plans several times. She becomes easily confused. When she asks me to clarify I may sound like I'm lecturing and my voice may be louder. Am I a wee bit irritated or impatient? I must be careful. The Lord knows she has every reason to be confused and I have every reason to want to help her understand things.

5/27/09
Things are going well. Jane's mood remains good. She jokes about her faulty memory and takes it more and more in stride. It is sad to watch her frustration trying to hold her world together. She is more accepting, less frightened, less desperate.

I believe the emotional storms are triggered by some small thing that is said or done, that in some way is often reminiscent of a piece of her early history of hurt and anger. The scene from the past is the fuel for the severity of the emotional reaction.

Case in point: we went to noon Mass yesterday. At one point the priest invites people to stand near the altar. We are usually two of the first ones there. The first few people step up on the raised area where the priest is. Yesterday two women went up ahead of us. They stayed near the edge of the raised area and there was no room for others to step up. Jane and I stood on the lower level with other congregants. Everything went normally through the rest of the Mass. Shortly before Mass ended Jane began crying. I put my arm around her and held her close. After Mass ended, Jane asked to stay.

I asked what was wrong. She was back in time to her First Communion when the Catholic school children got special treatment over the public school children. The Catholic school girls had veils, and "pretty white prayer books with a raised area inside the cover with a holy picture under it. They didn't treat us the same as the others."

Jane experienced the feelings attached to that earlier scene. Only now, the feelings were not restrained by childhood fears and the intimidation of adults. The two women at the altar were "better than we are," "closer to the priest," and "kept us from being on the platform." After several minutes the pastor came in to see how Jane was. She spoke about her First Communion experience. He embraced her and said, "You belong ahead of all of us."

It took time for Jane to acknowledge the two women ahead of us just happened to get there before we did, and not making room for others was just thoughtless. Then Jane became concerned others might think we expected a privileged position. She seemed to think the other people knew what was going on in her head.

Emotional storms are triggered by something insignificant. They pass rather quickly if I remain patient and loving. They are, after all, from some other time and some other place. I just happen to be the one who has to weather the torrent.

These days I continue to work on Jane's book. Our two readers have positive comments. One reader is a priest friend and the other is a social work friend. The latter had a very favorable reaction to the first three chapters. Jane is pleased by it all. I am anxious to get the book finished and find a publisher. It would please me so much if we could have a copy in Jane's hands "Before It's Too Late," the title of the book.

The book is described as the story of Jane's "emotionally isolated childhood, an unproductive education, and an unhappy first marriage. My deliverance came in the sustaining love of a second marriage and a rewarding life with my psychiatrist husband." It becomes an Alzheimer's story as "the emotional incontinence of Alzheimer's puts my peace, my love, indeed my life once again in jeopardy."

PART 6 (JUNE 09—NOV 09)

6/9/09

Jane is aware her memory is fading and more things are hard to find. When she is angry or sad, I remain with her. I hold her and talk about our love for each other, the permanence of our affection, the wonderful wife she has been, the great years we've had together, and how difficult I know life is for her now.

We went to Copper Ridge, an Alzheimer's facility. The doctor did an extensive neuropsychiatric evaluation. He raised the dosage of Razadyne. He said for someone who has had Alzheimer's for five years, Jane's illness is progressing slowly, suggesting it may continue slowly. That was good news because it would give us more time together.

We go to Laura's in three days. I hope we will have a non-traumatic visit.

(Laura 6/16/09)

First of all, it was a good visit. There were two or three difficult times with Mom when she wanted to "go home immediately," brought on by essentially nothing. She becomes so emotionally exposed when she is with someone she loves. It's like she's emotionally insatiable, and everything takes on an emotional context no matter how mundane and little it may be. But it was a good visit and worth it as far as we were concerned. I hope it wasn't too draining for you and the girls. Fortunately the trip home was an easy trip and without controversy until she began to focus on one thing.

This is a long story and difficult to explain but it gives some indication of how mixed up her thinking often is. On the way home she mentioned the silver necklace that was in the box of jewelry she gave you. Now she wants it back. I was not supportive of the idea and tried to say a few things to get her off the topic. That only strengthened her need to have it back. It was "the only necklace" she ever wore. Not true, but it was a favorite. She couldn't stand to part with it. She was heartbroken. She was going to call you last night to ask for it. I asked her to wait and think it over tomorrow. She said I was taking your side against her. I told her there were no sides. I finally mentioned this sort of thing has happened in the past with you, and I thought it might be difficult for you to accept it again. She was angry because I brought up the past and it only made her feel worse. I told her I was trying to protect the relationship the two of you have. I hoped if she thought it over she would decide it wasn't that important. Last night she was irritable and sad and talked about wishing it could all be over. She was angry at me but we finally sat down and watched a movie together.

This morning she brought the subject up again but more calmly and with clearer memory of what happened. She had a box for you near her jewelry and was picking out some pieces to give you. She picked up the necklace to put it aside to take on the trip for herself. When she saw you take it out of the box Sunday morning, she felt like it wasn't her necklace. I think she really didn't know what necklace it was. She first became aware of what had happened when we were on the way home. So she never had any intention of giving that necklace to you. It all sounds pretty strange but that is the convoluted way her head works at times. Something completely obvious to me escapes her totally or is seen by her to be something quite different. And believe me that can cause misunderstandings between us quite easily.

It is all disconcerting to her because when she sees clearly what happened, the possibility of similar events in the future frightens her. She says, "I can't be trusted." In fact she cannot be trusted to have things right because she often can't recognize what they are or if they are.

So I ask you to put the necklace in a mailer envelope and send it back when you get a chance. Just the necklace, not the silver piece. She definitely wants you to have that. She has had it a long time. This incident shows her confusion and how things she says or sees or does may not be what she intended. Things that others say or do may be just as easily misinterpreted by her.

(Laura 6/17/09)

Appreciate your quick response. It's amazing how big something can become after starting out just to be a simple little thing. Thanks for your understanding.

Mom has a nice silver necklace we are going to send you. Yes, she really wants to give this one to you. It is much more appropriate for the silver medallion you have. We have a sturdy little box we'll use to send it, and you can mail the other one back in the same box if you like. Mom appreciates knowing you only wear silver. She may have known it before but forgot it, and she'll probably forget it again by tomorrow. But I can remind her.

(Laura 6/19/09)

Your package with the silver chain came today. And believe it or not, Mom says this is not the chain. It gets confusing. On the way home she talked about the silver chain she mistakenly gave you. She kept saying it was the silver chain she wore all the time. But this is not it.

Now Mom says the necklace was gold and has rhinestones in a V shape at the bottom. I remember the necklace. That was a favorite necklace. It isn't in her jewelry here. I didn't see it at your house but I really didn't pay much attention. I suppose it is there. She has earrings that match it and they are here. Actually I haven't seen her wear that necklace in months.

When I opened the envelope with the silver necklace, at first she said she never saw it before. Then she got angry about the whole thing. I said I asked you for the silver chain because that is what she talked about when we got home. Nothing helped, because only one thing remains—she doesn't have the gold necklace.

Sorry about all of this. Things really get mixed up for her. If you have the gold necklace with the V shape rhinestones, will you put it in the mail when you can? Let me know if you have it. This has all been such a needless mess but it is the kind of thing we get into now and then.

6/27/09

I neglected writing for the past few weeks because I spent more time on Jane's book. I'm trying to get it in shape and off to some agents and publishers.

We went to Laura's for three day. Jane had a dreadful time getting ready. She bordered on hysteria for hours before we got away. The morning after we arrived she wanted to come home. She was irritated by things Laura did or did not do. The second day Jane insisted on going home. When I agreed, she quickly changed her position. We said goodbye the next day with loving comments between Laura and Jane.

The trip home was uneventful other than Jane mentioning "the silver chain" necklace she gave Laura. She took her usual number of gifts for the children. Jane is always disappointed with their expressions of gratitude, no matter how insignificant the gifts. After we got home comments about the "silver chain" continued and she worried Laura might "give it to someone because she didn't appear interested in it when she saw it."

I had several phone calls and emails with Laura over the next several days. It was a full week of irritability and sadness. Then everything settled down. The past week has been one of the best we've had in a long time. Jane points out the many positives in our life.

Jane is bright and interactive. I forget she doesn't know the state, the season, our apartment number, what store we are in, what meal we last ate, who she just talked to, or what we just did. Superficially she interacts as she always has. She is the Jane I have lived with, laughed with, and loved for all these years. It is easy for me to forget how much she does not remember and how much she does not know of what I know.

Sara Rubloff came yesterday with three chapters she finished reading. She is doing a magnificent job. She is enthusiastic about the book and the project is a positive venture for Jane. I continue reading the chapters to her. She enjoys them and recognizes most of what is in them.

7/9/09

A couple of rough days! Laura called Tuesday evening in a talkative mood. We talked about 20 minutes. Before I finished talking, Jane was in the background letting her wrath be known to both of us with loud comments.

When Jane took the phone she had difficulty hearing and before long she was shouting at Laura and gave the phone to me. I suggested Laura call tomorrow.

Jane was furious. She wanted to talk to Laura before I did because "I have been so worried and waited so long." While I was talking to Laura, "I thought someone may have died. Laura and you have always teamed up against me." She was loud and full of accusations.

An hour later, Laura called back. I answered and gave the phone to Jane. Laura must have been very loving and gentle and careful. Jane was pleased with the call.

The next morning Jane said she didn't want to talk about the previous evening except to point out I behaved terribly and said "the worst things you have ever said to me. Your attitude and behavior have to change for things to go well between us." I had tried to decrease the conflict. It seems necessary for Jane to review even settled matters. I said I don't rehash her angry comments and I am keenly aware of my failures. "Don't you know I have Alzheimer's and can't help what I do? How can you be so cruel as to mention in any way what I have done when I have no control over it or responsibility for it?" She certainly has a point.

The day was devoted to arguing. It was a short day because she woke after noon. I say "arguing." Jane kept finding things to be critical of and I kept trying to lessen her agitation. She threatened to leave the apartment. She threatened to kill herself. I was out of the apartment briefly. When I returned, one of the chairs on the deck was moved to the railing. She mentioned it to me later as if she wanted me to be aware of it.

My "not talking" is a repeated source of friction. It hangs over our relationship like a vulture. It was never a problem in our marriage. The rules have changed. I am expected to respond to any remark Jane makes. "I have to know you heard me." I feel like a school boy being taught proper manners. It annoys me. In a pre-Alzheimer's world we could have discussed this reasonably.

If someone does or says anything that makes Jane feel demeaned, left out, ignored, or discounted, it touches an emotional residue from her childhood that is highly explosive. She **needs** me to respond to everything she says; she **needs** me to compliment her on her appearance and her behavior; she **needs** me to pay attention when she is speaking; and she **needs** me to look at her when she speaks to me or when I speak to her. She is needy.

If I remain aware of her needs, I can respond to her expectations. But I forget, or I'm thinking about my concerns, or I just don't feel like doing it. At times it feels like I'm taking care of a "very needy child." I must remember our years together, our love, her completion of my life, her fulfillment of all my needs. **Her needs cannot be excessive.**

(Laura 7/10/09)
Thank you for the late call last evening. It was just what Mom needed. She was very pleased with the call and said you were so loving and so gentle. Last night was the worst episode she has had in a long time. While I was talking to you the first time, she was feeling left out. It becomes increasingly obvious that many of her childhood experiences and memories get played out in some crazy way in the Alzheimer's. Any little thing that gives her the feeling of being left out or demeaned or criticized or ignored can bring on this type of reaction. I'm very grateful that you called back. It really put out the fire. You were courageous and very thoughtful to come through the way you did.

7/14/09
Yesterday was an ugly day—beginning to end. I washed and dried Jane's hair. I thought the process was going well. Suddenly she attacked me. "You never said one word to me while you washed my hair. You never said one word to me while you dried my hair. Not one word." I apologized, although I talked as much as at any other time.

The only positive thing I can say about the day is I did not get angry or upset with her. I tried to placate and soothe her. I was accused all day of not talking to her, of abandoning her, of not being capable of taking care of her, of playing psychiatrist.

It was not a pleasant evening. She continued talking about how horrible her situation is, how cruel I am not to talk to her, how much she wants to kill herself, how we will never be close again. My comments are "defensive," "sarcastic," "belittling," "professional," or "ridiculous." I said I can't talk to her when she is like this. She hated me and God.

We made a semblance of peace at bedtime. This morning she begged me to forgive her for yesterday. I told her I do, and it is Alzheimer's that brings her to this point. She said I had not apologized for the way I behaved. I apologized to satisfy her neediness.

During breakfast she became angry and went to the bedroom crying. When I came in, she was in bed. I lay beside her and told her how much I love her and want to be with her. I massaged her feet and left her asleep. I anticipate she may sleep for a few hours. I wonder if I can take care of her through the duration of this illness. I pray I can.

7/20/09

We met Phil at the Mall for lunch about a month ago. It wasn't the best day for Jane but the visit went well. He has called from time to time, often saying he plans on coming up the next week but never setting a time.

(Laura 7/21/09)

Mom has been pretty difficult lately. She gets angry over little or nothing and sometimes quotes me as saying something I never even dreamed of saying. I think she thinks it in her own head and then decides I said it. We had some periods like this before and then they seemed to subside—or at least they have in the past. I hope this pattern changes before you come down. She has always been pretty opinionated, but it is much worse now. She can be critical of everything and anything. I never disagree with her other than sometimes to suggest another possible interpretation. Lying to her has become quite easy if it prevents difficulty.

8/06/09

Jane was edgy and irritable for the past two weeks. Several days ago it changed. She is more patient with herself when she loses things or forgets something. She is less self-critical and more relaxed. We can be together without fear of getting into conflict.

I have no idea what brought about the change and realize it could easily turn the other way. We recently talked about the illness and how it affects her memory and mood. She admitted that focusing on her symptoms and the anticipation of getting worse and "becoming a monster" aggravates her and contributes to her negative moods.

Laura and the girls will be down next week for a three day visit. It is important to Jane and to Laura that it goes well.

(Laura 8/9/09)

Mom had a really great week. One or two minor episodes of unreasonable anger but quickly contained. She got involved in doing more pictures to hang, going through art books, getting out frames, mattes, etc. It gets very confusing for her at times, but she sticks with it and I work along with her when I can. She wanted them all done before you get here, but so far we don't have even one done. I keep telling her the project can last for weeks or months; there is no reason to rush and no time limit. She is enjoying doing it. It makes her feel she is accomplishing something and there will be an end product. It keeps her mind busy and it feeds her interest and enthusiasm for art. It has been very good and I don't mind if it lasts for months.

On the one hand, she often approaches our staff or strangers and is friendly and complimentary. She always tells the mailman what a great job he is doing whenever she sees him. On the other hand, she is outspokenly critical of how people dress, how they behave, of fashions, of items on the news, etc., etc. She is often mixed up or just plain wrong about some of her criticisms but I just let it go or make some noncommittal comment, or even mildly agree at times. Rarely do I correct anything she says unless I feel it might be embarrassing for her if not corrected. She is embarrassed and sometimes angry if I correct something. It is very important for her that I agree with her ideas and opinions.

(Laura 8/17/09)

I was in the bedroom when Mom was giving the girls all the scarves. She seemed perfectly rational and happy to be doing it. Right after, she told me how much it pleased her to give them the scarves. A few hours later she told me she had to get them back and she was going to talk to you about it. I had doubts about her doing that but she was determined to get them.

Yesterday when we talked, it finally made sense. It has been clear to me for some time that emotion can totally govern Mom's reactions at times. Sometimes she can still deal with her feelings the way most of us do.

We have a variety of passing feelings as we interact with one another. Occasionally Mom gets caught up in one feeling and it dominates and controls everything. It crowds out all other feelings. When she gave the scarves to the girls, she was totally caught up in her affection for them. Nothing else was important. She was enjoying it. Yesterday when we talked about it, she said, "The girls could have asked me for anything at that time and I would have given it to them." The emotion of the moment was her love for the girls and her delight in pleasing them.

A few hours later she thought about the scarves we got at Nordstrom's when she worked there in Spokane. They became the most precious things she had, a connection to the past, a treasure she couldn't live without. That was the importance they suddenly had. Her affection and emotional attachment then was for the scarves and all they meant to her. The feeling dominated everything and she had to have them back. It sounds ridiculous but it so very true. I have seen this sort of thing in lots of ways and never fully understood it before.

Her head is in an entirely different place when one of these feelings takes over. When we talked about it yesterday, she understood it as well as I did, but of course it doesn't mean that will change anything. When it happens, it just happens and it can't be undone. What I try to do is listen to her, let her know I love her, not criticize what she is doing, and help her work it out or get through it all. She suggested I try to explain all this to you because she feels badly when these emotional things turn out hurtfully. Hope this makes sense for you. It's like her mind for a time has only one compartment and the particular feeling fills it.

9/8/09

I have not written anything for quite some time for a couple of reasons. It has been discouraging to find no takers to publish Jane's book, "Before It's Too Late." One agent said there are over 187,000 books published each year and publishers only take known authors or celebrities.

Another reason for not writing recently, I have been busy providing the finishing touches to Jane's book and getting if off for self-publishing. I could waste months looking for an agent or going directly to publishers. Jane is failing and may be unable to appreciate her book if it is not published soon.

The price for this choice is reasonable, and the book should be in our hands in four to six weeks. Jane will be able to enjoy seeing the finished product. We are putting her self-portrait on the cover.

Much has happened since I last wrote. Laura and the girls were here for a visit in August. It was a great visit except for a painful episode. Jane gave the girls a shawl and several of her scarves during a time of intense affection for them. Within a few hours she wanted them returned because "I love the scarves so much I can't part with them." She completely forgot she gave them the scarves. I had no way of knowing her behavior was driven by emotion without full awareness of what she was doing. It became quite an issue for Laura and the girls. Some email exchanges about it are noted above.

The night before Laura and the girls left for London, Jane and Laura talked on the phone. The result was disastrous for Jane. She mentioned the scarves again, and Laura "raised her voice." By the end of a horrible week, the story was "Laura screamed at me." Jane cried every day and fluctuated between hating Laura and fearing Laura would "never get over it." It became the focus of every conversation, every meal time, every bed time. When Laura returned, I alerted her to the situation and asked her to call Jane. She called that evening and they had a wonderful talk and all is well.

Saturday, Father Tillman gave a great homily about the imperfections we have and with death we will shed our imperfections and put on a new garment. I thought perhaps Jane will have a head start in heaven because she is already shedding much of who she is.

Jane's attitude has been positive this week and her mood is stable. She is truly a brave woman to face this illness with equanimity. I am filled with compassion and admiration for how well she handles the obvious dread that covers her life. Remarkable!

9/11/09

An interesting dilemma developed yesterday. Jane agreed to allow maintenance staff to enter the apartment if we were not at home. Staff came to fix a sink problem while we were at the Mall. On our return Jane entered the bedroom and began to examine things. We kept two plaster pieces about six inches long (like molding) on the bookcase. Jane said, "One of the three pieces is missing. Someone has taken it."

She continued to talk about it. At one point I said, "I only remember having two of them." "How could you disagree with me, argue with me, try to prove I'm wrong and make me look stupid?" I said I only remembered two but that didn't mean there were not three. She remained belligerent; although at one point she said maybe I was right. She slept poorly and told me she was up during the night looking for the third piece.

At breakfast she got into it again and I mentioned remembering only two pieces. "If you love me, you have to agree there were three. Why can't you be on my side for a change?" I finally said, "I'm sure you're right. There were three. I must have forgotten the third one." She remained sad and angry into the afternoon and told me to stay away from her. Later she said she was going downstairs to report the theft to the head of security.

I asked her to sit and talk with me. She was angry because, "You won't let me report the robbery." I said, "If you report it, you will force me to do something I am reluctant to do. I will go downstairs and tell them we only had two of those pieces. That is the truth and I cannot let them be suspicious of an employee without justification."

Things changed completely. Jane agreed there were only two pieces. She felt terrible for putting me through all the aggravation. Her remorse can be as difficult to deal with as her anger. She was angry that I lied and agreed there were three. I asked what alternative I had and reminded her of what she said. She never likes to hear things she says in anger.

I have no difficulty lying to Jane about things that might upset her, as long as I think she will not find out the truth. Perhaps I don't lie to her enough. I am deceived by her sound reasoning at times and believe I can tell her things that would be better off unsaid.

10/13/09
Jane's book will be finalized today. We should have the first printed copy (with dust jacket) in 10 to 14 days. I feared it might be too late for Jane to appreciate it.

A few days ago we had a lengthy talk. We talked about Alzheimer's and how it affects our lives. She spoke about her anger and the harsh and critical things she says. When I mentioned some of the things she said, it was like she was hearing them for the first time and could not believe she said them but at the same time she knew she had.

Sometimes Jane takes an unreasonable and ridiculous position about something and maintains it for days or even weeks. Recently the garden fence was moved to an area below our apartment. She was furious and wanted to "raise hell with them, burn it down some night, destroy it in some way." She will never go out on our deck again because that white fence "will be staring me in the face."

After three weeks she noticed the fence was not visible unless you went close to our window or to the edge of our balcony and looked down. Yesterday she commented the fence didn't look too bad. She admitted how wrong she was. She said it must be difficult for me to deal with her unreasonableness and how grateful she is I don't argue with her about her view. Now that's pretty insightful!

Complaints continue about the terrible sound of the TV especially during the news. I said it may be hard for her to keep up because Alzheimer's slows her thinking. Suddenly everything changed. Why hadn't I explained all of this to her before? She understood now and was embarrassed she had nagged me about it.

She says she is sad for what I have to "put up with." I say there is "to be happy with, sad with, frightened with, love with, live with" but not "put up with." She carries the real burden, and I want to help her in every way I can. That brings me fulfillment.

(Laura 9/15/09)
Mom is back on a pretty good track the past few days. She had been focused on the illness and what the future brings, and it just depressed her and made her edgy. But she's back to looking more at the days we have, and we try to make the best of each of them.

Mom got a nice card to send you two weeks ago and she often mentions sending it, but like many other things she doesn't get to it. She really has a difficult time getting to things she wants to do. We still haven't returned to working on a few more pictures to put up. It was something she was really happy to be doing but then we put it aside when you came to visit and she hasn't been able to get back to it. Like so many other things, she talks about sewing, making a pillow, maybe a skirt—but nothing ever happens. I know it is discouraging for her and frustrating. It's getting so she doesn't think of those things as often and that's good.

10/17/09

Jane's book came today, and it's beautiful: "Before It's Too Late" by Jane A. McAllister. We are pleased with the product. It is the story of her life, of our life together, and of the onset of Alzheimer's.

We had wonderful days the past week. Jane has been thoughtful and responsive in our numerous talks. We talk about Alzheimer's in a somewhat clinical manner. She asked, "Do I have dementia?" She doesn't remember prior discussions. I took a paper and made a sloppy pie-chart for dementia and the various illnesses that make the pieces of the pie. Jane does better when she can see the idea on paper.

Jane becomes frantic over losing something, condemning herself as stupid, becoming angry at God for punishing her, wanting to be dead. "I cannot live like this." I can usually turn her response around with careful comments and caresses. On the way to lunch she said she talks to God a lot and to herself. I often hear her mumbling.

(Kathie 10/19/09)

Fortunately your Mom seems to have a better attitude about a lot of the old issues. I'm not sure if it is because she has forgotten them or if she has sort of come to terms with them. She told me the other day things like "the cut down trees," the "garden fence out the window," and similar items that were major issues for a time are no longer of importance. She recognizes how unreasonable some of her attitudes were and thanked me for not trying to persuade her to think otherwise at the time.

It almost seems like her evaluation of things is more sound, but her memory (and losing things) is considerably worse. She doesn't talk about the past as much and gets confused in some of the stories she used to tell about the past, e.g. re grandfather and grandmother.

She is pleased the book is done, as am I. I took out a number of items that were more critical of your father. I keep a personal diary I may consider for a book sometime. Your mother is unaware of it because she would want to read it.

10/25/09

We went to Copper Ridge last Wednesday. The doctor told me Jane's insight regarding her angry episodes is quite remarkable. I told him we talk two or three times a day about the kind of thinking and feeling and responding that flows through her Alzheimer's mind. We often go over some past episode that seems to need clarification.

I wonder if most Alzheimer patients talk about how the illness affects their lives and everything they do. I suspect most family caregivers don't encourage such discussions. I doubt professional caregivers ask them about the inner workings of their impaired brains. Caregivers are more willing and able to talk about the food, the weather, visitors, clothing to wear, the schedule for the day—but not about how Alzheimer's affects their speech, colors their thoughts, influences their emotional responses, and turns the whole world from white to black and bleak.

We saw Jane's audiologist today. She decided he was going to try to sell us new hearing aids, recently advertized. He never mentioned them. She was tense and a bit argumentative during the hearing test. He increased the volume of her hearing aids and Jane was pleased with the adjustment.

When we got home I suggested we get our mail and go to our apartment. I would pick up our dinners later. Jane attacked me. "Why don't you speak words I can understand? You must know I didn't have any idea what you were saying! How can you do this to me? What is the matter with you?" I repeated what I said and she understood it, but she remained hostile for another two hours.

The next day she brought up the previous evening. She was apologetic and blamed herself for what happened. She said she did not understand my words in the car. It was like a foreign language. She felt I was not myself when I was speaking. There are times when I feel she can't hear me or doesn't recognize me. The experience was frightening for her. I believe the time we spend sorting through these reactions helps her be more comfortable with and more accepting of her illness.

10/31/09

Yesterday was a remarkable day. Jane was happy, relaxed, bright and philosophical. We talked for two hours over lunch. I said, "If anyone we know sat here listening to us, except for some memory difficulties, they would not think you have Alzheimer's." She was a wonderful companion, and I told her the day was comparable to any of the many wonderful days we have had in our life together.

My current opinion: 1. Our talks about Alzheimer's symptoms and how the illness affects us help her maintain some equilibrium and a calmer attitude. 2. The daily stress takes its toll and additional rest is important to maintain her stability. 3. There is a great deal of mystery and unpredictability in Alzheimer's.

The last few days I wonder if we are the benefactors of some special blessings. That may sound far fetched to many. I have enlisted a chorus of about 100 saints whom I call on daily to pray for us. There are also my parents, brothers and sister, and about 100 deceased relatives and friends whom I petition every day.

Jane's current state brings me to an ever deepening admiration for her spirit and courage. She is loving toward me, warm and gentle with others, comfortable and reassuring to all. I am in awe. I am aware this will not last. We cannot escape the outcome. I pray the course will be peaceful for her and her contact with God will remain firm and our bond of love will always remain a comfort to her.

11/13/09

If I've written some stories that sound strange, this will outdo them all. It will be difficult to make it understandable. Convoluted is the best term for it.

Four weeks ago Jane shopped alone in the Midget Market in this facility. An hour later she returned with a necklace she bought. A Market clerk called and asked if by chance there was a second necklace in the bag, one Jane looked at in the store. I checked and called back with a "no." Jane was irritated the woman called. "What does she think I am a thief?" She mentioned it angrily several times the next few days.

In November we went to Rehoboth for three days. Packing was a nightmare. Jane can't decide what to take, so she takes everything and then feels like a failure for doing so.

Rehoboth was a strain. When I said she acted like she was being tested, she agreed and said she had been unable to put the feeling into words, although she knew it was there.

The day of return I began packing her things. In a large handbag I felt a hard object in one of the pockets. I opened it and found a small box containing three pieces of jewelry with price tags from our Midget Market. I was startled. It was unbelievable. I moved the box to another compartment of the bag thinking I would take it out at home before Jane found it. I thought, "Jane stole the jewelry, hid it, and forgot where she hid it." If I could get it back without her knowing, she would probably not remember it.

On the way home we stopped at a familiar antique store. Jane mentioned things she would like "if I had the money and room for them." The trip home went well. Jane insisted on doing her own unpacking so I had no chance to recover the jewelry box.

What should I do about the jewelry? I decided never to confront Jane about it. I could talk to the woman at the Midget Market, tell her what happened, and give her $30 to cover the cost of the jewelry. I had concern she might not keep it confidential.

The next afternoon Jane said, "There is something I have to tell you. I did a bad thing at the beach. I'm ashamed of it. At the antique store on the way home I took three pieces of jewelry." She said she reached in a jar of jewelry and took three pieces. She had no idea why she did it and not one piece of the jewelry was to her liking. I was sympathetic and associated the behavior with Alzheimer's. I asked her to give me the jewelry tickets and assured her I would take care of it and she need not worry.

She delayed giving me the tickets for several days. Then she said she had given me the jewelry and the tickets. She insisted she had, but when I persisted, she finally agreed she maybe had not. Two days later she found the box with the jewelry and gave it to me. She was concerned the theft could be traced to her if I contacted the antique store. I said I would give the jewelry to charity and give $30 to another charity to make up for the theft. She was pleased with the suggestion and agreed.

I gave $30 (to cover the cost of the jewelry) and the tags to our Midget Market. If the jewelry were returned to the store, Jane might see it and recall the whole event. I didn't want her to suffer unnecessary embarrassment. The matter is settled. Jane's limited sense of self-worth is preserved, which was my primary goal. I put the jewelry in a charity bag.

What does all this mean? Jane is not a thief. Jane is not a liar. Jane has Alzheimer's. Did she know she took the jewelry from the Midget Market? Why did she think she took the jewelry from the antique store? Who knows? I know I do not want her to be hurt by anything she does or says or by anything others say or do! She has already been hurt too much! And she hurts too much now!

(Paul 11/17/09)
Jane's mood has been more stable lately and her attitude and acceptance have been rather remarkable. She and I talk a lot about things that go on in her thoughts and in her feelings and she seems to benefit from the opportunity to discuss it. Her memory continues to fail and she can often have difficulty understanding comments made or conversation. Much is subject to misinterpretation. In casual brief conversation, people would still doubt she has Alzheimer's.

Many of the old wounds don't seem to fester as they used to. Childhood memories no longer are prominent, even though at least three of the women who read her book have mentioned how they cried when they read about her childhood.

(Laura 11/24/09)

Am wondering what we should do about Christmas. If we come up, I'm not sure how it will work out. There are no guarantees these days. Mom has been more emotionally stable over the past several weeks, maybe even months. But there are times when she is "just gone." It's like she is someone else—angry, bitter, depressed, threatening to kill herself, totally unreasonable. Sometimes it seems there is no way out of it and then suddenly she changes, is remorseful, apologetic, and clearly sees how unreasonable and hostile she was. You have seen a bit of that during past visits. I hate to expose you and the girls and Mom to any scenes of that kind at your house. She makes promises about how much better she will behave but it is beyond her control. When she goes, she goes, and some days it just seems that's the way it's going to be.

She wants desperately to come up for Christmas and I want very much to have the time with you. I don't mind the drive. The train would be confusing for her. Packing is the worst part of every trip. She gets anxious and almost immobilized and then wants to throw everything in at the last minute. I can't imagine we will be coming next year but I've thought that and said it the last couple of times we were there. I am concerned our being there puts an emotional burden on you, as in the past two or three years. Not to see you and the girls at Christmas would be difficult.

At your house there is more room and more flexibility than here where it is confining and limited. "Here" also puts the burden on Mom to "take care of everybody and everything" and that is stressful for her. Of course, she tries to do that at your house too.

PART 7 (DEC 09—MAY 10)

12/3/09

Since Jane's book is finished I have not been in much of a writing mood. Perhaps I don't want to face the changes that are taking place. Changes are gradual, almost imperceptible. But Jane is slipping away from me day by day. She is less aware of things and less likely to talk because she can't find the words. She refers to feelings that "do not have words." She is not withdrawing but is less communicative.

She is as loving as ever and expresses regret if she shows some brief irritation with me. Sometimes she has difficulty hearing, especially the television. She says, insightfully, "It isn't that I don't hear; it's that I don't understand." She still attacks the television as "a piece of junk," and "if I ever have the money, I will throw it away and get a new one."

12/14/09

The last week was difficult. Jane is easily confused. Anger is ever present, under the surface or full blown. She is very angry at herself, at me, at God. I know she is frightened. She mentions her forgetfulness all the time. She wants me to "realize how bad it's getting." As if I didn't know! I see it! I hear it! I live with it!

I am tired today. I wonder how things will be—later today, tomorrow, next week. We go to Laura's in ten days. Can we possibly do that? I pray about it. Should we make the trip? Is it too risky? Will it spoil their Christmas? I feel very alone.

I promised Jane the other day I will always talk to her and always do all I can to console her and let her know I am with her. Then I wonder: will I be here to do that, can I keep the promise if I am here? And will I be able to keep her here with me?

This past week I had the grace not to get angry but to maintain calm and to continue talking during her angry, irrational, threatening periods. Yesterday we talked for two or three hours on two occasions. Does it help? How would I know? She becomes calm, apologetic, rational and then warm and tender. Ten minutes later I say something that offends her and the whole thing is undone.

Jane wishes she were dead and threatens to kill herself. She threatened to jump over the rail of the stairwell near our apartment. There is an opening, probably less than 24 inches wide, from the 13th floor. She said she put her leg over the rail but was afraid she would not be killed if she jumped. Other times she wants to live as long as she can. I sometimes pray for a peaceful and early death for her. Or is that for me? I usually tell her she will go in God's good time. I reread these words and wonder what my life has come to, what our life has come to?

(Laura 12/17/09)
Mom had a rough week last week. Last couple of days was a bit better. Her memory is very short. I remind her often of anything we plan. Her "executive functions" (as they call it) are close to non-existent on most things. She recognizes this and allows me to get more involved in some things she needs to do—up to a point and then she may get irritated by my "interference."

We are pretty well set with a range of presents that goes from the ridiculous to the acceptable and possibly enjoyable. Mom has forgotten past issues over jewelry and scarves. So there is a scarf for each of the girls that may be ones they liked. I don't think there will be any "I need it back" this time but no guarantee. Mom is determined to make this as wonderful a visit as possible. She sees it as her last and that may very likely be true. But in spite of her determination she does rather poorly in controlling her irritability and volatility.

(Laura 12/30/09)
Don't know what to comment about the visit. Sorry it was so trying for you and the girls. It seemed to be almost a constant stress for Mom through no one's fault. As usual, the only thing she remembers about Christmas

morning is you collecting wrapping paper and ribbon. No memory of girls and presents. So sad.

The trip home was tedious. Mom had a hard time going to bed that night. Made it about 1 a.m. and then slept until 5p.m. yesterday. Continues to mourn the lost necklace. That at least gave me ample time to check our luggage carefully before we left and after we got home. No necklace! It's probably in one of your drawers somewhere, where she put it so she "would remember it". Hope you find it. Now, as usual, it was the most important necklace she ever had.

1/1/10

Christmas at Laura's was a disaster. Jane was confused most of the time. One day she thought it was someone else's house. She asked why Laura and the girls were there. She wondered why so many of our things were there.

Christmas morning she focused on Laura picking up the wrapping paper and crushing it in a trash bag. Jane wanted to save it. Her memory contains nothing about the gifts, only Laura retrieving the paper and ribbons to discard, which Jane regards as being deliberately hostile toward her. The same thing happened the last two years.

Packing to come home, we could not find a necklace she wore Christmas Day. When we arrived home, I carefully went through our luggage. It was not there. Laura and the girls haven't found it.

Jane has been irritable, depressed. Last night we went to bed about 11p.m. I was exhausted and fell asleep. I woke about 2a.m. Jane was writing a letter to Laura, which she is now unable to find. She returned to bed. I woke her at 5 p.m. again today.

This week Jane is irritable but mostly sad and, I believe, frightened over her marked deterioration. She loses things all the time. She forgets what she started to say. She mourns the loss of the necklace. It is "the most precious necklace I ever owned. I wore it every day." In fact, she rarely wore it.

The trip was not a pleasant experience for any of us. The effects are lasting and devastating. I hope we get back to the rhythm of our lives and Jane gets

141

back to the level of two months ago. The four weeks prior to Christmas were anxiety provoking for her. She anticipated the enjoyment of wrapping gifts but it became necessary for me to do it. She was "too busy" to get to it and I doubt she could have done it.

The last three weeks were trying but I maintained a calm and supportive attitude. My patience wears thin at times, especially in bed when Jane repeats the grievances of the day. This goes on 30 minutes or more. I am obligated to respond in some way so she knows I am listening. At some point she drifts off to sleep. Then it's my turn.

(Laura 1/2/10)
Mom is having a difficult time getting over the trip. I keep reminding her of the good things which she doesn't remember—the popcorn and cranberries, the cookie making, the girls' concert. She doesn't remember what we gave the girls or you, doesn't remember opening gifts—just the wrapping paper and the ribbon. It is so frustrating at times not to be able to get her to recognize and appreciate the nice things that happen.

(Laura 1/6/10)
Our Christmas trip seems to hang like a dark cloud over our current life. I truly regret having exposed Mom to the confusion which occurred for her and the aftermath for both of us. She is just not able to deal with the complexity of some situations and the results are devastating. It frightens her to be aware of how different life can become under stressful conditions, and it frightens me to see it and know there is nothing I can do—except avoid it as much as we can.

I live with her Alzheimer's thoughts and words and behaviors. They sometimes frighten me. They always make me sad. I have learned there is no reason to be angry over them or to confront them or to have any idea I can change or correct them. Those who love her need to know she is not accountable for them and there is no value in a negative response to them. This is not who she is. Who she really is doesn't show up very often and it is hard to know whether she is really there or not there. She can be there one minute; and then some remark, some happening, some random thought takes her away to another place—even though she is right there in front of me.

I think I have spent a good bit of time trying to explain your mother to you. I think it's time I quit doing that. It may be a burden to you and I'm sure it just sounds defensive of her. She doesn't need anyone to defend her. And neither she nor I need to make any excuses or any explanations for her thoughts or her words or her behaviors. It is all covered under the heading of ALZHEIMER'S. I've sent you a couple of books about Alzheimer's. There is more material available. If you want to know some specifics of what it does to your mother, read and think about the last two chapters in her book. Those chapters report on how she was before the deterioration that occurred in the past two or three months and which will continue.

I know it is difficult for you to deal with your mother and it has been for a long time. But she is the way she is and the only change will be for it to get worse. You will have to find your way as best you can. That's what the rest of us do. And you can make clear to the girls what Alzheimer's is all about.

Your Mom loves you and always has. She has a difficult time finding you as she used to know you because her memory serves her poorly. Sometimes I think you have a difficult time finding her as you used to know her because you may not want to go back that far. For me to sit on the sidelines is painful but that's what I feel I must do. You and your mother will have to work things out between the two of you.

(Laura 1/8/10)
Thanks for writing what you did. I needed that. I am now aware of how inappropriate and critical my email was. I do most humbly apologize for my words and my attitude. It was totally undeserved on your part or the children's. The three of you did a great job and put a great deal of effort into trying to make it a good visit for us. Mom and I talked about it afterwards and agreed it was the best visit we have had with you in a long time. You three went out of your way to make it nice. The popcorn and cranberries, the concert, the cookie making, Casey's cooking and your own, and Tara's thoughtfulness with Mom.

I obviously took out my frustration on you. I felt tense most of the time, attentive to how Mom was doing with it all, knowing she was confused and unable to take the good things in, wondering what things meant for her and how she would react. I do know it is something we should not do again but not because of anything you or the girls did wrong. For Mom to be away from here for any length of time is too disorienting for her. I doubted we should go, but she would have been very disappointed and angry if we had not.

The worst part was after we got home. She went over things that had happened—the table cloths she took, the napkins, the necklace she lost, the things she brought to you and the girls and now says she never meant to give this or that to you (things she had definitely picked out, talked about giving, and insisted she wanted to even after I might say "are you sure you want to do this".) Every time we sat down to eat she would get into it and she could spend two or three hours repeating the same things over and over. When we went to bed at night she would go over it again for an hour or more and even then had a hard time sleeping.

I do not offer any of this as an excuse. There is no excuse for what I wrote to you. I can only say over and over how sorry I am. No one could deal with Mom and not come out on the short end lots of times. You were loving and thoughtful and the girls were too.

I have encouraged Mom to be more open with you and tell you more about her Alzheimer's and how she thinks. Over the past week she said she wanted to get on the train by herself and go to see you so the two of you could be together and talk. I suggested she ask you to come down for a short visit so the two of you could be together for some time.

I feel I am losing her as the weeks go on. Our conversations become narrower. She drifts away more easily. She has a difficult time focusing on anything for long. And she is so, so slow in everything she does. That tries my patience. But I really have no basis for complaints.
Again let me tell you I am sorry. I was thoughtless, unkind.

(Laura 1/10/10)
Last night it felt like you had come back home. It was great to talk to you and your long talk with Mom certainly was good for her and I hope good for you. I know she felt very reunited with you and I reminded her there were times at the beach, in Grants Pass, in Spokane and in London when

the two of you were very close and spent great time together. I told her if the necklace had not been missing this wonderful event might not have happened, and although the necklace was precious to her this was more precious. And she agreed.

I usually mention the problem issues when I write to you about Mom but there are certainly positive ones. When we talked after your call, she was perfectly clear and recounted what she could remember of the call. She is like her old self at times like that—thoughtful, caring, sensitive, logical, and all the rest. I never mention to you how courageous I think Mom is through all of this. I dreaded how it would go when we first knew she had Alzheimer's. With all the negative ideas she has had about herself, I thought this would be overwhelming for her and utterly impossible for her to deal with. She has been brave about it and expresses a determination to make the best of it, which she usually does very well. She deals with the memory loss well. Losing things and getting confused can be devastating at the time but she pulls out of it and recognizes how limiting those things are but she will still forge ahead. I think she has done well to keep her spirits up. Her emotions drag her around mercilessly once in a while.

1/12/10

It is difficult to capture the fluctuations of the past ten days. At times Jane functions well. She visits appropriately with other residents. She and Laura were on the phone for an hour and a half the other evening. Jane reported on the conversation with clarity and ease and mentioned insightful comments she made. It was a reunion for the two of them.

For no apparent reason, Jane may suddenly become perturbed and accuse me of "changing." "I see in your face you have changed." She decides I am upset or angry at her. She insists I have changed but won't tell her why. She said, "Maybe this occurs when I am talking too much about something. I know how I go on and on about things." When Jane mentions a past disturbing incident, I worry it will become major. I probably look uneasy or worried and Jane interprets it as anger or irritation. So the battle begins. "Why have you changed? What are you angry about?"

Jane moves more slowly and wanders in her activities as well as in her thoughts. She starts to get ready to go out and I find her sorting rubber bands, paper clips, and hair pins. She begins doing one thing and ends up trying to do several others unsuccessfully.

I get impatient and have to be careful not to show it. I am a clock watcher, and these delays and wanderings irritate me. I realize I am fortunate she can do what she does.

(Laura 1/14/10)
All in all Mom seems to be recovering her pre-Christmas level. She is cleaning out her bathtub and doing a remarkable job. She threw away a bag of Kleenex boxes and a lot of her collected shopping bags—about 70 of them. She is throwing away a lot of the nonsense stuff she saved.

I am not critical of all the things she saved. They were ridiculous but not to her. She always planned on "doing something" with them. I think she came to terms the last couple of days with the reality that she was never going to do anything with them. She had a difficult time "retiring," not having jobs around the house, not keeping busy and not feeling needed.

(Laura 1/19/10)
Mom was distraught after your call. Not because of you!! She felt she didn't say the things she wanted to say and told you some story that didn't make sense. She fussed about it the rest of the evening. She struggles with things of this kind—did she do or say the right thing or didn't she? Her judgment is poor about it because she often isn't sure what she said.

I told her I would tell you and Kathie, "sometimes if Mom thinks it isn't a good time to talk on the phone she should let me know and I will tell you." I told her she could just say to someone on the phone, "I'm having a difficult time and this isn't a good time for me to be trying to talk." She worries someone might think she's crazy. There is really no good solution but to "play it by ear." She is concerned these days about how poorly she is functioning.

I continue to be grateful for the closer relationship you and Mom have. It is very meaningful to her. She was pleased with what you said to her about coming down anytime if we needed you. I appreciate it too and hope there will never be a crisis that demands such a response.

(Kathie 1/19/10)

Things have continued a bit rocky for your Mom. Her moods fluctuate quickly and markedly. Memory seems much worse, but when her mood is stable her thought processes are remarkably clear, often poetic, and sometimes quite philosophical. It almost seems like she is a student of her own illness. She told me the other night, "There must be a little piece of my brain that deals with time. Well, that piece is gone." She said so clearly what I have noticed. Mentioning a time of day to her has no meaning. If I tell her we need to leave by 11:30 to go somewhere, it means nothing. I need to say it is time to get ready to leave. When I add, "We'll leave in ten minutes" it means nothing. I have to say, "It is time to get your pocketbook and your coat so we can leave."

(Paul 1/23/10)

Wanted to thank you for your gentle caring for Jane the other evening. She has continued to criticize herself for the outburst in front of you. I was amazed she got herself back together as quickly as she did. I thought it might just be an end to the visit. The evening visit was pleasant and I am glad you were able to come down.

Jane's episode was not unusual but was perhaps the first time with someone present. It was unusual it ended so quickly. They typically last for hours. Your presence helped end this one. I always worry something like that might happen in a store and get pretty complicated. We had a similar episode twice while shopping before Christmas. Christmas turned out to be a destructive time for her. I'm kidding myself when I think we might get back to where we were a few months ago. We don't ever get back to any prior level.

(Laura 1/25/10)

Just wanted to let you know Mom was sorting through some of her stockings last evening and found her necklace in one of her socks. It was as big a surprise to me as to her. I went through the suitcases before we left your house and again when we got here. I was as certain as I could be the necklace was not here. Well, I was wrong. We have it, and all is well. I have no doubt Mom put it in the sock in preparation for packing and forgot all about it.

1/28/10

Yesterday was the first good day in quite some time. The 24 hour period before that was hell. Jane was irritable, unreasonable, arguing, pursuing endless discussions of my "behavior." To say anything is being defensive, critical, and putting her down. Not to respond is "the worst thing you can do to me. You know it drives me crazy."

She was more physical than usual. She pushed over the coffee table and another table. She shoved me against the wall. I left the apartment briefly. On return I felt cold air in the living room. I asked if she opened the balcony door. She said she went out to jump but was afraid she wouldn't die on impact. She spoke of going to an upper floor someday and jumping from someone's apartment. She shouted, "I wish you would drop dead right here at my feet." Later she begged me never to mention that to her.

Am I afraid she will try to kill herself? It is a possibility but I don't think it is likely. I think it is a threat to get a reaction from me. Would I feel responsible if she did? I would feel terrible. I would wonder if I let it happen so it would be over for both of us.

I don't know how to prevent or lessen these episodes. I can't prevent them. Can I lessen them? "They" say the caregiver should not feel responsible for things. Usually I don't feel responsible for them occurring. But can't I do more to keep them from escalating?

Jane is extremely obsessive and compulsive. If she goes to get something, she gets lost in little items she needs to straighten, to look at, to put somewhere else. Going to bed has its endless rituals and frays my patience. In bed she may talk for 30 minutes. I get up at 6a.m. and she sleeps until 9:30 or later. I think she is thoughtless to keep me awake. Sometimes I think a little clearer. "What difference does it make when she gets in bed? It's no great sacrifice on my part to be awake a little longer. I'm really not a martyr if I miss a half hour sleep for her sake. I need to be more generous. If talking brings her some peace of mind, so much the better."

I feel more alone these days. It is difficult to have meaningful conversations. Jane forgets. She doesn't understand. She questions comments and then I have to clarify and she can be impatient and irritated when explanations aren't clear to her. I know she is aware of her deficits and that they are getting worse. Will there be some period when she is not so aware? Will that time be less painful for her?

1/30/10

Last evening Jane brought something to show me—three pieces of jewelry wrapped in purple tissue paper. The jewelry looked familiar but neither of us remembered where we saw them before. She couldn't remember buying them. I knew we didn't buy them. I thought we saw them in our Midget Market. She "knew" she didn't steal them and I agreed she had not. Stealing requires intent, awareness, choice. These were not stolen but were taken by a person with Alzheimer's.

I'll suggest she might have taken them from some store without being aware of it. Then I'll suggest we "donate" them to the Midget Market to sell. If she is disturbed by the idea she took them, then I will secretly pay the Midget Market for them. In the future I'll go to the Midget Market with her and watch her carefully. I cannot confront her. She already has too many harsh and negative thoughts about herself.

I know life is increasingly difficult for her. She slips farther away each day. Even when I hold her in my arms, I sometimes feel she is not really there. What next? How will things be next year? Next month? Next week? Tomorrow?

(Laura 2/1/10)

Mom mentioned the baskets to you. I encouraged her not to bring it up but she couldn't resist. That's another topic which she has brought up repeatedly since we came home from your house. The fact is she picked out three baskets to give to the three of you at Christmas as presents. She was very clear about it, deciding who would get each one. We were on the way home when she said she never intended to give any of the baskets away. I was totally surprised. She never wavers in the position she never intended to leave them there. At times she decides she can part with them. At other times they are the most precious baskets in the world.

Mom says you told her it is hard for you not to be able to help her. That is the hardest part for me. I see her so sad or so angry and there isn't anything I can do to change it or to help her with it. Holding her or talking to her often doesn't do any good and sometimes those things annoy her because "that doesn't help one bit." I think you and I are the two people closest to her and we both seem to get the brunt of her anger and pain. Please, don't be upset over these things. You have been very affectionate with her and I know you wouldn't do anything to upset her.

Wanted to let you know I think you are doing great with Mom and I realize how difficult it is to know what to say or how to say it. Even the tone of voice is important to her. My further difficulty is "my face" because when she is upset she sees "in my face" I am angry or mean or disgusted or something bad. Probably what she sees is that I am sad.

(Laura 2/2/10)
Email is my best way to communicate with you, at least in a freer way. Mom is not very interested in emails and doesn't really understand them. I occasionally say I emailed you or someone else. She rarely asks about the content. When I get one, especially from you, she may ask the content and that leaves me reading it to her or showing it to her. I don't usually tell her when I receive an email I wouldn't want her to read. Deception comes easily to me these days.

2/8/10
We woke without electricity two days ago due to deep snow. It was a confusing day for Jane and resulted in marked anxiety. She was easily irritated and tried to keep busy "sorting things," bringing them out of the dark bathroom.

Kitchen staff delivered a nice lunch by noon and said power would soon be restored. Power returned by 2p.m. and the kitchen provided buffet only for dinner. Lisa in the dining room kindly put together two carry out dinners for us.

By five o'clock Jane agreed to a nap and woke two hours later feeling "much better." The energy she expends must be tremendous. I can't imagine how she manages to put together fragments of the day and bits and pieces of the past, including yesterday and a few minutes ago, and bring them all together to make a meaningful picture.

When I showed the manager of the Midget Market the jewelry Jane found a week or so ago, she told me the jewelry is not from there. I can now only assume she took it from the antique store on the way home from Rehoboth last November. She must have hidden it some place and then found it just before she brought it to me. She has not mentioned it since the night she told me about it. I will put it in our next charity bag.

We have not been to the Mall for three days and snow is predicted for the next two days. It will give us some sense of what it would be like if we could no longer go to the Mall. What would keep us from going? If I could no longer drive, we couldn't go regularly. That does not appear imminent. Poor health of either of us could prevent it. Currently our health is good and walking is never an issue. If Jane became too confused or too irritable to manage, that could be a problem. We just have to pray that doesn't happen.

I'm reading Jane's book to a dear friend here who has poor vision. Jane comes with me and listens attentively. When she talks about the book, she refers to it as "my book." When she talks with people who read it, she is comfortable accepting the high praise they give her. I am happy everyone praises her work and my contribution is not mentioned.

We talked yesterday about who might die first. She thought it better if I died first because then I would not be alone, and she would probably not even know I was gone. I thought it better if she died first because I can care for her and it would be easier for me to live alone than for her to live without me. We each have fears about the future. Jane's unbridled emotions make her fears much more destructive to her sense of peace.

In final analysis it is in God's hands. She talks of wanting to "die now." In response I recently said to her, "In God's own time." She became angry at such a "stupid, religious comment you might say to a patient."

2/15/10

A few days ago Jane became paranoid about Laura. She said Laura "screamed at me" during a recent call. Jane called Laura back that evening and resolved the problem and had a good talk. Later she recalled the earlier phone call and again became irate that "a daughter could talk to her mother that way." Jane repeated her claim several times each day. I don't agree when she says, "Laura doesn't love me and never did love me." My comments were not acceptable nor was it acceptable for me not to comment.

On Friday Jane called Kathie. Kathie mentioned she talked to Laura on the phone. That set things off! Jane didn't want anything more to do with Kathie or Laura. She didn't want to talk to either one "ever again." "They have one another to talk to. I don't need to talk to either of them." I listened attentively but kept my comments minimal and neutral.

Laura called on Saturday. Jane had a good conversation with her. After the call Jane said how weird her mind was the day before and apologized for "putting all of that" on me and expecting me to respond. She recognized how far fetched her conclusions were. She is back on good terms with both her daughters.

Last night Jane woke me to say she was thinking how anger fills her head sometimes. She talked of evil and hate in the world and she has to learn not to let anger get to her.

2/20/10

Today is day three of anger, paranoia, hostility, threats, and verbal abuse. I wonder if I can stay the course. I am dedicated to Jane and her care but I wonder if my skin is thick enough for the job. My patience runs thin. I usually contain the anger. But her viciousness gets to me and hurts. I want to run away. I get hostile feelings I would never act on. I thought of leaving some morning before she woke and staying away for the day. What would she do then? Maybe she would realize it wasn't so bad to have me around. I thought of discontinuing my exercise and my blood pressure medicine. Pretty childish!

Obviously I want to hurt her when I think this way. She threatens to kill herself. Sometimes I think, "Well it would be over then." When she is so angry and vicious I feel like I don't really care about her, myself, or anyone else. I guess that's what happens sometimes with the care of an Alzheimer's patient. Pretty self-centered!

She criticizes Laura several times a day lately. This morning, she repeated her list of grievances. Later she was on the bed crying and wanted me to be with her. I lay down beside her. She said everything in her head turns green and purple when she is angry.

She talked about Laura. I responded carefully, trying to acknowledge her anger and sorrow and not criticizing Laura. I thought my response was appropriate and more than I usually say. She told me to go away because "you won't talk to me."

Jane continued to "rant and rave" for three hours. It is impossible to talk with her, to quiet her, to console her. I try to embrace her and she pulls away. She abuses my comments. "That's what you say to patients. I'm sick of this textbook stuff you give me." If I say less, her fury continues, "I have put up with this all our life." At one point, she professes her love for me and I am the only person who makes her feel good about herself. The next moment she hates me and doesn't want me around. I maintain calm.

But I am frightened. Where will this end? How will it end? I don't want her to harm herself, but I know she might, and I cannot prevent it. She is not only smart; she is clever. Recently when she threatened to leave, she took money from the desk drawer. Two weeks ago she put our change jar money in a plastic bag in her purse. She was going to take a cab and "go as far as the cab would go for the money."

I'm not afraid of her wandering away. I fear her running away during one of these episodes. Two days ago when I stepped into the living room, she slipped out the door. She went to the clinic. She spent time with the social worker there. The social worker called me and recommended Jane see the mental health nurse who comes to Vantage House. I'm fine with that. Jane agreed to see the therapist but I doubt she will.

Perhaps we are too close, too much in love. She depends too much on me for affection, security, and her sense of self-worth. I love her, and though I am not as dependent on her, my feelings of attachment make it more difficult not to be hurt by the vicious things she says and does. Sometimes I fear I might stop loving her and sometimes I feel I have stopped. When calmer times return, the love returns. It's never really gone. Today, I wonder if she still loves me. I know she did but she has changed so much. What is left of her love? What is left of mine?

(Laura 2/20/10)

Things have been very bad with Mom the last three days. She gets angry, unreasonable, hostile toward me. Threatens at times to leave the apartment, to kill herself. She recently showed increased hostility toward you, Kathie, and others. It is totally irrational with no basis, of course. I'm sure she distorts conversations she has with you, as she has with mine. She doesn't remember what people say and makes up what she thinks they said or what she wanted them to say. She is crying this morning and accuses me of not talking to her—which really means I don't agree with everything she says—and there isn't much I can say to make her feel better. She insists my words should make her feel better. Today she never wants to talk to you again. But she goes through these episodes with me, with Kathie, and with Paul. So you are still in good company.

2/21/10

Yesterday was despair and desolation. Today the sun shines and all is well. I sometimes think I can see Jane building up to the horrible emotional episodes. I know some of the items that contribute to the fire. The match that lights the fire may be a minor thing.

I never know how these episodes stop. They play themselves out, run out of fuel, are simply over. Laura called but Jane wouldn't talk to her. We had not eaten since 10 a.m. It was 5 p.m. and Jane wanted to go to the Mall for dinner. I expressed weak enthusiasm but we went. Things changed. I can't pinpoint just when or why.

We had a good time at the crowded Mall. There were no vacant tables except the table where we prefer to sit. We both saw it as a special gift—perhaps a deceased loved one, perhaps an angel, perhaps one of the hundred saints I pray to—but a blessing.

Today I went to 8 a.m. Mass and brought Communion to Jane. The darkness is gone. The psalm at Mass was: "Be with me Lord when I am in trouble."

(Laura 2/21/10)

Mom gets irritated when I talk to anyone on the phone for an extended period. I think she feels left out and alone. She gets a bit paranoid after a while, no matter who it is. I email you because then I feel free to go on and on if needed.

Last evening Mom gradually changed back into her pleasant and companionable self. Everyone was forgiven. I'm never sure what starts these episodes and I surely don't understand how they stop. The fire burns out and she is herself again. She told me the day we opened the Christmas presents at your house the room was so dark she couldn't tell who was there because she couldn't see them. Most of that time she was in a dense fog and I had no idea how bad it was.

She still craves the two blue tablecloths she gave you sometime ago. They were the most precious, etc., etc. she ever had. I don't imagine you use them. Would you write her a note and say you thought about the tablecloths and decided you would really like her to keep them and enjoy them. She will never use them but they have become a centerpiece for her happiness.

(Laura 3/1/10)
Thank you! Thank you! Thank you! Your email to Mom said it all. You did it so thoughtfully and so lovingly! I am grateful for your response. My only regret is I did not suggest this weeks ago.

At lunch today we talked about all kinds of things. She was pleasant, agreeable, rational, interested and interesting. She was like she might have been ten years ago—except for the memory. Today she said the illness is not a problem for her. Alzheimer's is so strange. She is a different person than she was Saturday night and Sunday morning.

I may need to get someone in at a later time when Mom is worse. I know it would be difficult to do that now and there really isn't a need. It would be nice if I could have someone come in for a couple of hours during a "bad spell," but that would be frightening to Mom (she would have all kinds of paranoid delusions about my leaving her), and no one is available on short notice.

(Laura 3/8/10)

Mom has had Alzheimer's for almost seven years now and continues to have a positive attitude most of the time. When it is bad, it is terrible—but at other times she really puts a great deal of effort into interacting with others, keeping calm when she loses things (which is constant), maintaining her interests, and not getting irritated with me. She feels she should be doing creative things or producing something. I tell her to get dressed, do her hair, and do her cosmetics is a challenge every day and truly an accomplishment.

3/22/10

It is a month since my last note. It is difficult to summarize events. Jane started on Prozac three weeks ago in addition to the 225 mg. of Effexor. Has it helped? How can one tell since her course is so changeable and unpredictable? She seems to have better control over anger, how bad it is and how long it lasts. Dare I hope this could continue?

Memory continues to deteriorate. How many times have I written those words? What day it is, what plans we have, where we are going, all need repeating. I remind her of many things to keep her in contact with our life. She rarely mentions anyone here. She forgets them until she sees them and then she responds readily and affectionately.

We boxed up winter clothes to put in storage. Jane was overwhelmed, although she cooperated and picked out clothes to store. She says she will not be here to see them again. "What will happen to all my things" is a major concern for Jane. To say it is not important after a person is dead would lack understanding of her feelings. She insists we must decide it all while we still can. She believes I would be unable to make those decisions if I outlive her. I cannot tell her I think she is already unable to make those decisions readily and prudently.

Jane tells me I am patient with her. It surprises me she is aware of it. She takes more time with everything. She gets lost in totally unimportant side issues. I refrain from saying things I think because I recognize the jumbled world in which she lives.

(Kathie 3/24/10)

The lady you met at the Mall, "the diamond lady", became a bit too intrusive. She and her mother joined us for lunch on two occasions and another day she came and sat with us for about two hours while we ate our lunch. Not very comfortable! Your Mom is very taken with her and seems to view her as "the only friend I've ever had." She talks to your Mom like Mom is a child. I laid awake a couple of hours yesterday morning thinking about it and finally decided I must do something. I wrote her a lengthy email explaining how important our time in the Mall has been to us and gently (?) suggested she might drop by for 10 or 15 minutes to visit. She responded appropriately and seems to get the point. While your Mom enjoyed her company it created a good deal of tension for her to keep up in the conversation.

(Laura 3/28/10)

You will notice Mom is more confused in her speech. She tells stories that are quite different from what actually happened. When she talks about things from the past, much of it may be totally inaccurate. She keeps saying little things to me during the day and at night when we go to bed, things that really don't require an answer or to which there really is no answer. But if I don't respond, she gets irritated because I "don't talk to her." I think she worries about being alone and about being unable to talk someday. She is very sensitive to being ignored or feeling ignored. If I just look away when we are talking, she is insulted. She tries to keep up in conversations with others and will ask me if she "did all right." She is so afraid she might look "stupid" to others.

3/29/10

Laura is coming for two nights. Jane promises "to be good." I know her intentions are good but her responses are not always under her control.

I worry about her. She is more tired these days, less energetic, with little enthusiasm. She complains of stiffness in her legs. Aches or pains frighten her. She always anticipates the "next stage." Will she be able to walk, to talk? These questions are in her mind. She fears she is dying. She will not be here next Easter. She doesn't expect to see her winter clothes again. What a fear filled life!

She continues to recover quickly from episodes of anger. I wonder if it is the result of adding Prozac. I wonder if her new physical problems result from the added medication. I'm uneasy about all of this and recently have not felt as cheerful as I usually do. That too wears on Jane and probably has an affect on her mood.

Laura called and said she will leave Thursday morning because she wants to visit Phil on her way home.

4/4/10

Our friends, Sara and Gary, visited yesterday afternoon for about four hours. Gary helped me change my email address and gave me some pointers regarding the computer. He's one of those genius types. Jane and Sara had a good visit while Gary and I worked on the computer. After they left I realized Jane was tired. With a little encouragement she slept for two hours and was refreshed.

What if an Alzheimer patient was unable to nap? I believe there would be increasing confusion and irritability. In a care facility it might be time for dinner or an activity or a meeting. We have no schedule. We do whatever we want when we want. The freedom is helpful to Jane, especially at a point of exhaustion and confusion that can happen so quickly and so unpredictably.

Jane slept twelve hours last night. After breakfast we had a long talk. She was philosophical and spiritual about her illness. She no longer resents the illness, acknowledging she was angry at God about it. She talked calmly about the future and the expectations she has. It must be good for her to talk so frankly and deeply about her thoughts. This kind of exchange must be a positive exercise for her frontal lobes.

It is remarkable Jane responded so well to the visit yesterday but was so fatigued and confused afterwards. We have times when she is utterly worn out for two or three days and then her vitality and spirit return. I dread the possibility that each of these periods may be leaving her a little more deeply in the dungeon of Alzheimer's.

Today was Easter. I went to Mass and brought her Communion. I wonder how it will be next Easter. I'm sure she wonders too.

(Laura 4/5/10)

Last Friday we had several episodes relating to Diane, the woman in the Mall. I told Mom I did not dislike her but I didn't want to have her join us for lunch. That became, "You want me never to see her again and you hate her." It came up again today and is always a source of anger for Mom. We went to lunch today and Diane came by. I went for ice cream and let them talk. Diane told Mom I contacted her by email and indicated I felt she was too intrusive. I had emailed Diane before you ever came down and told her Mom and I went to the Mall to be together and I would prefer she just stop to visit for 10 or 15 minutes. Mom seemed to have it all settled by the time we left the Mall today. But who knows? It may come up in full bloom at any time.

(Laura 4/11/10)

Bless you! Bless you! I want to thank you for the kindness and love and wisdom you showered on your mother last evening when you talked. She was thankful for all you said to her. You seemed to say exactly the right things to her to help her straighten out her head regarding Diane. She said you were not critical or judgmental in any way and you helped her so much in understanding what happened and she is no longer blaming herself for it all. You really put her mind at ease and I am grateful for your help. You knew the right things to say and the right way to approach it all. It showed much about your ability to understand people and to talk to them in a helpful and careful manner. I am very proud of you for what you did. I could never have straightened things out for Mom because she wants to talk about details with me, and she has them all mixed up. You could talk about situations and ideas and people. Thank you so much.

4/15/10

The two day visit with Laura went very, very well. Jane was relaxed, and we enjoyed our time together.

We had given Diane one of Jane's books and from reading it she knew about Jane's dolls and her affection for bags and boxes. She began bringing Jane a present in a pretty bag each visit. Presents included two dolls from Diane's baby days, pretty boxes, gifts one would usually give a child.

She became quite intrusive with encouragement from Jane. She and her husband had lunch with us at his suggestion. She and her mother ate with us twice, suggested by them, encouraged by Jane. Diane talked to us for two hours one day during our lunch.

In addition to these intrusions, she treated Jane like a small child. "Now you be a good girl until I see you again, and I don't want any bad reports from Robbie." This attitude was pervasive in their relationship and the gifts were demeaning.

I told Jane I felt our time in the Mall was important and special for us and I preferred not to have lunch with Diane. Jane understood and was in total agreement. Later she forgot the discussion and was angry if I referred to it because then she feels stupid. The subject of her relationship with Diane has been a source of conflict for the past two or three weeks. I feel Jane had something of "a school girl crush" on someone she regards as a mother figure. Diane is probably 20 years younger than Jane.

Kathie met Diane one afternoon at lunch. She was not impressed. When Laura was here for a visit, Jane was anxious to have her meet Diane. When Diane stopped at our table Jane asked if she and her mother would join us for lunch. Diane looked at me, and I shook my head "no." Laura and Kathie both felt Diane treated Jane like a child.

I worried about Jane's attachment. Diane was the "dearest friend I've ever had and the only friend I have now." Each day Jane focused on seeing Diane at the Mall. I sent Diane an email telling her we desired more privacy during our lunch time. When Diane told Jane about the email, Jane's attitude varied. "You had no business contacting Diane behind my back," or "You did the right thing because I could not see it myself."

Our conflict lasted about two weeks. I told Jane I did not want to have lunch with Diane with or without other family members and I said it was demeaning the way Diane treated her like a child. Laura phoned one evening and her talk helped change Jane's attitude about the whole affair. Jane acknowledged she had been impressed with Diane's clothes and jewelry and the gifts she brought. She felt she had been "taken in."

Now a week later, Jane is embarrassed by her behavior and wants to get the gifts from Diane "out of the house." I hope the episode will soon be forgotten. It is a good example for me and the children how Jane could be taken in by someone.

(Kathie 4/15/10)
I think your Mom is really slipping. Her memory is very bad. Doesn't remember something we just talked about, doesn't remember much of anything from yesterday. Gets very confused even at home. Very aware of how much is gone from her head and is sad and irritable at times. Tells about something we've said or done and the story has all kinds of confusion.

The unsavory attachment to Diane has been broken but Diane is still "the only friend I've ever had, the only person who cares about me. I have no one I care about here." But when we see some of the people here, they are like long lost friends to your Mom. She also acknowledges Diane was "buying" her with gifts and is very self-centered

(Laura 4/18/10)
The other evening "out of a clear blue sky" Mom brought up the baskets we brought to your house at Christmas. I thought they were out of her mind. I suppose she was looking at the baskets in the bedroom and suddenly the others were back center stage. She said she was going to ask you for them, and in return she has other baskets to trade for them and would also like to give your girls the little dolls and other items Diane gave her. She is now looking for a way to get rid of all the things Diane gave her.

4/25/10
We put the winter clothes in storage. Jane is terribly confused sorting through her summer clothes. She says she needs someone to help her but knows no one could. When she opens her closet or a drawer, her mind seems to go blank. She doesn't have the slightest idea what to do. I dare not touch anything because it would be interfering in her work and telling her what to do. She is obviously unable to make any decisions.

She is critical of herself for buying so many clothes. She is unwilling to give extras to charity and she won't put them in storage. "I would never see them again." There is the dominant theme of dying. When we put the winter clothes in storage, "I will never see them again because I will be dead." If some summer clothes are put in storage, "You will have to take care of them all after I am dead."

It is sad to see Jane overwhelmed by something that was simple for her in the past. She realizes how hopeless it is but she would feel defeated if she gives up. Today she planned to "work on my clothes." She was in the kitchen for well over an hour before she went to the bedroom. She is aware she accomplished nothing. She can't help but feel a failure.

Before she takes a nap I massage her feet and talk to her for a while. I bring a chair into the bedroom and read while she sleeps so she won't be lonely when she wakes, or perhaps so I won't be lonely while she sleeps.

Our conversations are narrow. Her interests are limited. The news is forgotten soon after she hears it. We were never much for "small talk" (whatever that is). I find myself talking about the weather of today, of yesterday and of tomorrow. I talk about the traffic driving to the Mall, the number of people in the Mall, etc. I guess that's "small talk." Jane repeats childhood stories. They are all sad and disturbing for her. We talk about the children. We go over things we have said before. For Jane it is probably all new.

Topics we used to discuss—religion, politics, art, philosophy—are rarely available to her. Her fashion interests continue strong and critical. The Mall provides her with clothing on store racks and on people to comment about. I avoid topics that have bad memories for her, that stir up anger and resentment, or that she may not follow well.

The bad times aren't as bad as they used to be. The good times are not as good as they used to be. Jane is slipping away; little by little I am losing her. It is so hard to reach her these days. Is it because I am tired? Because I am sad? Or is it because our love is unable to span the distance between us? She speaks often of death. Is this what she is talking about? This void between us? This space that touch and words and feelings cannot seem to cross?

4/27/10

Last evening Jane said, "Where are we going this week and how should I pack?" She was sure we had a trip planned. As we talked she seemed uncertain about where she was. She did not welcome my embrace. Was I a stranger? Later she said she felt "out of it, disconnected." As we talked her focus improved. But then as we got ready for bed she was different, distant, unsure of herself. She went to sleep quickly.

During the night I woke with Jane calling me. She was on the floor of the bathroom. She had fallen twice trying to get to the toilet. I helped her up. I bandaged a scratch on her knee. I helped her back in bed and she was soon asleep. Her hip is bruised.

She showed poor judgment two days ago, getting up on a chair to clean the top of the refrigerator and the cabinet above it. I chided her and she promised never to do it again. She made the same promise the last time she was up on a chair.

Yesterday morning Jane complained of chest pain. There was tenderness over the sternum and in her back. Her pulse was 60, strong and regular. Her temperature was normal. I thought the pain was likely from muscles she strained cleaning the kitchen the day before. Throughout the day she mentioned the chest pain and thought it might be a heart attack. She is preoccupied with dying, so I am not surprised about her concern.

(Kathie & Laura 4/28/10)
We saw Jane's internist this morning. He ordered some lab work plus a neurological exam and a brain MRI. Have neurologist exam tomorrow, and brain MRI on Monday. Your Mom's gait is very poor, shuffles, and speech becomes very slurred at times. She has been complaining for several days about her body being sore in different places and her legs not responding to her brain. I'm glad we could get in to see the doc today and lucky to get the other two appointments so early. Internist is not really sure about what is going on. Tests may give some answers. The most likely answer I would think is advancing stage of Alzheimer's.

Will let you both know outcome of tests and exams as soon as I have any info. Your contact with Mom should be as always. She does seem hypochondriacal at times but there is obvious and genuine impairment in both gait and speech.

5/3/2010

The past week was a significant week. Jane's deterioration is increasingly obvious. We were in bed about an hour Tuesday evening when Jane started to get up. I woke and asked where she was going. She said she had to find something for the next day. About two hours later she came in the bedroom and woke me. "Where is little Laura? Where did she go? I can't find her. Is she with Bonnie? Why did you let her go without telling me? I didn't get to say goodbye." She thought our daughter was four years old and she had looked in all the rooms, the closets, and the balcony for her. I could not convince her that Laura is an adult, has two children, and teaches school in New Jersey.

I held her and talked to her. Finally she slept. In the morning things were no better. She demanded to know where "our little Laura" was. I showed her a picture of herself with Laura taken four weeks ago. She finally accepted the reality of Laura as an adult.

The next afternoon I woke Jane after a two hour sleep. She asked who called. No one called. She said she heard me talking on the phone so loudly she heard it in the bedroom. Later she asked again who called. I said there was no call. She was unsatisfied. I asked what she heard. She said, "I heard you say, 'I love you.'" I took her face in my hands and said clearly to her, "There was no phone call. And you know that I love you and no one else. That's the way it is, the way it always was, and the way it will always be!" She seemed satisfied and the "phone call" was never mentioned again.

Last Friday we went to the University of Maryland to see an art exhibit. Kathie works there in the art department and invited us. It was a pleasant interlude for both of us.

(Laura 5/10/10)

It is interesting how Mom seems to be reliving so much of her childhood . . . . maybe not reliving it, re-feeling it may be better. It seems like she craves expressions of affection and comments of praise. Something she never had as a child. Bob called her yesterday and so did Paul to wish her happy Mother's Day. It was great for her. And your call Saturday night pleased her a great deal. She just can't seem to get enough of hearing that someone loves her. I've become more aware of that and have increased the love words I say to her . . . . things I've always said but just more often now. And when I praise her for something she did or said, she is delighted. I tell her often how well she is doing with the Alzheimer's and it pleases her.

5/10/10

We talked about Alzheimer's again yesterday and I described the following. Each Alzheimer's patient has a different course, although some things follow the same pattern. First is increasing memory loss accompanied by losing things and not being able to find them. You will probably recognize the world around you for a long time but, as time goes on, you may not know who some people are and eventually what some things are used for.

You get confused and that confusion gets worse over time. Decisions may become increasingly difficult. At some point you may need help finding your clothes, deciding what to wear, and eventually dressing. You may also need increasing help in doing simple things. You will find doing ordinary things more and more complex.

You may find it difficult to control your emotional reactions even toward little things. You may do things and say things you will later regret and feel guilty about. These reactions do not mean you are a terrible person or that you are going crazy. These emotional changes may become less problematic as time goes on. We can expect the person you have always been will continue to be the center of your being and of your behavior in spite of the decreased functioning.

The things which are happening to you do not indicate stupidity, laziness, neglect, or craziness, nor do they indicate loss of your own integrity, dignity, or value. You will remain the kind of person you have been all these years we have been together during which I have known you so well and loved you so tenderly. At some deep level, you will remain a caring, tender woman with a marvelous sense of humor, a quiet courage, keen observational powers, and a fascinating response to all of the life we share.

But the years will be hard for you because life is becoming increasingly confusing and mysterious, thus disheartening and frightening. Every day is a challenge and becoming more so with each dawn. I believe in your courage which I have witnessed through the years. I believe in your faith which you have nourished from a feeble seed planted by your grandmother and which you have clung to with determination through difficult times. I believe in you because I have been part of your life for almost fifty years and I have known first hand and with certainty the kind of woman you are.

5/17/10

I have been reading the pages I wrote two and three years ago. How many times have I said: "Jane's memory is definitely worse," "Jane has been depressed," "Jane was angry?"

This disease appears to be cyclical with a gradual decline in function. Because of shuffling gait and slurred speech Jane recently had lab work, a brain MRI, and a visit to a neurologist. There were no new findings. The neurologist recommended physical therapy "to evaluate gait and treat." The physical therapist tested Jane for balance and muscle strength. She will return for leg exercises which she can continue on her own.

Is this episode the result of the despondent, angry mood she recently had? Or is it some neurological deficit that occurs and then improves? Is that possible? Or does she have a decrease in function she gradually accommodates to and then shows improvement?

During that three week period Jane was very tired. She slept poorly and took two or three hour naps almost daily. This past week the situation has markedly changed. We go to the Mall daily for lunch or dinner. She walks well and speech is not as slurred. She is not napping in the day and sleeps better at night. More importantly her mood and attitude have improved. She is a congenial and delightful partner. It is clear she is determined to respond in a better manner to the symptoms of her illness. She repeatedly tells me she dreads hurting me or upsetting me and she is trying not to do so.

I'm doing a lot of thinking, prompted by the pages I wrote months ago. I rededicated myself to serving God through my care of Jane. I try to put her needs and her desires ahead of my own. This is not a great sacrifice or duty on my part. It is my love and appreciation for all this lovely creature of God means to me and to my life.

5/21/10

I recently read some of the notes written last January. They do not describe Jane now. She is doing remarkably better the past two weeks. We have a rather uniform schedule lately. She gets up about 9a.m., has breakfast, and gets ready to go to the Mall. We have lunch in the Mall and talk for an hour or two. We get home about 4p.m., play some gin rummy and eat about 6:30p.m. We watch a movie and go to bed about 10p.m.

Jane had two physical therapy sessions this week to strengthen leg muscles and improve balance. She was cooperative during the sessions and reacted positively to the opportunity. After two more sessions we will continue the exercises on our own.

She has been insightful and interested in the details of things we talk about. Yesterday she asked why Alzheimer's research was not making more progress. I explained some principles involved in doing research on diseases and their treatment. She was attentive and eagerly took in what I was saying. She understood it well.

Today we talked about phone calls from Laura and Kathie and how Jane worries about their tone, what they said, or what she said. I told her about my dislike of phone calls, which are not nearly as satisfactory as face to face contact. We agreed that misunderstandings can easily arise in phone contact. It was a great conversation and left us both feeling we had discovered something important to remember.

Jane is struggling not to harbor anger. She said today, "I owe it to you to do better; after all you do for me." My attentiveness appears to motivate her to remain calmer. She is not frantic when she loses something or forgets something.

Does all of this represent a change of direction in her illness or will she revert to some of the behaviors noted previously? What is really happening? I believe avoiding stressful situations, maintaining routines, and talking often about what is going on in her head is making a marked difference in her illness. We wait to see what the future brings.

PART 8 (JUN 10—NOV 10)

6/5/10

Jane did remarkably well the past three weeks in spite of severe memory impairment. Her mood was stable and generally pleasant.

Two days ago we were watching the news during breakfast. The reporter had a strident voice, talked rapidly, and moved quickly from story to story. Jane seems to wait for an opportunity to criticize the sound. She hates the TV, wants to throw it away, get it fixed, etc. "No one in the building puts up with this kind of TV." Material from her audiologist reports how difficult it is for older people to follow television, especially the news.

She was angry for three hours. Finally we made peace and went to the Mall for lunch. She looked at a scarf on a kiosk and thought it was beautiful. I said, "Get it, if you want it." I didn't think it was beautiful and I was certain she would never wear it. She decided my tone meant, "Don't get it." Maybe it did, because I thought it was a foolish purchase.

Except for minimal replies to my comments, she said nothing until we got home. Then she voiced her anger loudly and clearly. All the money comments of old were repeated. In the midst of this Laura called. Jane wouldn't talk to her and left the room. I let Laura know the essentials of the argument.

Laura said she would like to try to talk to her mother. I took the phone to Jane and surprisingly she accepted it. They talked for an hour. Afterwards Jane was calm and told me about their conversation. Laura was supportive and worked in some good counsel. Laura apparently used some of her own experiences and philosophy of life in talking with Jane. We both praised Laura's wisdom.

All went well until a couple of hours later Jane insisted we talk more about the afternoon. This led to anger and tears on her part and helplessness on my part. She prepared the sofa to sleep there but I persuaded her to sleep in our bed. We both slept well.

Everything was fine in the morning. But she wanted to talk about yesterday again. In no time she was screaming and accusing me of all sorts of wrongdoing. She sat out on the stairwell for almost an hour while the housekeeper was here.

We made up and went to the Mall for lunch. When we returned home, I suggested we play cards. She said she had a couple of things to say about yesterday. There are never a couple of things to say. There is everything to say about everything she thinks happened, right or wrong. We were back again to the rancor and ridiculous accusations. Even the distortions change as she remembers less of the few facts she had before. After a couple of hours, peace returned. What brings peace? It just happens, the way the anger happens. It's like a thunderstorm that moves in quickly and may stay for the day or be gone in fifteen minutes. The rest of the evening was fine.

When something happens that seriously disturbs Jane, e.g., garden fence, pool Mary, the trees, the event stays in an active part of her brain and seems to force her to talk about it often and for some time. Is it any wonder when I do something that causes anger she needs to talk about it over and over again? And I'm the available one! But I don't listen as calmly and as sympathetically in this case.

(Laura 6/12/10)
Your phone call Thursday was providential. I am so thankful you spent the time with Mom. It is remarkable how quickly Mom could convert to a reasonable person as she talked with you. She was very pleased and I think proud of all the wisdom and good advice you so delicately passed on to her, and apparently without being too direct or lecturing her. You have a marvelous way of talking with her at times like that. Thank you so much.

I have to say again that you have remarkable ability to be insightful and so appropriate in your conversations with Mom. Kathie and Paul both do very well with Mom but I think you are the only one who can "talk sense into her" as people used to say. You have a gift, some talent in that regard.

You are quite a remarkable daughter and I am grateful for all your years in our lives.

6/13/10

Jane is focused on "what will happen to our things." She is preoccupied with how I will manage when she dies. She doesn't want to leave all these things I won't be able to manage. When I mention Laura, Paul, and Kathie helping, that means nothing. She is determined to decide on and dispose of most of what we have in the apartment now.

I said I want to keep the apartment as it is as long as she is alive. I want her to enjoy it, to be comfortable in it, and to have the things she cherishes still around her. I see no reason to make changes now. I told her I want our things to be here. If she dies first, I will move to a smaller apartment, and the three children will help me.

Two days ago everything was going smoothly. Jane asked me to explain something I said and I did what I sometimes do. I raise my voice, I use gestures, I over explain, I may sound harsh. She became angry, and in no time it went from bad to worse to worst. Jane and I talk two or three times a day about the kind of thinking and feeling and responding that flows through her Alzheimer's mind. Three or four times a week we go over some past episode that seems to need clarification.

She refused to eat dinner. She went out on the bedroom balcony and pulled a chair over by the rail. She got on it and had one foot over the rail. I went out, took her arm and pleaded with her to come down. She finally did. Was she getting my attention? Would she have jumped? My fear was more that she would fall than that she would jump. She has been clumsy and unsteady lately. In any case it was not a safe place to be.

She threatened to leave the apartment several times but never prepared to do so. I said, "I am afraid I might be unable to take care of you in this apartment." That frightened her. I said I could not care for her here if there is danger she might kill herself or run away. She accused me of deserting her and insisted I said I would not take care of her.

She prepared to sleep on the sofa. I went to bed and went to sleep. I was exhausted. About 4 a.m. she came in and got in bed. I kissed her and told her I loved her. We slept.

This morning we tried to keep everything calm and friendly. After breakfast she was in her bathroom and I was in the studio. I went to see what she was doing. She showed me she had cleaned everything out of the bathtub. She crushed the tissue boxes she saved and put them in a trash bag with many of her other "treasures." I complimented her for her work. She said she hoped I was pleased because she did it for me. I said it was her bathroom and I didn't mind how she used it. Not a helpful comment.

She was furious, saying I always nagged her about it and that's the only reason she did it. "I put my precious things in the trash, and it's all your fault. Now they are gone!" I said I did not press her to do it. She told me to get out and leave her alone. A short time later Laura called. I told her briefly what was going on. She asked to talk to her mother. They talked for half an hour.

After the call Jane was calm and friendly. She said what a wise woman Laura was and how helpful it was to talk to her. We went to 4:30 Mass. The rest of the evening was like old times. We talked about her bathroom work but there was no mention of my pressuring her to do it.

6/18/10

I cannot describe the feelings I have or the thoughts that go through my mind today. Perhaps I dare not describe them. Is this the end of our time together as friends and lovers? How can I love someone who is as hostile as Jane has been for four days?

She says she loves me, admires me, etc. Inside I say, "Bullshit." She says it from memory, not from current feelings. Odd she should remember how she loves me, when she behaves like she can't stand the sight of me. I join the long line: mother Grace, stepfather Ed, husband Tom, Olga Brown (some brat in her neighborhood), and all the other enemies of her life.

These days have been much, too much. Jane is gone and I don't think she is coming back. But she is here to be cared for, and I'm wondering how I can fulfill my promise, my obligation, my need not to abandon her.

I have doubts whether or not I can successfully care for her in the apartment. She walked out last evening and sat in front of the building. Security alerted me. She finally came back with the insistence of a resident-friend and escorted by security. Two nights ago she put a chair by the balcony rail and put one leg over the rail before I pulled her back down. I'm not sure it's safe for her to stay in the apartment. The assisted living unit is the only alternative. She would hate it. I would hate it.

She verbally attacks me every time I come near her and try to talk to her. She picks on words I say or on things I don't say. Her mind functions well in her hostile state. She makes clever remarks which are critical and caustic. She mocks what I say; she criticizes what I say; she misinterprets what I say and gives it back to me in its distorted form. And she makes up things she thinks I said. Her confusion abounds.

I recognize her illness but today it doesn't move me. I pity her confusion but her anger only makes it worse. I try to embrace her at times but she probably "knows" it lacks what used to be there. She hears my words for what they may really be—not highly affectionate empty sounds. Can this be the last chapter in the life we had together? Is this the shipwreck of what was so wonderful? Was I a fool to believe that Alzheimer's could not destroy what we have?

(Laura 6/23/10)
When we watched news last evening, Mom got angry again about the TV and why I don't do something about it. I told her Alzheimer's makes it difficult to understand and older people especially with hearing loss have difficulty understanding news programs. She seemed to accept that Alzheimer's accounts for most of the problem. She often tells me, "It's loud enough, I can hear them, but I can't understand what they are saying." I thought the problem was over. By bedtime it started again with the same hostility about the TV. She got up and stayed in the studio writing until she returned to bed about 3a.m. She began talking about it again. I gave her another sleeping pill and she finally slept.

This morning she is apologetic for it all. Yesterday I remained calm and kept talking with her, saying how I love her and reminding her of good times and whatever else I could think to say. I have done some thinking and praying about it. I recently read the autobiography of St. Theresa of the Child Jesus (the Little Flower). She felt "left out" and picked on by school mates and even by other nuns when she was a Carmelite. I thought she would have some sensitivity for Mom, and I guess I sometimes feel picked on. I've asked her to be my patron and mentor and help me get through these times with good spirits, as she was able to do. If I don't sound too much like a religious nut, I will say I have been able to keep my calm and feel complete sympathy for Mom.

6/24/10

I wrote the last page five days ago. It was angry, bitter and despondent. Those feelings are gone, were gone the day Jane came back to the apartment and made peace. She was full of apologies for the next several days. We picked up our life as it had been. I tell her, "Nothing is broken, no one is injured, we are together and always will be." She became angry at me later over some insignificant, now forgotten matter. I talked to her and embraced her. She relaxed and dropped the onslaught of words.

She woke me during the night to say, "I can't remember why we were angry when we went to bed. Why were we angry?" I assured her we had not been angry. I held her and she soon went back to sleep.

Yesterday she was anxious and mildly confused most of the day. In the morning she talked to the psychiatric nurse whom she now sees on Fridays. In the afternoon we were playing cards. Jane mentioned driving to Philadelphia to see our friend who lives there. I said, "I don't care to drive in unfamiliar areas with heavy traffic." Jane decided, "We'll never go to Laura's or Rehoboth again. I'll never be able to ride in a car again."

She was furious. "Why did I say that? Did I have health problems?" I asked her to repeat something. "Why don't you get your ears checked? You need hearing aids. You're always saying 'what, what, what.' I'm tired of it." I had a hearing test a month ago (she was there), and there was no recommendation for hearing aids. "Then get another doctor. You need them and you're just too proud to wear them."

Confusion dominated the scene. She claimed I told her I didn't want to drive because of severe health problems. She insisted I tell her about them. She decided I could not drive due to brain damage causing hearing problems that hearing aids could not remedy.

It was a tortuous path she walked. I held her and told her over and over I love her and I know she loves me. I answered questions as best I could without aggravating her. I reminded her I am 91 and reluctant to drive in unfamiliar, busy areas. I maintained a soothing tone of voice and comforting words. She gradually became calmer and recognized I was not angry, but "You'll be angry before the night is over and you'll shut yourself off from me. Just wait and see." It sounded like she wanted to force me to do just that. I was determined not to feed the pathology that destroys her.

She talked for a while in bed, wanting to get back to the same issues. I resorted to the same response pattern and before long she agreed we should get to sleep.

Why was it different this time? How could I avoid the quiet, withdrawn, subtly hostile behavior these episodes usually provoke in me? I thought about St. Theresa of the Child Jesus. Something stirred inside me. Theresa went out of her way to do difficult and self abasing things. I have suffered very little in my life. I need to accept these painful situations calmly, quietly, and (like Theresa) gratefully. I will pray daily to St. Theresa and ask her to be my mentor and guide in caring for God's waif.

6/25/10

When Jane is speaking and thinking calmly, she thinks rationally and soundly. She is focused on what is being said and is quick to respond, often with appropriate humor.

When negative emotions appear (anxiety, sadness, anger, fear, loneliness), they don't just appear, they take over, they run rampant, they dominate her thinking so that reason and modulation are gone. Anxiety becomes panic. "The lost object will never be found. It is gone. It can never be replaced. I cannot live without it." Sadness becomes desolation. "There is no reason to live. Nothing will ever be good again. This is what life will be. I want to be dead." Anger turns to hate. "That's the worst thing anyone ever said to me. How could you be so mean to me? I hate you for being so cruel." Fear becomes terror. "This is the monster I will be some day. I am terrified of the future. I'm going to die soon; I can feel it. God is punishing me." Loneliness becomes isolation. "Everyone in the family has left me. I can't tolerate being by myself. You desert me when I need you and someday you will leave me totally."

These negative emotions are triggered by minor things: a word of mine, a memory from the past, a lost pencil, a misplaced dish, an unreturned greeting, a bad dream—a myriad of possibilities. These incidents unleash a storm of statements and behaviors far beyond what Jane could ever have imagined or produced. This runaway has no bridle and must expend this surge of energy before reaching control and calm. I have learned not to goad, not to challenge but to try to soothe with a soft voice and a warm touch, as one might do to a distraught animal. It seems animalistic, like our more primitive selves.

I write of negative emotions above. Positive emotions also emerge but are more regulated and controlled. Jane is as loving toward me as she ever was and we are united with the same intensity as always. Toward those who are friendly, she is cordial and quite affectionate. She is always friendly toward strangers and willing to help others if she can. These emotions are genuinely felt, appropriately displayed, and suitably controlled. Are these less primitive emotions supervised by a more mature part of the brain? There are many mysteries. One thing I know, reason and negative emotions cannot occupy the same playing field at the same time in an Alzheimer's patient.

7/1/10

Yesterday was a difficult day. I don't understand what is happening. Jane went to bed after breakfast, after lunch, and after dinner. She slept 6 or 7 hours during the day after a ten hour night. She slept through last night as well.

Jane is eating poorly and not taking adequate fluids. She was confused all day yesterday and kept insisting "something broke in my brain. It doesn't work the same. I know it has changed and it's not going to change back." She was desolate and certain this was the beginning of the long dark night of oblivion. "Maybe I've had a stroke. I never felt like this before." She was not argumentative or hostile, just sad and terribly frightened. I am not surprised she is so fearful. She feels she is going into a coma and is desperate.

175

I tried to console her. There was little gain in doing so. She was distant and rejected attempts to quell her fears which she repeated throughout the day and evening. We ate lunch in the café. She didn't want to see people. The loud voices were aggravating. She didn't finish half a sandwich. She ate no breakfast and a few bites for dinner. She went to bed, got up for an hour, then back to bed.

I am worried. Has she "slipped over the edge," as she describes it? This was a longer period of confusion than ever before. There were no inroads to the place her brain had taken her.

I acknowledged something major seems to have occurred. I said the brain is a complex organ and finds other channels when some routes are blocked. Is it possible that can happen in the Alzheimer's brain? I told her we will sit in the Mall in a couple of days and I will remind her she insisted she would never return to such a good level.

This morning Jane was brighter and more herself. During breakfast she faded away and ate very little. I was thinking, "Another day like yesterday." Then her indomitable spirit took over. How? She said, "I think I'll wash my hair."

She finished her shower quickly, put her hair up, did her make-up, and got dressed. I helped her find a couple of items. Otherwise she did well on her own. Yesterday none of this would have been possible for her. We got to noon Mass on time.

Talking at lunch in the Mall I reminded her of what I told her last night about sitting at lunch and telling her the horrors have gone away. She remembered what I said. I wish she could remember it when she falls into that pit of despair.

The rest of the day went well. The return to her previous level was remarkable. We know similar episodes will occur and we wonder how readily we can emerge next time.

(Laura 7/7/10)
Mom is easily confused these days and I don't think that is going to improve. When she is upset, anxious, worried, it is much worse. I tell her when

anyone is anxious or worried, their thinking can get screwed up. But even on good days her confusion is obvious. It is hard for her to accommodate because it makes her feel "stupid." Her lack of self-confidence has always been easily destroyed and now is pretty much non-existent.

One very good thing, I've started reading "A Woman Wrapped in Silence" to her while she does her hair and cosmetics in the mornings. She follows it very well and loves it, and it is a very inspiring book.

(Laura 7/16/10)
Thought I'd drop a line to keep you up to date. It has been a pretty good week. Mom continues to be confused and forgetful but her mood has been more stable and her attitude considerably better. She remembers bits and pieces of things and often puts them together in very strange ways. She continues to work on her bathroom and the drawers but has difficulty making any real progress. It is frustrating for her most of the time. She expresses concern she will never see you and the girls again, though I remind her you are coming in August.

7/22/10
I have not been writing lately and don't know why. I'm not depressed but I've lost my enthusiasm over the past few days. I've written some emails to Laura and Kathie about what has been going on. I've felt lonely and burdened. Maybe I didn't want to write. Writing is lonely and reminds me I don't have anyone to talk to.

Jane is not the companion she used to be and I'm not sure she can be any more. She is caught up with Alzheimer's and how it affects her life, her day, her moment. She talks about it: how bad it is, how much worse it will get, how often she forgets or loses something, how she is unable to do things, how useless she feels, how frightened she gets. It weighs heavily on us. It shadows us. It brings sadness and fear into our life.

Maybe I don't write because writing makes me face what is happening. I've started playing solitaire on the computer as an escape. It takes my mind off other things. I note how useless it is, how wasteful of time. I run off a few games waiting for Jane, who gets lost in the smallest and briefest task, and a few minutes quickly is half an hour or more.

Jane is often very confused and misinterprets what I say or can't understand what I say. She became quite angry several times yesterday. She would get over it, apologize for things she said, and before long would be angry again. She threatened to walk out and never come back but didn't make a move to actually leave.

I do better responding to her anger. I don't disagree. I am more patient than I used to be. She is so terribly slow at everything. She dawdles. She is off somewhere in her head, or perhaps lost in her head. It is difficult at times but I keep my peace and get through it.

I find myself wondering how long Jane will live. I look in the obituaries to see the age of people who die with Alzheimer's. I'm disappointed to see it is often around age 86. I find myself thinking of changes I would make in my life if Jane died. It seems so wicked, so unfaithful, so unloving to have such thoughts. Jane would be devastated, feel betrayed, deceived, if she knew. When I see her torment I sometimes pray for a peaceful and early death for her. I would be lost without her. I don't know how I would manage. I continue to ask God to let me care for her as long as she is alive.

I believe my life would likely have deteriorated in major ways had I not met Jane. My demons might have got the upper hand and destroyed any good accomplished prior to meeting her. I will be forever grateful she joined me nearly fifty years ago and made these years far more fruitful and blessed than they would have been without her presence.

(Laura 7/23/10)
We are anxious to see you and the girls. Hate to say it, but it may be the last visit with good recognition. Mom's short term memory is pretty much gone. And she gets confused about things that have happened or she thinks have happened. There was something yesterday she told me about and when I asked more about it, she realized it had not happened at all. Her world is mysterious and threatening. Even in the midst of all the devastation she is thoughtful and caring toward others and she enjoys talking and having a good laugh. It is amazing how perceptive she is about her condition and her behavior.

(Laura 7/25/10)

Yesterday was a fiasco. Mom left the building and went into the woods nearby. She apparently fell in a hole and couldn't get out. She called a workman in the area who helped her out. I went out looking for her on foot and later got the car and drove around the neighborhood. She got back in the building on her own and then the guard found her. She had a bloody arm from scratches. The nurse from our health center cleaned it up, checked her over and took her vitals. The guard had a policeman with him. It was a pretty frightening experience for Jane and for me. This all occurred in the heat of the afternoon when it was 105 degrees. She could have had a heat stroke. At times like this I have no idea what she might do. It is truly like she is another person. Today she is completely remorseful and sad about it all.

(Laura, Kathie, Paul 7/28/10)

I address the three of you because you represent our "lifeline" so to speak. Wanted to alert you to what may be a need of ours at some time.

Last night when we were talking about Mom's problems with memory and confusion, I mentioned Alzheimer's. She asked, "Does everyone know about it?" I replied, "All the kids know you have Alzheimer's, but I don't know how much they know about the illness." Mom was immediately angry. "I don't have Alzheimer's. How can you say such a horrible thing to me? I don't have that terrible disease and I never even say the word." I told her we often talk about it and she often tells people she has it. She grew increasingly angry and volatile and threatened to leave the apartment. The more I tried to say, the more hostile she became. I told her I was going to call Kathie. She said she didn't care. I called Kathie and told her briefly what was going on and asked her to talk to Mom. She did and Mom became calmer. (THANK YOU KATHIE) After the conversation, Mom said she believed she did not have Alzheimer's and attacked me for not being able to convince her she didn't. Later she calmed down and we got to sleep.

This morning Mom got up about eight. She wanted me to tell her what happened last night because "I know I did something horrible to you." I told her as gently as I could, and after talking about it for an hour she said she would take a sleeping pill. She is terrified now that "something like this will happen again anytime and we can't go anyplace anymore." She is sleeping now.

I wanted to alert the three of you that I might call you sometime and ask you to talk to Mom—if it is in the evening or on a day when you might be available. Talking with you, Laura, has been very soothing and calming for Mom at critical times, as well as times she has talked to Kathie. She is always very able to talk easily with Paul. It was a godsend for Kathie to talk to Mom last evening because it certainly turned things around. The three of you are a great source of comfort and affection for Mom and a great source of support for me.

(Laura, Kathie, Paul 7/28/10)
Since the episode Sunday when Mom left the building and fell in the hole outside, she has been more irritable and easily reaches an angry level. She talks about wanting to kill herself, leaving the building and walking into traffic. I am uncertain if I can continue to take care of her in our situation. I don't know how they would manage her if she were moved to the nursing unit. I believe she would deteriorate rapidly and would never forgive me for doing it. And I don't know if I could live with that arrangement.

(Laura 7/29/10)
Thought I'd bring you up to date on Mom. Last evening she got very angry after we went to bed. She was talking and at one point I said, "Let's try to get some sleep." That did it. "Too tired to listen to your wife who is dying of Alzheimer's." I held her and kissed her and we said goodnight. She began talking about how mean I'd been, etc. After several minutes I suggested we talk about it in the morning. Another explosion. She got out of bed. I suspected she was dressing. I had a chair by the outside door when she came out dressed and carrying a bulging purse. I said she couldn't leave the apartment at 3a.m. She began screaming and pounding on the inside of the door. I called the front desk and asked them to send someone up. Security came up in a few minutes and took her to 3rd floor of the health center, purse, jacket and all. Mom called Kathie from there, and Kathie called me as to how to respond. I encouraged her not to come up. About a half hour later they brought Mom back.

I felt utterly exhausted and not very enthusiastic about her coming back. I embraced her but didn't say much. She said it was like being in jail. She wanted to know why I was not more welcoming. I told her I was "worn out" by her anger because it had been so frequent in the past several days. I said I knew it was not her fault but due to the Alzheimer's, but nevertheless I was "worn out." I told her she has three pet peeves that fuel her anger. One is that she doesn't have any money. I said I'd give her fifty dollars each time we go to the Mall, but she would have to return whatever is left when we get home because I don't trust her not to leave and get a cab to take her "as far as it will go." Two is that she complains about the television. I told her the TV is going to stay just the way it is. Three is that I need hearing aids. I told her this is the most ridiculous of her Alzheimer's stories. I had a hearing test two months ago and I do not need hearing aids. I told her I will do everything I can to prevent her from leaving the building alone.

This morning she has everything twisted and says I embarrassed her in front of several of her friends by making fun of her for the things she does. We went to lunch in the café. I apologized for my remarks and told her I was very tired and should not have said them. After lunch we slept—me for two hours and she for three. So we are getting back on track. It was a frightening night for both of us but especially for Mom. I'm sure this is all some kind of blur for her and pretty distorted. There may have been some benefit if she got a sense of limits. I come away feeling pretty lousy about it all.

Mom got up a while ago and seems to be calm and relaxed, and we are back on good terms. I don't know what we learned from the experience. I hope she can remember there are some limits about walking out. At one point during the night she got the butcher knife and stood by the bed saying "You can watch me die." I hid the butcher knives today.

Hate to burden you with all this grim and sad stuff. Maybe it unburdens me a bit to do it. I pray and hope for the best and certainly feel more optimistic since I got some rest this afternoon.

7/30/10

My writing has shifted more to emails than to these notes. I don't feel dedicated to this writing because it is not as fulfilling as it used to be. It is so much easier to just slip into playing solitaire. Emails have a new meaning for me since I involve the three children in our life through them. There is a sense of personal contact when I write them.

As I write today, Jane and I have recovered our loving, sensitive relationship. She wonders why recent things happened as they did. "Alzheimer's" brings the answer.

It is unbelievable how warm and loving Jane is, how bright and vibrant she can be, how charming and sensitive in responding to others, and then can change to someone who is fiercely angry, threatening and belligerent.

Jane is apprehensive about Laura's visit in two weeks. Will this be Laura's last visit before Jane dies or loses contact with the world? Yesterday she said, "Maybe Laura and the girls shouldn't come down. I don't know how I will be by then. I might be much worse."

Next week we have an appointment at Copper Ridge with a new female physician. Jane didn't like the prior doctor and says he was a fool who never said anything to her and didn't even look at her most of the time. He was not the most personable man but I thought he was acceptable. She also views the facility as "very uppity" and that makes her uncomfortable. It is our best contact with someone who specializes in the field. All our other doctors seem uncomfortable with the subject.

(Laura 8/1/10)

At Mass yesterday afternoon Mom sat by a cranky looking woman who seemed a bit irritated when we passed in front of her to get a seat. I didn't realize the situation was irritating to Mom but she kept thinking about it all during Mass. Last evening she was on edge. At bedtime she told me it disturbed her deeply. It is remarkable how some minor thing can irritate her, and she has no control over it. I tell her if any situation annoys her let me know so we can leave. I would have left Mass yesterday if I had any idea she was upset.

The idea of death hangs over her all the time. Yesterday morning she had pain and tenderness in her shoulder. There was a bruise on the shoulder, probably from a fall she had a couple of nights ago. During breakfast the shoulder was terribly painful and the pain went all the way down to her wrist. She was moving the arm as little as possible and protecting it. She sat on the sofa and I brought breakfast in. We put her arm on cushions to be comfortable. It kept hurting. I got her some Tylenol. Then I got her a hot pack. No relief. It kept getting worse.

I talked about going to the ER. I really decided it was not a serious matter but I treated it as one and tried to be reassuring. Mom panics now when anything is wrong. Physical symptoms or pains are frightening to her. Whatever it is, it is an indication she is dying. I got her a tranquilizer. By the time we finished breakfast she was starting to use her hand to eat and before we finished breakfast the whole thing was forgotten.

(Laura, Kathie, Paul 8/3/10)
Plan to keep the three of you informed regarding Mom's condition as much as possible and as much as necessary. We are grateful for your affection and support. And I gain support by keeping in touch with you.

A couple of days ago as I was talking on the phone I heard the apartment door close. Mom left from the living room in her stocking feet. I didn't think she would go outside. I went through the stair wells looking for her. I informed security. When she returned after 90 minutes, she said she was afraid I might be gone and might never see her again or ever speak to her. She had locked herself in a bathroom on the ground floor where she put paper towels on the tile floor and sat there all that time. We made up in no time and all was well.

I talked to a staff member yesterday about the possibility of some respite plan for Mom. The staff said several people thought I should have some help and were concerned about both of us. She encouraged me to talk to the administrator. Over lunch I asked Mom what she would think of talking to Meriann (the administrator) about a plan so she could leave the apartment and have a safe place to go sometimes. To my surprise she agreed.

Before we left for the Mall yesterday Mom was uneasy. Several times she asked if we were just going to the Mall or were we going somewhere else. Before we left the apartment she said,"Are you planning to take me somewhere and have them lock me up?" I reassured her.

(Laura, Kathie, Paul 8/5/10)
We spent 5 hours in the ER last evening with Kathie joining us there. THANK YOU AGAIN KATHIE! When Mom was on the phone with you, Laura, the phone went dead, and Mom lost it. She shut herself in the bathroom with a towel tied to the door so I couldn't open it. I tried to talk to her. "Get out. Go away." After an hour she came out dressed to leave. I said she couldn't go. I called security. He came. She wouldn't let me open the door to let him in. She agreed to get her nightgown on if I asked him to leave. He left. She went back in the bedroom. There was a knock on the door. Two from nursing service were there, probably called by the guard. Mom thought I lied to her about security. She shut and locked the bedroom door and went out on the balcony. I tripped the lock and the two nurses came in the bedroom and saw Mom standing on a chair by the balcony rail. They talked her back in. Mom said she was only trying to get my attention. The nurse called the administrator. I talked to her and she was pretty insistent Mom go to the hospital for an evaluation.

The nurse called the paramedics and police. Four paramedics and two police came to the apartment. Mom was vicious toward me and frightened. She agreed to go in the ambulance to ER. Kathie met us there. Labs, CAT scan of head, physical and psych eval. Found urinary tract infection. Kathie stayed with us and talked to Mom while I left the room, which was extremely helpful. By the time we got to psych eval, Mom was calm and reasonable toward me. So that's the story of last night. This is about the fifth episode in two weeks.

I'm concerned the administration may try to move her to an assisted living unit. She would deteriorate rapidly. I'm strongly opposed to it at this time. Have to see what the future brings.

No fault of yours, Laura. It was going fine till the phone went dead. Paul had called just before you called and there was a brief problem with phone. Mom was condemning the TV just a while before the phone calls. Actually the TV, the camera, telephones, computers and all such gadgets threaten her. My need for hearing aids gets mixed in. She kept telling the medics I need them.

8/8/10

Most of what happened during the past couple of weeks is in the emails above. Not everything is there because much goes on I never get to write about.

Since the hospital visit there are no additional difficulties. The visit made a deep impression on Jane which, in spite of her memory loss, may be lasting. It is clear her behavior over the past three weeks has caught the attention of the administrative staff. They could ask to transfer Jane to the Assisted Living Unit. That would be a disaster for both of us. Jane would not do well there and I could not tolerate it.

The director of Building Service is a kind and helpful man. He suggested keyed locks on both patio sliding doors. They put a separate alarm on our outside hall door that alerts the front desk and security when the door is opened. The alarm will be set from the hours of 11p.m. to 5a.m. If the alarm sounds, the person at the desk will call us and send security.

Jane's therapist, a psychiatric nurse, asked me to join them on Friday. I noted every incident apparently is entered in Jane's chart. I gave the therapist a clear picture of the events of Wednesday and of last Sunday. It was a helpful session and very supportive. She and Jane have a good relationship.

We went to the Mall for lunch. We talked for three hours. Jane was insightful, completely focused, bright, and thoughtful. She spoke of her pattern of criticizing others and letting one incident or item affect her complete attitude. She can feel herself getting angry over what people wear or how they look. She said she did this all her life and wondered how I put up with it. She has exhibited that attitude at times and I altered my responses to accommodate. She would like to stop it. After dinner we talked for another two hours.

Yesterday Jane was in good spirits but thoughtful and sad. We talked about her concern about dying. She said the least little ache or pain makes her think she is going to die. Sometimes she is afraid she'll die before we get home.

She was relieved when I talked about our apparent good health. I assured her Alzheimer's does not cause sudden death.

We went to the Saturday Happy Hour in the lounge. We haven't done that in over three years. At least a dozen residents went out of their way to speak to Jane and many greeted her with a hug and a kiss. One woman told her what a magnificent writer she was and said she couldn't put her book down until it was finished.

When Jane gets angry it usually begins with an attack on me for something I did or said or failed to say. When it happens I begin to feel like a different person. I feel like a little boy being severely reprimanded, and it is frightening. I feel she doesn't love me and I feel isolated from her. She seems unreachable. When I think about this I know it is a good description of my feelings and probably explains my behavior of withdrawing, hiding, being silent, like she says I do.

This is a strange reaction for me. My parents were gentle people and never punished me, other than my father may have spoken harshly to me on occasion. I was "the baby" of eight and close to my mother. She was a gentle, quiet, loving person. My father was also quiet, slow to anger, and never volatile. The frightened boy I become seems like someone in a movie. I never knew or witnessed children who were frightened.

(Laura 8/10/10)
Mom now wants the baskets back. I shouldn't be surprised. We brought three baskets up at Christmas. Two of them match. Those are the two she would like to have returned. They are now a critical factor in the arrangement of her shelves. It is difficult to see her get into these things and be defeated by them. Please, bring the two matching baskets if you still have them.

Copper Ridge went poorly. The doctor made a mistake in seeing me first while Jane was occupied with a staff member. The doctor is a young, attractive female who "batted her eyes." Mom didn't like her and was quite angry before we left. She settled down later.

(Laura 8/15/10)

I am very sorry but we have a new problem. I hoped this would not happen. Mom and I discussed what she would and wouldn't consider giving the girls. After they got here, anything we said went out the window. Now we have another "I didn't mean to give them that." I felt angry and frustrated yesterday when she came up with the news. "I gave Tara my favorite necklace that I wear all the time." Mom went on and on about it. Finally I told her I would let you know about it. It is a silver necklace with individual squares of silver and a clear stone in each one.

I told her to put the jewelry she wanted to keep separate from anything she gave the kids to look at. We had agreed, etc., etc. It was meaningless. She was showing Tara the jewelry in her drawer, and Tara admired the necklace. Mom gave it to her. It is not Tara's fault. Of course, it really isn't Jane's fault either because she isn't responsible for these crazy things that happen.

Here we are again with Mom losing one of the "most important pieces of jewelry I ever had." She hasn't worn it in years and probably never will. She has a story about when I got it for her and times she wore it. I don't remember any of that and I don't think she does. Please, put it in a padded envelope and mail it when you can. Probably just as well not to bring it up on the phone. I told her I would take care of it, even though my first impulse was to stay out of it completely.

Yesterday was a bad day for Mom. She described it as being "disconnected." It felt like that to me too. She talked for two hours at breakfast—eating gets put aside—and it irritates her if I suggest she eat. She kept telling me all day about the thoughts in her head and thus reinforces them. She needs to repeat them, maybe with the hope they will go away or change. I felt it was difficult to "connect" with her. She was snappy and critical. She started the hearing aid thing and I told her clearly how it is and that her thinking is delusional. She seemed to accept what I was saying.

(Laura 8/16/10)

Last evening Mom began to obsess about the jewelry. She does not remember the scene of the jewelry on the bed and inviting the girls to "take whatever you would like to have." She doesn't remember us watching the girls play with the jewelry. She says, "Why didn't one of you know that I wasn't in my right mind?" At one point she said, "Why did Laura let me give all the jewelry to the girls? Didn't she know I wasn't in my right mind?" My reply was, "I know you better than anyone and I didn't know, so you certainly couldn't expect Laura to know." That made sense to her. Now she is frightened to realize she did all that, and no one recognized she wasn't herself. I reminded her if I had intervened and tried to stop her, she would probably have become very angry. She accepted that as true. So it's damned if we do and damned if we don't.

This morning Mom was onto the jewelry again. "All my precious jewelry. Every piece was special to me. I remember where we got it and why you bought it, etc, etc." I finally asked if I should ask you to bring all the jewelry back when you visit. She was greatly relieved. She was hoping I would say that. Just set it aside and bring it when you visit. "Are you sure it is okay to wait until Laura can bring it?" "Yes, yes," she replied. I don't know whether I'm angry or embarrassed to ask you to do this, but I know there is no reason to be either one. I hoped nothing like this would happen during this visit. I urged her not to spontaneously give things to the girls but she can't help herself.

This morning Mom brought me a note she had just written about her thoughts. This is her note: "God, how quickly comes your love to me. Can I join with your pain and suffering? Could I? I do not feel any words are needed to explain to you. You are with me. I know I must think and learn about my condition. I want to carry it well for myself and my loved ones—and for you. I pray to go to heaven to find the creator of love and the mother of peace." A rather remarkable piece!

It is amazing to remember how "with it" Mom was during the visit and now realize she remembers very little of the morning with the jewelry. She probably remembers little about the visit. But know your visit wasn't wasted. It was good and it was wonderful. It brightened our days and our life.

(Laura 8/17/10)
Will you please put the jewelry in a box and mail it? We spent three hours this morning talking about it. She ruminates and obsesses and repeats

the same things over and over. It gets to me when it is so useless to talk about it. Maybe having it here will put an end to it. She hasn't been horribly angry. She admits we agreed not to get into any jewelry when the girls were here.

8/20/10

It is difficult to capture recent changes and events without writing several pages. Nothing is stable enough to comment adequately. Calm days take a lot of effort.

Laura and the children visited three days last week. Jane was furious with me when they arrived, so I went alone to greet them. When they came in, Jane locked herself in the bedroom. I tripped the lock and Laura went in. She handled it beautifully. She was gentle but firm and loving. She embraced her mother and spoke of her love and how great a Mom she has been.

Yesterday we went to the Mall for lunch. Jane felt overwhelmed. Dresses in store windows offended her. People were "not the same." She decided I should take her home. At home she would not lie down because "if I go to sleep, I'll die." She wanted to see our doctor. I got an appointment for late afternoon. Blood pressure was normal. No examination was done. The doctor talked with her briefly after an hour wait. He recommended we see a psychiatrist. The visit was reassuring to her.

When we went to bed Jane wanted to talk to me. "Something has been on my mind all day. It will only take a few minutes and you need not reply to anything I say." Sounded simple enough. "You have not talked to me all day and made no reply to things I said. I felt separated from you, totally alone. It was not only today, but it has been going on for weeks." Then she said I have done it for years. I apologized and said I will try to do better. Nothing assuaged her anger. Each comment was going to be her last and "I need not reply." It was never her last and I did need to respond or I proved her right.

She finally turned out the light and agreed to sleep. But her words kept coming. She decided she could not put up with my "silence," so she went in the studio. I slept for about two hours, woke and went to see what she was doing. She just finished a note to me saying how much she loved me. I said I thought she should come to bed. "What no kiss? No expression of love? No response?" She came back to bed and continued talking for an hour before she fell asleep. Then I slept until exercise time.

I dreaded this morning. What mood would she be in? What would she say? What would I say? I exercised, went to the grocery store, and then sat down to read. I was dosing when she woke me. She was very loving. She apologized for the previous night and said she didn't know what she said but knew she gave me a bad time. If it was okay with me, she would rather not talk about it. Miracle of miracles!

She has been content not to mention it again. I believe she has little or no memory of what it was about. Finally, some real benefit to memory loss!

8/26/10

There has been a distinct change in Jane's responses the past ten days. Is this really a change or simply a better phase we are passing through? Are we just being set up for major disappointment with a return of the volatile angry periods?

Jane has "peace of mind and heart," something we both pray for every day. I mention it each morning when I go through my ritual of prayers during exercise. I beg the Triune God to give Jane peace of mind and heart these remaining years. She has a remarkable sense of calm and inner peace considering the constant reminders of her illness as memory deficits confront her in every conversation.

She became irritated about a Netflix movie last evening. I tell her, "If there is anything you don't like about a movie, please tell me and we will stop watching it." After awhile I asked how she liked it. She was hostile and said she was avoiding looking at it. I was able to calm her and it did not become a major issue. Instead of more movie, I cut her toe nails.

Jane started on Risperidone 0.25 mg. twice daily. Although she has achieved this peace of mind and heart, I thought the additional medicine is worth adding. It may solidify the better mood and help her be less obsessive in her thinking and behavior.

(Laura, Kathie, Paul 8/23/10)

We have had three good to very good days. Talking today, we agreed that on good days her focus and attention are directed outward and on bad days are directed inward. Looking inward either makes a bad day or makes a bad day worse. Or maybe it's the other way around. A bad day comes of itself and demands that thoughts and feelings turn inward. Good days make us both feel so positive that the bad days seem worse when they come. But these days are restorative. We both pray Mom will have peace of mind and heart.

Mom saw the oncologist who has been following her breast cancer for the past five years. He reported no pathology, a great relief to Mom who fears dying from breast cancer any day.

(Kathie 8/23/10)

I should let you know that your "droid" was rather disturbing to Mom during your visit. I think this digital age is overwhelming to her and she has reached the point where she is intimidated and perhaps frightened by it. I sometimes get something on the computer I would like to show her, and she either doesn't want to see it or in a short time says, "I'm not interested in the rest." The television controls are a mystery to her and she doesn't want to learn about them. Even the phone is daunting sometimes, and on occasion she has lost it completely because the phone shut off or she tried to make a call and couldn't or she just didn't hear well. She wants to use our simple camera and has on occasion, but it too is intimidating to her.

(To our friend, Harriet Lerner 8/31/10)

About ten days ago Jane reached a place where she seems to have peace of mind and heart. It is something we both prayed for, that the anger in her heart over the past more than over the present could be quieted, although never to be resolved. It seems that is happening. Her indomitable spirit has wakened again. She is accepting of the memory loss which is quite inclusive. She is happy to see people we know and she engages with them in her usual warm manner. She and I talk for hours about what is happening in her head and in our life and in the lives of the few she can remember. She is well focused when we talk and responds with her typical insights, humor, and affection.

People sometimes ask how I am doing. Jane remains a wonderful companion and my best friend. She is truly a delight to be with almost all the time. I ask myself, is this just a phase or will things stay this way emotionally and socially and between us? I feel this change will be permanent but at the same time recall the ups and downs of the past. You are kind to keep in touch with us. Jane always remembers you.

9/4/10

Considering the possibility that all I have written may someday be read by others, there is an area I have hinted about but never wrote about directly, i.e. our sexual relationship.

After years of study and psychiatric practice and my own spiritual journey, I have come to believe the principal reason men, and perhaps women, wander from their commitment to their partner is a notion they are missing some sexual experience or sexual pleasure that might still be found with someone else. Whether or not that is true, I believe the sexual relationship and experience Jane and I have had and still have could not be improved, because it is so complete and satisfying.

With that as prelude I will say our sexual relationship has not suffered in any major way with the onset of age or the presence of Alzheimer's. We continue to enjoy that aspect of our relationship. We arrange a period of two or three hours when we will not be disturbed and we leisurely spend time caressing, talking of our love, and completing our longing for physical intimacy with each other We talk about God's presence in our lives and the gift we have in our love for one another and for God. It is a deeply spiritual time.

Jane's peace of mind and heart continues. At times she is on the verge of an angry episode, caused by a small event that brought horrible anger in the past. She avoids the hostility and we talk about it and she recognizes what is happening and remains calm. It is truly remarkable to watch this "control" occur.

A few days ago Jane began being angry with me. She said she had suggested a sexual interlude on three successive days and I ignored her invitation. She said she was awake two nights crying over my rejection of her sexually. I recalled we talked of a rendezvous one day but agreed to a postponement for a good reason. She agreed not to discuss it further. We played cards and before long she was relaxed. Later we agreed to arrange several hours the next afternoon that would be "our time." The time was spent with the same love and satisfaction as always.

Jane is a delightful companion these days. She is alert, focused, witty, and relaxed. It feels like times from past years. Her thinking is solid, valid, regular, and real. She refers to "that period when I gave you such a hard time. I'm so sorry. I know how I used to follow you around screaming at you. It must have been so hard for you." What amazing insight! Where does this come from?

We both recognize her immediate memory is essentially gone. The other day she said, "Tell me something and it's gone in ten minutes." I said, "How about ten seconds?" She laughed and agreed. She wonders where things she hears or sees go when she doesn't remember them even when reminded. She often talks about cameras and pictures. I said it may be like taking pictures but being unable to develop all the film.

She seems comfortable with her forgetfulness and refers to it with good humor. "We need not be sad about it." I tell her how I admire her courage and the grace with which she handles these things. She is a remarkable woman! I am unable to find words to voice my love, my admiration, and my gratitude for all she is and has been in my life. Sometimes I think she has achieved this level of dealing with her illness to please me.

I begin to believe Alzheimer's will not separate us because we are so close, so dedicated, so able to communicate with each other. Only death can break this bond we have.

(Laura, Kathie, Paul 9/7/10)
When anger surfaces, Mom is aware of where it can go and makes a genuine effort to ward off escalation successfully! I do not suggest she might have been able to do this in the past and just never tried. I think something has changed so she can accomplish this.

I should also mention the TV seems to be working much better with even an occasional comment about how good the sound is. In addition, I no longer need hearing aids. Mom says much of the change is due to her love for me and her desire never to hurt me again.

193

Mom seems to have poor recall of past difficult times. She mentions, "I know I used to be very difficult to deal with and very hard on you. I don't know how you put up with it all." She never gets into specifics and I am happy it is fading. Past things pop up with the usual distortions I have tried to correct numerous times. These too become less significant in her mind.

She is for the most part cheerful and interested in everything we see and do. Our conversations are narrower than they used to be but she participates with thoughts that are usually cogent, clear, rational, and appropriate. Her humor continues sharp, and of course, her criticism of various things has never dulled. All in all, she is a wonderful companion these days and I have to say currently our life is very pleasant.

9/14/10)

Jane continues to do well. She shows remarkable spirit and patience. On occasion there is a bit of anger and a harsh remark but in a short time she recovers her good mood and often says how sorry she is for sounding "that way." She says she wants to be good to me because I am so good to her. She puts things aside for minor sewing and never gets to it. I sew on a button, patch a pocket, or fix a tear. She is grateful for these things. She is gradually giving up more of the little things she used to do in the apartment.

We saw the neurologist last week. He said to Jane, "Will you spell 'home' for me?" She did. Then he said, "Now will you spell it backwards?" Her immediate but pleasant response was, "Oh, no. I don't spell words backwards!" He mentioned she did one on her last visit. She replied, "Not today. I don't spell words backwards today." The neurologist accepted it well and went on to ask her to do some addition. She immediately said, "I don't do arithmetic either!"

I complimented her later on how she handled the situation. She thought she might have been too brash. I told her I thought she did exactly the right thing. Trying either task would have increased her anxiety and been of no benefit to her or the neurologist. We avoid situations that create anxiety and tension and are of no significant value.

A couple of days later, she showed her keen and quick wit. When I asked her to repeat some word she used, she said, "Do you want me to spell it backwards?"

9/17/10

The days pass slowly. It feels like we are just waiting, waiting. I don't know what I wait for. The wife of a friend here died suddenly last week of a brain hemorrhage. She had a rapid onset of dementia in recent months. Another resident lost his wife a few months ago. She had Alzheimer's and died suddenly. A stroke, I believe. And there is another male resident we know whose wife died a year ago with Alzheimer's.

Am I waiting for Jane's death? Or my own? I am 91 but my health seems very good. I find myself wondering about our demise. When? How? Who first? Jane has death on her mind frequently but it is more disturbing for her. Last night she said she asked God when she was going to die and it was like she heard God say, "Don't expect an answer to a question you should not be asking."

A few nights ago Jane became anxious and irritable. Her left breast is getting bigger, is very hard, and has an obvious lump. We saw her oncologist a month ago and everything is fine. Jane had cancer in her left breast and had a lumpectomy followed by radiation treatment and chemotherapy. She remembered the surgery but believed it was on her right breast. It is so logical for her to be frightened. She thought her cancer was in the other breast, so "this is a new cancer." All the facts were not in her memory bank.

She kept her fears unspoken for several days because she didn't want to worry me. What a nightmare! No wonder she thought she would die soon. When she spoke about it, it was difficult to convince her of the facts relating to her previous cancer.

There have not been any extended periods of sadness, anger, or volatility for several weeks. We went to see a different psychiatrist last week, a man who works closely with the psychiatric nurse Jane sees here. His office was very hard to find. I was tense because we were 30 minutes late for the appointment. It was trying for Jane.

She was angry and didn't want to go in, wouldn't sign the papers on admission, wouldn't talk to the doctor, wouldn't go in his office without me. He saw us for 20 minutes because of our late arrival. I summarized quickly and explained why Jane was disturbed at the moment. He was patient and kind. We discussed her medicines and the Risperidol which he recently added to her regimen prior to our visit.

Before we left Jane apologized for her behavior and for embarrassing me and him. She was very appropriate. She apologized to the receptionist and signed the necessary papers. She criticized herself for her behavior the rest of the day. I assured her she had not embarrassed anyone and I could understand what a strain the trip had been for her.

The point in reviewing these episodes is to say Jane is recovering much differently than before. The event does not spread over hours or days. It does not destroy, even temporarily, the loving relationship we have. This is truly different from the several months, the several years preceding. As I write those words I can't help feel some doubt it will last. Is it too good to be true? Is it a doubt of faith on my part?

9/27/10

We washed Jane's hair today. Once she closes the shower door she can't remember which way to turn the faucet for hotter water. She is also afraid of falling if she lets go of the grab bar. After she shampoos and rinses, I put a conditioner on which she rinses out. I towel dry her hair, comb it out, and dry it with the dryer. It is an ordeal for her

She kept up her spirits with effort today. After lunch she was confused and asked, "Is this the beginning of a downturn?" I suggested a nap to which she consented. I darken the room and prepare the bed. I sit by the bed and massage her feet as she goes to sleep. Then I move to a low hanging light, get my detective story and read until she awakens.

This sort of freedom and flexibility we have in our life becomes a major advantage for Jane. A nap at unexpected times can be of tremendous value. The flexibility of our day, our eating, our sleeping, our going and coming are advantages in dealing with her illness.

(Laura 9/29/10)

Mom continues to have a difficult time getting to things she plans on doing. But I keep telling her if she can do her make-up, find her clothes (even with some help), fix her hair and dress herself, she is doing more than one can really expect of her, and that is already a full day's work. I try to keep her from feeling pressed to do something. All in all things are going well.

Mom is an emotional woman and responds strongly to her emotions. I think that has been part of her problem in dealing with Alzheimer's. Her emotions are strong, and without much cognitive control they get out of hand easily. But her emotional strength has always been appealing to me and has made our bond more complete because I have learned to respond to it and admire it even if I don't have the same strong feelings. Life certainly becomes more colorful for emotional individuals, but it also has some sadness when it cannot be shared with someone who either lives it or at least understands and appreciates it in someone else.

(Laura 10/5/10)
You have the gentleness of heart and the generosity of spirit that your mother has when you are at your best (as she does when she is at her best). No one is always at their best. And I think you both have a poetic soul (whatever that is) I can only appreciate and perhaps not fully know. I believe Mom is close to God. I know she talks to Him often in her own way and her own time.

I'm grateful Mom acknowledges quite directly that we will not schedule any more trips. That is a kind of wisdom and acceptance that she displays more often these days.

(Laura 10/20/10)
Mom continues to do okay. Going to the Mall seems a bit like taking a patient for an outing. Conversation is limited. We talk about the weather, the trees and how they are changing, the people in the Mall, the clothing, etc., etc. She borders on being irritable much of the time but she is much more able to calm down once she gets angry.

Mom just came in the studio and we talked for over an hour. She was perfectly logical and reasonable. We talked about why she doesn't carry her own money or credit card, how we could hem her skirts with tape, about the future and the plan for me to take care of her here as long as I'm alive, and if I die before she does, she will go to the Assisted Living Unit, and we talked about what that is like. She was amazingly clear on all of it and quite agreeable to all the things we discussed. It always surprises me when we have these periods where she is completely lucid. Later today I'm sure she will not agree to tape the skirts and will not understand why she does not carry money and will not understand what the plans are for the future.

Every once in a while Mom comments she will never see you again and will never see the girls again. When I say I'm sure we will see you, then she wonders why you can't come any weekend you want. She has little appreciation of the necessities and complexities of your life or that of anyone else. Time has little meaning for her. When I told her you and the girls were here two months ago, she couldn't believe it. Thought it had been a year or more.

10/22/10

It has been a month since I last wrote a note. I don't even know if the time was good or bad. We are losing ground to the Alzheimer's but I'm not sure how to describe it. Jane had peace of mind and heart for about two months. She was at peace with her illness and its limitations. She wasn't thinking about grievances of the past. She showed minimal irritation with people and situations that previously caused negative responses.

Lately she recalls the past frequently and with bitterness: Ed throwing away her dolls, trips to funeral parlors with her mother, Tom leaving a pan of ice cubes when she was about to deliver her first child. She has been more irritable with me, picking up on what I say or should have said. She is unreasonable and distorts things, claiming I said something or did something that in reality never happened.

One night she insisted I said something about Alzheimer's that I never told her before. She was irritated because I had not told her. As I tried to get some understanding of it, she began telling me that two of the characters in the movie we just watched had been talking about Alzheimer's.

This kind of confusion occurs more frequently now, especially in the evening. At times she is aware of it and is disturbed by her realization of "how bad I'm getting, how far gone I am." I try to avoid some topics in the evening because, if they come up, we are likely to take them to bed with us.

Jane gets irritated and asks, "Why don't you talk to me? Why don't you do something to help me?" I am more patient than I used to be and less likely to feel angry. Whatever I say she will find faulty and irritating. I try to be gentle and comforting. These episodes do not last for hours as in the past. I am grateful we get through them without her screaming or threatening to kill herself.

If I tell Jane how much better she is doing in these emotional storms, it suggests a comparison with the past. I have no desire to recall that pain for her. She never mentions times she left the apartment or the night she went to the emergency room. I am grateful she does not remember them.

She fears I cannot care for her, I will leave her, Alzheimer's will separate us. She believes she is becoming a "monster" and will be angry and volatile and impossible to live with. I talk about Alzheimer's storms. She gets caught in the storm, but when it passes she is with me and it is over. There is no damage done. She will never be like this all the time because this is not who she is or who she was. She will always be my loving, sweet, gentle companion. I say this and pray it will be true.

I find myself less cheerful these days. I know I am gradually losing this woman who means everything to me. I don't feel as close to Laura and Paul and Kathie as I did. It seems harder to keep in touch with them. I know it's a bit of depression. But it isn't bad, and I'm sure I'll pull out of it. Caring for Jane is not a burden but life sometimes is.

(Paul 10/28/10)

I realize how important the computer is to me these days. I would feel lonely and lost without it. Email is important because it allows me to keep in touch with a number of people easily, privately, and regularly. Strangely enough Mom never asks what I'm doing at the computer. She seems to see it as "my work." On the other hand, I always feel uneasy when I'm talking on the phone to someone, because I feel she is left out. And I think she feels that way. I can tell her I got an email from someone and summarize it and she is content with that. It is a world in which she has no interest. Email is a godsend to the caregiver.

(Laura, Kathie, Paul 11/5/10)

Mom has shown increasing confusion, especially evenings. We went to the Subway party Sunday evening and with Kathie's presence it went very well. It was tiring especially for Mom but she held up well. Tuesday afternoon she began looking for clothes to wear to a party she thought we were going to. She thought all day we were going out but couldn't remember where and was reluctant to ask because I would "think she was stupid." I had no idea this was going on in her head until late afternoon when she finally said she was looking for clothes to wear to the party. She had a hard time believing there was no party. Wednesday was a pretty bad day with confusion. She was argumentative, quarrelsome, and sad. It was a very trying day for both of us, one of those days when I wonder how we can maintain living here. But there were no threats of violence toward self. We just had a difficult time maintaining harmony for any length of time.

By contrast yesterday went very well. Then last evening Mom started making a list for "our trip." When I told her we had no plans for a trip, she was surprised but subdued. When she spoke about our trip again and I said we had no plans, she let it go. Confusion has definitely increased. She told me last night there was a period earlier in the day "when my head was just blank."

11/09/10

I am weary these days. Jane wears me out sometimes. She has asked me at least eight times today where a certain book is. I tell her and 30 minutes later she asks me again.

We're changing from summer clothes to winter clothes. This seasonal change was always difficult for Jane but now it is catastrophic. There is concern about "never seeing them again because I will be dead by spring." There is concern about keeping summer skirts out to shorten. "I will shorten them before spring comes." There is concern about putting them in storage. "I will never be able to find them."

The skirts are good skirts she made or bought years ago. On several occasions she agreed to take them to a tailor. She acknowledges she would be unable to hem them. "I couldn't even thread a needle these days. I would be totally at a loss if I tried to hem them." I tell her, "I think it would be difficult for you. I don't think you should take time from our activities to do it. Please have them hemmed. It would be a relief to both of us."

We agree but within hours Jane says, "I'll never pay anyone to hem a skirt for me. I've made clothes for myself and my kids. I've made dresses and skirts and suits. It will take me an hour to hem one. I can do it while we watch television." And so it goes. We had this same exercise when we brought out the summer clothes. She is unable to mend a pocket or sew a snap on her pants. I have done these minor repairs and later she talks about them as if she did them.

Jane was "cleaning out" her closet. She became utterly confused and was angry when I tried to help. She said I told her she had to hem all her skirts so they would be wearable. I am "being defensive" if I deny the comment.

She is very sad this evening. We talked about her fears and confusion. She said, "I'm afraid I will lose you. I'm afraid you will leave me. I'm going crazy. They will have to lock me up. I've always been afraid I would go crazy someday and now it is happening. I'm dying. I'm afraid you will be by yourself and I can't stand to think of you being alone." Changes in her veins that come with aging are indications of her imminent death.

While we were talking I leaned over to pick up a tissue she dropped. She became furious. "Little do you care about how I feel or what is happening to me. You can't even pay attention when I'm speaking to you." She was angry briefly and then apologized.

Jane couldn't find something in her bathroom and was feeling hopeless. She said it damages her self esteem when something is lost. I told her these things are going to continue. They will get worse, not better. She cannot overcome them. She must live with them and accept them. She must get around them or minimize them by calling me when something is lost rather than continuing to look and come away defeated. She was thoughtful and understanding and agreed with everything I said. She won't remember it.

The skirts will not get hemmed again this season. And Jane will wear black pants and white shirts throughout the winter as she did last year. We'll put a few summer clothes in storage and the rest will remain in her closet and be confusing for her.

I accomplish some "cleaning out." I take garments she will never wear and never miss and put them in a large plastic bag hidden in my closet. When I go to the barber, I sneak the bag of clothes out and take it to a charitable drop place near the barber shop. I take "junk" Jane has in her drawers and hide it for a week or so. If she never mentions it, I throw it away. Perhaps I should feel badly about deceiving her like this. I don't.

11/13/10

I get annoyed at myself for wasting time playing solitaire. I'll write. Things are changing for Jane but how many times have I said that? She reports "times when my mind is just blank." I have to say she looks "blank" sometimes.

We walked in the Arundel Mall for two hours yesterday. She enjoyed the day but talked very little except to comment about different pieces of clothing. Once when I failed to respond, she said I act like I'm not interested. I'm interested to a certain extent but I don't have a lot of enthusiasm for looking at women's clothing for long periods.

Jane was very quiet last evening. She seemed reluctant to talk. I asked what she was thinking. She was concerned about all the clothing she had given Kathie. I told her she had not given Kathie any clothing. She recognized she was confused.

This morning Jane had a terrible pain in her left breast, "the worst pain I have ever had." We talked about her visit to the oncologist and his comment that the breast was firm and painful at times because of prior radiation therapy. I said she is getting a mammogram in two weeks and we will check with her doctor if the pain continues. During breakfast she said, "My breast doesn't hurt any more now. I think I was dreaming." She provided this assessment of the pain without further comment.

Jane has been withdrawn the last few days. Perhaps this is how peace of mind and heart will come. And with its coming we will be separated more. Perhaps she will not be as aware of the change as I am. I will be grateful if she is spared that. I pray God will relieve her of the emotional pain she endures.

(Laura 11/16/10)
About Christmas presents, so far I've kept Mom from buying all kinds of odds and ends for the girls. She often wants to buy some of the cheap jewelry we see on the kiosks or in stores. She likes it and decides the girls would like it and wear it. Or she wants to buy a stuffed animal she likes and give it to the girls. I tell her we have no idea what the girls like at this time in their lives. Shopping in a store like Joann Fabric or Target is just too overwhelming for Mom. She wants everything and can't decide what she really wants and is confused by the whole thing. I'm not too comfortable going to the Mall with her these days because she looks in the windows and either hates things or would like to have them.

(Laura 11/26/10)
Mom suggested the other day we might eat in the dining room sometimes. We plan on trying it tonight. I hope it works out. I think it would be better if we had a little more contact with the community. So when you are here we may plan on eating a couple of meals in the dining room. It would be nice to show off our elegant daughter and two granddaughters.

11/29/10
Jane had two good days. She seemed calm and at peace. They were pleasant days for us. Yesterday she began worrying again with frequent comments about how much worse she is, how bad things are getting and how terrible they are going to be.

Last evening Jane focused on something she said she read in a book that afternoon. She obsessed about the book. She was unable to find it or describe it accurately. She wondered if she left it in the Mall, in the car, or in the apartment. We had been in the dining room for dinner. She wondered if she left it there. The reality was she didn't have a book at any time during the day. I said we would look for it tomorrow. That satisfied her.

Jane chided me for not accepting how bad her illness is and how bad it is going to be. "Either you don't know anything about Alzheimer's or you just don't want to face what is happening." Somehow we shifted to a very reasonable and coherent discussion of her illness. I told her having a headache does not mean she has a brain tumor, having a period of confusion does not mean she is going crazy, and having a bad day or a bad afternoon does not mean she is going to become a "monster." I said I am well aware she may reach a point where she does not recognize anyone, although I believe she will always recognize me. I said she may at some point be confused most of the time but I think there will still be times when she is in contact with what is going on. I said she may need more nursing care than I can give her and then I will hire someone to come in and provide the additional help we need.

Jane sees other residents who are "out of it" and assumes it is due to Alzheimer's, and often it probably is. I said seeing them makes me grateful she has the awareness she has. Seeing people with walkers and canes and wheel chairs doesn't make me think that's going to happen to me, although I am well aware it could. Seeing them makes me grateful for the strength and health we have now.

Jane accepted all these ideas as valid and said it was important to hear them and she will take them to heart and remember them. Does any of this really help? I don't know, but it might. Her rational brain still functions and can influence her reactions and behaviors.

We went to the dining room for dinner last Friday and again yesterday. Many people greeted Jane warmly, came and embraced her as we entered and said how happy they were to see her there. Jane was comfortable with the arrangement. We sat at a table for two. It was a good thing to do. It was evidence for her that many people here love her and care very much about how she is. I hope we can do this more often.

Today has gone quite well. We had a wonderful visit with Paul. Jane followed most of our conversation, and she contributed many appropriate comments. It is obvious Paul is aware of what things must be like for Jane. I think he spends some time trying to imagine what it is like inside her world.

PART 9 (DEC 10—MAY 11)

(Laura 12/1/10)

We've eaten in the dining room twice at a table for two. Many people responded warmly to see Mom there. I am hoping we can continue to do that two or three times a week. Mom comes up with stories about things she thinks have happened recently and there is just no basis for them. I can sometimes tell her directly I think she is confused and sometimes I say maybe she dreamed it. She usually accepts quite readily that she must have been confused.

(Paul 12/1/10)

I have a theory that some conversations with Alzheimer's patients can be very therapeutic and even though they may not remember the content, their brain works with the information in some way. I think all the money and effort is being used to find medications to treat and perhaps to cure or prevent the illness. But changes in the thinking and feeling are being ignored—or just considered symptoms of the illness. Maybe a good deal could be done without medication to prevent or partially modify or control or undo some of these changes.

12/01/10

We ate in the dining room this evening. When finished, Jane asked how far we were from home. I thought she was joking. She said, "We must be over a thousand miles from home." She was serious. I said, "We live here. We've lived here for seven years. This is our home." She accepted it well and said it was an example of how mixed up she is. She thought we were on a trip but knew we wouldn't take our furniture on a trip. How does she do it? How does she live with it? No wonder she says she is crazy. Her world is crazy! How does she achieve any peace in this kind of turmoil and uncertainty?

Last August we reached a peak in her volatility, her threats toward self, and her vicious anger. Jane says she came to realize how much I was suffering from her behavior. I'm sure I could not hide my distress from her. She became determined not to continue behaviors hurtful to me. What a gentle, sweet woman she is and desperately desires to be! These thoughts apparently helped bring about the change. I believe our prayers fostered those thoughts and gave her strength and resolve to make the changes. Could she, because of her determination and courage, have quelled these tempests on her own? I doubt it even though I know what a strong woman she is. Every morning I pray to the Holy Trinity to help Jane come to peace of heart and mind and to have periods of clear thinking in the midst of the overwhelming confusion. Will this respite of the past three months continue? Only time will answer that. If the old behaviors return, will I doubt God's intervention? Not for a second!

Jane seems to be slowly accommodating to the confusion, as she previously did to the forgetfulness. It is less disturbing to her to realize she becomes confused at times. She talks about it more easily and with less self criticism. We talk about it openly when she is mixed up about something. It rests more easily with her these days.

12/6/10
I don't know whether I'm depressed or just tired. It is clear Jane is leaving me. I see her drifting away and sometimes it is so painful I could sit and cry.

She gets terribly confused. She talks about people and events as if they really happened. Of course they did in her mind. Usually I can say, "Sweetheart, I think you're mixed up about that. I don't remember that happening. You may have had a dream or you may have had a thought about what could happen, and then you got confused and you thought it really did happen." She usually accepts this well and acknowledges the error.

I think Jane is frightened most of the time. She is afraid I will leave her or "lock her up somewhere." I assure her I will take care of her. Deep inside I wonder if I will be able.

Our conversation is slowly dying. She can't follow news on television. She no longer blames the television. She knows she can't comprehend what they say. One advantage of the Mall, we can talk about things we both see, displays, people, styles, etc. We talk about the weather, the changes in the trees outside our windows. We talk about the kids and grandchildren, all pretty superficial. We talk about our apartment, how much we like it, all the things we have done to it. I bring up stories from my past or our past. Jane follows them at the time but cannot contribute. She brings up stories from her past, stories she has told over and over through the years. Her stories are often distorted now.

Sadly enough she is as aware as I am of most of this. She mentions "things are going to get much worse." I assure her we will be together and she will always know me. She often speaks of her love for me. And I reply in kind. The words are true, but they seem like a formula to get through the day, a need of hers to which I reply. She is sad and frightened and I feel so sorry and helpless to alter the course.

12/9/10
We saw the neurologist today. He suggested we get a big calendar showing the day of the week and the date, so Jane will have it to reassure herself. What good would it do to look at the calendar when she won't remember for 30 seconds what she saw? He really isn't worth the $103 he gets paid for a 15 minute visit.

Jane told the neurologist she is going crazy. He said, "You are not going to go crazy." Does she remember he said it? Of course not! I asked him to examine a slight dent on her forehead which has worried her for months. She thinks it is cancer. He assured her it was normal. If she remembers either comment, maybe it was worth $103.

At dinner, Jane said, "I put the ironing board away. I got a lot done today. I just have two more shirts ready to iron." The ironing board was not used. Where does this come from? A dream? A fantasy? Will she realize it didn't happen? No, she forgets she ever said it. But where does it come from? Wishful thinking maybe.

12/13/10
Last evening Jane told me she sat with Rachael earlier today in the auditorium. Other residents were there but the two of them were talking and Rachael

asked Jane to be in the program she is preparing for New Year's Eve. Jane was surprised Rachael asked her and told her she would think about it.

Jane has not seen Rachael for over a week. A couple of days ago I reminded Jane of the programs Rachael used to present on New Year's Eve. We both participated. Jane's idea about meeting with Rachael was a memory of a meeting that occurred four or five years ago, just as Jane presented it. When I told her we had not seen Rachael in several days, she accepted her "mixed up head" quite readily.

This evening she asked if she had seen Laura today. When I told her no, she asked if she spoke to her on the phone. She had not. Laura called yesterday and Jane chose not to talk to her. I have encouraged her not to talk on the phone if she doesn't feel like doing so. She calmly accepted my statements about Laura. She later mentioned it has been a good day "although I got mixed up a few times." We looked at some pictures of Laura earlier in the day. I said that might be why she thought she saw or talked to Laura today.

Last week our neurologist referred Jane for a physical therapy evaluation. She will have a few sessions of PT to improve her gait and her balance. The therapist sees her gait problem much as I do. Jane becomes very focused on how she is walking and has lost her spontaneity. Balance is reasonably good and the therapist thinks she can do much better with some help and some continued exercises. I emphasize the importance of maintaining her ambulation so we can continue to go to the Mall.

12/21/10

Today we went to noon Mass. I told Jane several times it was a funeral Mass for a man. As we left, Jane spoke about the woman's funeral Mass. I told her it was the husband who died, not the wife. Several times during the afternoon Jane mentioned the funeral for the woman who died. Each time I said it was the husband who died. It was an indelible idea in her mind, "We went to a funeral Mass for a woman." This is how her mind works. She hears something, formulates her understanding of it (true or false), and it becomes a clear memory that automatically pops up whenever the subject is mentioned.

This explains ideas that lodge in her mind and seem impossible to correct or obliterate. This mechanism must be neurological, microbiological, whatever. She has a memory and holds onto it desperately, sometimes passionately. Sometimes the lodged memory is her own idea, for example, that I need a hearing aid because she can't hear me, or that we need a new television because she can't follow the news, and countless other memories that are blank walls to me but active, living realities for her.

We saw Jane's plastic surgeon today, primarily to reassure her that the pain and swelling and hardness in her breast are not unusual following the implant surgery of ten years ago. She listened carefully to his explanation of capsular constriction and for the moment was reassured. She will remember little he said but she may remember we were there and believe what I tell her about it.

Coming home we were passing a restaurant we frequented for fifteen years, until we quit going three years ago. We stopped going because I no longer had an income from work and also due to Jane's worsening illness. The idea came to me, "Do you want to go to the Candlelight for dinner?" It was after 4p.m. and we'd had a light lunch. Jane hesitated and asked, "Do you really mean it?" We had a celebration dinner—for good news from the doctor, for Christmas, for us. Jane was alert, talkative, and appropriate in every way. She was her sweet, gentle, thoughtful self.

Now she is getting ready for bed and all the demons return. She can't find anything, she can't remember anything, she can't do anything, she can't live like this. But we had our evening! And I'll think about it and wish it could happen again.

12/23/10
"I had no face. I had no person. I had no place. It's the most frightened I ever was." Jane told me that happened this morning as she looked in the mirror to do cosmetics. She was irritable all day, criticizing everything I said. She was argumentative, belligerent, fired her physical therapist and then returned to apologize.

This morning she was looking for me when I came back from exercise. "I didn't know where you were." Later she said she saw the note I always leave and knew she could call me on my cell phone. She wanted to be up so she could be with me when I returned. This is the recurring theme of why she gets up in the morning after I leave to exercise.

I have decided to give up the morning exercise for sometime later in the day. She will stay in bed if I am there. When she doesn't get enough rest, it is invariably a bad day. I don't want to give up exercising. It is important for both of us that I maintain my health.

(Laura, Kathie, Paul 12/31/10)
I need not update you on Mom because you have all visited since Christmas and you are aware that she is slowly leaving us. She remembers very little about your visits, although she remembers each of you was here and that we had grand visits, not much about details.

I wanted to thank each of you for the strong support I received from you during the difficult times of this past year. I would not have survived so well if I had not had regular and frequent communication with you and if you had not been as available as you were both in person and by phone and email. Each of you played an important part in helping to comfort and stabilize Mom. Your visits, your contact with her, and your love for her have been a continuing boost to her indomitable spirit and a comfort in her sad times.

12/31/10
Laura and the girls came on Tuesday and left Thursday. It was the most peaceful and fulfilling visit we have had with them here. Laura was in good spirits, warm, and her charming, loving self. The girls were at ease and comfortable to be with.

We had dinner in the dining room with Laura and the girls on Tuesday and Paul joined us on Wednesday to make six. Both evenings were pleasant. Jane was comfortable throughout the visit.

Jane is calm and peaceful today. During lunch she said, "Where has my 'unhappy' gone?" We decided to wash her hair. She was at ease throughout the process, which is a change. She was satisfied with the outcome and completely cooperative. When she did her hair by herself, it would take three or four hours, and she often ended up in tears.

This is noted as the best and calmest Christmas we have had in several years. Jane is back with me today, my companion, my love, my soul mate. She was less interactive with the visitors but maintained contact as best she could. She responded with her heart if not her mind, and that is gratifying to us all. She has not said, "This will be my last Christmas and the last time I see them." I admit those thoughts came to my mind.

1/10/11

We have changed our schedule since before Christmas. Jane began waking when I got up at 6a.m. to exercise. She would promise to stay in bed but when I returned she would be up "straightening" drawers in her bathroom or doing some other unproductive task. She did not get adequate sleep and was agitated by her fruitless efforts to do some work.

This early awakening became a pattern so I decided to try to change it. Her reason for being up was "I want to be up so I can be with you when you come back. I don't want to be alone, and I don't want you to be alone." I decided to stay in bed in the mornings and exercise later in the day. Jane was agreeable to the plan. Now we go to bed around 10p.m. and get up together about 8:30 or 9a.m.

There are some losses and some gains. I no longer have the three hours I had to myself in the mornings. No more spiritual reading time, no more detective stories, no more writing time on my own. I am sleeping more than I want to and perhaps more than I should.

On the other hand, I'm not as concerned about when we get to bed and get to sleep. Jane is not as prone to talk in bed and is ready to go to sleep. There is another benefit. After I began exercising during the day, Jane said she would come down to exercise with me. She joined me New Year's Day and has been there most days since. She does the NuStep while I do the tread mill and upper body weights. Three or four days a week we do the exercises at home which the physical therapist gave us. Jane seems pleased with the regimen.

Since our pastor left, we do not have a priest who speaks intelligible English. As a result we go again to the Shrine of Saint Anthony once or twice a week. Our new pastor will be here in early March. We'll wait and see how well he fits our need.

(Laura, Kathie, Paul 1/21/11)
Wanted to send the attached document to each of you. Just finished it today and I think I will feel more comfortable with it in your hands.
Attachment:
Some Requests—Addressed to Laura, Kathie, Paul
I've been thinking about a lot of things lately and have decided it is important to give the three of you some information that should be helpful at a later time. I need to face the reality that Jane and I are not going to be here forever and the three of you need some information to handle things.

First I will say, as you must already know, Mom will be pretty helpless if I die before she does. In that case you will need to take over, and so some requests and recommendations now. If Mom dies before I do, I'm not sure how I will be or what I can manage, so these will serve as some guidelines for the three of you.

There is a folder in the big desk drawer to the left of my computer marked "Funerals." There is information there about services at the church and I will try to leave a few pictures to have at the evening prayer service.

As you know, we both plan to be cremated. The funeral Mass and prayer service the evening before can be arranged without any pressure of time. As things are now, we want the funeral Mass to be at St. John's. * * * * * *

With cremation there are, of course, the ashes to take—probably after the funeral Mass. There is no need for an urn; a simple box will be fine. At Jane's death I will take the ashes. If I die first one of you should take the ashes. We will want our ashes finally put together. Laura would be the one to have the ashes, but perhaps Paul would be more comfortable having them. Mom and I have talked about final disposal. We considered the ocean but not sure we feel right about that. I'm sure Mom would agree to my wish that our ashes be sent or taken to Montana and buried in the Geyser cemetery near my parents and Don and Helen. I'm sure Jim (my nephew) would be willing to take care of that if the ashes are sent to him. If Laura feels otherwise about where the ashes go, that is her decision and we respect her wishes.

Mom worries a great deal about "what will happen to our things." They are not just "things" to her; they are treasures. She wants to decide now where they will all go but she runs into the reality that we live with them and treasure them now. We have discussed this many times and have agreed on the following ideas.

If I die first Mom will have to go to Assisted Living on 4th floor of the health unit. You should have 30 days to clean out the apartment. I believe Mom could take and should take some furniture for her room there. If Mom dies first I would move to a one bedroom apartment or an efficiency apartment as soon as possible. I would take whatever furniture I needed. All that being said, there will need to be some emptying out of the apartment and our "things." In our estate plan Laura inherits all our real property. When we are both deceased I ask Laura to take any and all things she and her girls might like to have. Then I ask her to let Kathie and Paul make their choices. Mom was concerned that others not come in and "pick through our things." I agree.

The marketing office here has contact with persons who will come in and buy whatever has not been taken by family. I am fully aware that the vast majority of "our treasures" may be disposed of in that manner. That is always a painful thought for Mom but it is the reality of life and times. The proceeds of selling things should, of course, go to Laura. * * * * * *

These are thoughts I have put together the last few days. I feel a need to pass them on to each of you. I hope they are not disturbing things for you to read and know. They are things I face calmly enough, and thankfully Mom needs face them only as passing thoughts that hopefully will become less frightening as the weeks go by.

I will leave you the name of two good friends who would be willing to help out with any details you might need taken care of. I will also leave a list of various people we would like you to notify when the time comes to do so. The list will be in the funeral file.

(Laura 1/25/11)
Mom had a great birthday. She received 18 cards. Many residents sent cards or wished her happy birthday when they saw her. We ate in the dining room with another couple. They ordered a birthday cake and the servers sang happy birthday when they brought it. Mom did very well the whole evening. We went to noon Mass at the monastery and then to Subway for lunch. I told Nandi it was Mom's birthday and lunch was on the house. We went to the counter after we ate and they all wished Mom happy birthday.

Mom was especially pleased with your card and with your email message. I printed it out for her. Those were wonderful words you wrote, and the cards from the girls were beautiful. Mom of course said she would write to them, but that's not likely to happen. Tara's card was beautifully done.

1/25/11
We celebrated Jane's 81st birthday yesterday. I have described most of it in an email to Laura. Jane had good days the past week. She thinks Alzheimer's is starting in her feet and working up her body causing decrease in function as it moves upward. She walks normally at times but then becomes conscious of it and takes small uncertain steps. I don't see any evidence of physical deterioration. She exercises with me some days.

Jane looked tired after lunch today. She wanted to lie down for a nap. I suggested I go exercise while she was asleep. She was agreeable. I pulled the shades and turned the bed down. I massaged her feet until I thought she was asleep.

I left to exercise. I take my cell phone and leave a note saying I am exercising and call my cell with the number in large print. I was on the treadmill when my cell phone rang. Jane asked if Robert McAllister was there. I answered and told her I would be right up.

When I reached the apartment, she was angry and semi-hysterical. "You thought I was asleep. You couldn't wait to get out and leave me. I didn't know when you would be back. I thought maybe you wouldn't come back. I have never been so frightened in my whole life. Don't ever leave me in this apartment alone again. It was horrible. I went around turning on all the lights. I called and no one answered me." She insisted she didn't hear me on the phone. Her hearing aids were out but I think it was sheer panic that kept her from hearing my voice.

We talked about it. I told her I won't leave her alone again and that is probably the safest approach to the matter. I will stop going to Sunday 8a.m. Mass. I can take her with me to the grocery store, although that will not be a pleasant venture for either of us. I can take her to the barber shop and she can wait for me. I can skip exercise when she is unable or unwilling to go with me. I am not pleased to have to change these things.

A couple of days ago Jane said, "I have to tell you something bad I did. The other day when we were in the bookstore I took a book and didn't pay for it. It's not even a book I want. I just felt other people can go to the bookstore and buy a book if they want it, because they have money. And I don't have any money so I took it. Now I'm frightened and don't know what to do about it. I was afraid to tell you because I was afraid you would be mad at me."

I was truly sympathetic and understanding and I said this sort of thing happens with Alzheimer's patients. Jane worried she might be arrested and was quite distraught. I said I will return the book tomorrow. She was uneasy, so I said we would return it now.

I asked her to get the book. She began looking and couldn't find it. She described the book size. We began to search the apartment, but as I looked I began to wonder about this book. How did she get it out of the store without me seeing it? From her description it was too large to fit in her purse. We have not been in a bookstore since before Christmas. She said it happened just a few days ago. She described a bookstore that is not the one we go to.

I told Jane I thought the "stolen book" was from a dream. I told her why I doubted it ever happened. The whole thing seems to be resolved and has not been mentioned again.

(Laura, Kathie, Paul 1/27/11)
Once more I have another page to send you. I've had this funeral thing on my mind lately so I went ahead and completed some details that might be helpful for you at a later time. I will attach this latest and I hope last note about the subject. Not the best reading for a dreary day, but here it is.
Attachment: Additional comments—Addressed to Laura, Kathie and Paul
I don't want to burden the three of you with too much information, but I decided I would try to complete what I started a few days ago about our funeral arrangements.
* * * * * *

I want to give you more information about the funerals. There will be no viewing. Cremation will take place probably within the first 24 hours. The vigil or visiting the night before is described as a time to gather, to pray, to read scripture, to tell stories and to support those who are grieving. There could be a eulogy and/or a sharing of memories. The ashes will be there. If pictures are put up, several should be of the two of us together—and at least one with Laura.

The Mass is considered a Memorial Mass rather than a funeral Mass since cremation has occurred. The cremated remains are brought to the church. It is suggested that a picture of the deceased be placed beside the cremated remains for the Memorial Mass. I have selected the hymns, the readings, and the petitions for each of our funerals. A brief eulogy may be given after Communion. It is recommended it be no longer than five minutes and be written out and given by only one person. Ten minutes should be fine.

I have not discussed any of this information with Mom. A long time ago we talked about planning our funerals but her preoccupation with and fear of dying means this is not a time to talk about any of these things.

I have placed the folder for funerals in the back of the drawer to the left of my chair. It might be too obvious in its alphabetical order. There is a file for Mom, a file for me, and a general file about funerals. I hope this will be all I need say about the subject. Now perhaps I can stop thinking about them.

(Laura, Kathie, Bonnie, Paul, Bob 2/1/11)
Mom and I had a long talk recently about her problem with phone calls. She has a hard time with them. I think she is sometimes uncertain about whom she is talking to. Calls probably provoke anxiety and doubt and fear rather than having any great benefit. After the call she is always uncertain about what you said and what she said. She typically decides she didn't say the right thing or didn't ask the right question or didn't answer the right way. I am certain she often distorts much of what was said. She gets pretty obsessive about it and her usual response is to think she was "stupid" on the phone. I'm at a loss to correct any false impressions other than to say you love her, you know she has Alzheimer's, and you don't have any high expectations.

Jane readily agreed that talking on the phone rarely if ever turns out well. Even if she felt it was a nice talk, a few hours later she wonders about it and doubts it was as good as she thought. I suggested I just don't ask her to come to the phone. I told her I would explain it to each of you. She was relieved with my suggestion and agrees that talking on the phone brings no satisfaction or sense of love or peace to her.

So that is how I will respond to your calls in the future. I am sad her illness has reached this point because I know each of you is important in her life. This might be easier for you because I know it must be hard to weave your way through the cloudy conversation as you try to handle what is said. You know she appreciates visits when those are possible. If you would like, you might address a brief email to her once in a while or drop a brief note. I print out emails and give them to her. I keep her informed of contacts I have with you. Of course she rarely remembers the phone calls for very long.

She is losing more and more contact with the world we live in even though we keep that world pretty small. We talk about each of you quite regularly so you will remain clear in her mind. I should mention she might decide to call one of you someday. Occasionally she gets worrying about one of you and says she must talk to you. On occasion when she was terribly upset, she talked to one or the other of you on the phone and found it very helpful. That too might happen.

2/1/11

Jane tells me fifty times a day (without exaggeration) she loves me, in three or four different phrases she uses. I think it's because she feels increasingly separated from me and because she can't think of other things to say. It is a strain to respond each time, not because I don't love her but because the whole exchange seems so artificial, so sad.

We continue to plod along day after day with little that is new and an increasing loss of what is old. What's down the road? Jane's picture of the future is "being crazy, being locked up somewhere, being a monster." I don't have a picture of the future. Is it because I don't see it, can't see it or because I don't want to look?

Jane talked yesterday about hemming skirts for summer. We'll soon go through the change of season again and it becomes more problematic and more distressing each time. I hate this cold, gray winter but I can't say I look forward to spring and the turmoil it will bring to Jane's wardrobe and more importantly to her mind.

I'm ashamed to say I'm feeling sorry for myself these days. I'm ashamed because I have some idea of how frightening and destitute life must be for Jane. In comparison I have no reason to complain. But the man with no shoes still has cold, sore feet and seeing the man with no feet brings him little comfort. It may stop his complaining. I feel increasingly lost and lonely, somewhat like I did when I left the ranch at age eight to go to boarding school. I missed my parents and my home and wanted to be back on the ranch. Homesickness is a special kind of sickness, like no other. It returns now when the person I love more than I ever loved anyone is "no longer home" some of the time.

Eight of our residents died within the last two months. It becomes increasingly obvious as I look around in the dining room, that's why we are all here. It's a matter of waiting to see whose name will be next on the black edged card on the bulletin board. The English TV show, "Waiting for God," is no longer funny. Will Jane go first or will I? I pray I will outlive her and be able to care for her. Sometimes I wonder if I will outlive her and not be able to care for her. That would be the worst fate of all.

2/3/11

Jane and I had a minor tiff last evening. She distorted something I said and made an issue of it. An hour later I went in her bedroom to see how she was doing. She said, "Come and sit with me. There is something I want to tell you." We sat and talked for over an hour. She said she suddenly realized she sometimes tries to make me mad. She was quite clear about it. There is nothing I do or say to provoke her, but she hears words coming out of her mouth she knows will irritate me. "I don't mean them. I don't know where they come from. I don't understand why I want to make you angry."

I told her it feels like she wants me to be angry at her sometimes. And it feels like I am someone else at whom she is angry. We talked about her childhood. I wondered if she was so accustomed to having someone angry at her that she deliberately provokes me at times. As a child she always worried someone would be angry over something she did. Is it a familiar feeling from childhood she wants to know again? A kind of repetition compulsion, the soothing presence of a familiar situation or feeling, even a painful one?

2/10/11

I mentioned Jane's story about the book she thought she stole. I thought it was forgotten, but the other night it came up full force. She was thinking of it for sometime and was afraid to tell me. I reminded her she had told me and it seemed certain the event never happened. She was satisfied with my comments, although a few minutes later she said, "I wonder where I put the book." I insisted there was no book.

Some brain cell grabs it and won't let go of it, I guess. We wonder how these stories come about. Did a dream come vaguely back to her as dreams do, and she thought it was real? Or do fragments of other experiences show up on her empty screen of consciousness and pretend they belong together? She took some pencils from that bookstore a long time ago. (We never confronted that issue.) She has admired books there and possibly thought of taking one. About three months ago she brought an art book from our library to the apartment, which is a "no-no." She hid it in her bathroom until she agreed to let me take it back. Did these bits and pieces find one another in her memory bank and build a story?

We had an interesting discussion a few nights ago. Jane often says she is stupid and makes many mistakes. I have been searching my mind for some way to approach that issue. She is afraid of making mistakes others will see. We talk about her being "mixed up" and "confused." She accepts these words and is comfortable with their reality. We spent an hour talking about how she is "mixed up" when she does things she thinks are stupid. I explained that all the people we know are aware persons with Alzheimer's get mixed up and confused. As a result, she is living in a safe world where "mistakes" or "stupid" things she does are seen as evidence of her illness. Jane was relieved and appreciative of the insight. If only she could hold onto it!

(Laura 2/15/11)
Thanks for the long and beautiful email of last week. I decided to copy your email to Word, then make adjustments (others might call it censorship) and printed out a copy for Mom. In that way she has all the news and feels it was addressed directly to both of us. That works quite well and I will probably do it occasionally in the future. Then Mom has a copy she can read anytime. She really doesn't fully understand email so she ends up thinking we got a letter from you.

2/19/11
Three days ago Jane fell in the deep pit again. I'm not sure how it happened. She seemed preoccupied throughout the day but was generally affable.

Before going to bed she commented, "I thought all day about you dying and leaving me alone. I wouldn't know the first thing to do. There is no one I could call." She talked about our "things," a word which includes everything from her underwear to the furniture. We have discussed how our things will be taken care of or disposed of by the three children, Laura, Kathie, and Paul. I believe we reached an agreement about it.

This time she stated, "I don't want to hear any names about kids and what they will do. Not one of them is capable of doing anything." Not an auspicious beginning to a reasonable discussion. There was nothing I could say that was not disparaged or dismissed. Jane's anger increased as she became more confused and irrational. The conversation became more amicable in bed but it continued until after midnight. Our final agreement was to discuss it all at a time when we felt calmer and more rational.

I began the next morning with kisses and statements of my love. The issues were still there. Jane was irritable and despondent. "I am much worse. I'm not going to get better this time. I won't come back. I'll be crazy soon and they will lock me up." I attempted to console her, being cautious not to aggravate the situation.

Jane slept four hours in the afternoon but did not feel better on waking. It at least gave us both some respite. We got through the evening without any hostile exchange.

Yesterday the same dark thoughts filled her mind and left room for nothing else. I suggested we go to the Mall for lunch to get her mind out of the narrow channel. As we talked at lunch she brightened up. By bedtime she agreed it was a good day.

This kind of episode is usually easier for me to deal with now. I am more patient with Jane. Usually I don't feel angry at what she is doing or saying. I feel helpless and sad for her and I worry about how difficult things may be in the future.

Jane was in a good mood this morning. We planned on washing her hair. She prepared to wash it in the sink. When I intervened, she refused to wash it in the shower. She was confused. We sat down to talk. She was exhausted. She is sleeping now. When she wakes I'm sure she will wash her hair in the shower as we have been doing for months.

I've contemplated some of the recent changes in my life. Since I don't exercise early, I'm sleeping ten or eleven hours each night. Occasionally I miss a day of exercise because I don't make it a daily priority. If Jane is unwilling to come with me and is not in a favorable state of mind, I skip exercise.

2/24/11

Last evening Jane said, "You are thinking about my death, aren't you?" I was completely startled. I have been thinking about her death and mine. Our funerals have been in my mind. But this was a shock. I have no idea where it came from but it did introduce the topic of dying. I pointed out if she dies first she will still be with me in my mind and my heart so I really will not be without her. If I die first, I would still be with her in her heart but her mind might have a difficult time holding onto it. She cried and said she does not fear dying but dreads leaving me alone.

Since I last wrote there were a couple more days of bitterness and anger, but Jane has achieved a calmer state now. She asked why she is so focused on her illness lately, thinking about it all the time. I said it may be a lot of things: her increased confusion, her increased forgetting and losing things, the people in the dining room with canes and walkers and wheel chairs, the grey, cold days of the past two months, the recent eight deaths here, and a change of season is coming.

Jane said she has been thinking a lot about the things I mentioned. I suggested she has gone through difficult periods in the past when these same things happened. Each one of these holds out a big sign for her that says "Alzheimer's and death."

She is struggling with the idea of not talking with the children on the phone. I explain how we arrived at the decision and she agrees it is better this way but it makes her feel more cut off from the children, so I wonder about the wisdom of it.

Last night she said she wants to get rid of the angry feelings she has had throughout her life. She said she has no more animosity toward anyone including those who were difficult in the past.

(Laura 3/7/11)

You mentioned "sensitivity" yesterday. Being sensitive does make life a bit problematic at times, because a sensitive person is bound to feel things more than other people do. And feeling things sometimes is great and wonderful and full of happiness and life. And feeling things sometimes is full of pain and hurt and sadness and anger. But if I had a choice of being sensitive or not, I would take "SENSITIVE." Being sensitive is like being a bird, and being insensitive is like being a fish or a stick of wood. That's why we have the expression, "He's a cold fish."

Mom's first husband was a pretty insensitive person. He wasn't a bad guy but he was not responsive to Mom's sensitivity. Consequently he blamed all the problems on her because she was "too sensitive." Give me a sensitive person any day. At least they "live."

3/8/11

During the past few weeks I reread all these pages. I edited some of the writing and eliminated some of the repetitive information. The reading was enlightening. It gave me a clearer picture of Jane's gradual but persistent decline. I gained information about my behaviors over the period. The end result is to be grateful for where we are at present.

Jane does remarkably well to cope with the illness as well as she does. I suspect many Alzheimer's patients find it difficult not to give up, not to quit. Jane has not done that and is not doing it now. Oh, yes, she talks about quitting, about wanting to die. "I can't live this way. I want to die now." But she does not behave that way. She can talk in the morning about all the negatives in her life, all the impossibilities, all the mistakes, all the sadness; and by noon she can say, "I'm going to try harder, the afternoon is going to be better, and it will be a good day." And it happens! Of course it doesn't just happen. Her spirit, her determination, her faith, her devotion to me provide a force that turns things around and they become as she says they will be.

It sounds overstated, egotistical to say "her devotion to me." It is not really a positive statement about me. It is rather a statement of the power of Jane's love for me. She often says if it were not for me she could not do what she does. Above all, she does not want to hurt me or bring pain into my life. Sometimes I think she worries more about the effect Alzheimer's has on my life than on hers.

Reviewing these pages gives me some view of my passage during these past several years. My patience has improved and increased from what it was. I'm glad I have made adjustments to respond to the inroads of Alzheimer's.

I wanted to practice psychiatry a few more years. I wish I could still be teaching at Loyola. I believe I could still do a good job at both. I miss the early morning exercise. I miss our trips to Laura's and to Rehoboth. I would like to go to Montana again with Jane. I miss the detective stories I read before Jane was up in the mornings. I miss going out to dinner with Jane and close friends. I miss going to Sunday Mass.

These are not great and noble sacrifices. I am content to be with Jane and live the simple, somewhat ritualistic life we live. We recently heard a homily about not being here to live for ourselves but being here to live for God. Living for God comes down to living for others. Life has become simple for me. God's will is obvious every day. God lives in Jane. There lies my answer to present happiness and to eternal happiness.

It seems so simple it is almost frightening. When Jane gets harsh or shows some unprovoked anger, I think about God being present in the situation. I rarely have any feelings of anger or resentment these days toward Jane or toward anyone else actually.

Life is not always pleasant. There are still difficult times when Jane is irritable or sad or frightened, and I'm at a loss to make the world right for her. I try not to add to her distress but to hold her, speak calmly and reassuringly, and tell her of my love, our love, and our life together, past, present, and future.

There are lonesome times for me and for Jane too, I'm sure. For her it is probably an emptiness which she cannot describe. She misses me when I'm not with her. I miss her sometimes when I am with her, because I find an emptiness that I dare not mention or try to describe. "Being without the other" is a feeble expression of the loss which even now must be the greatest pain for each of us.

3/9/11

Last evening watching a movie, Jane had a response characteristic of similar episodes. Turn offs have occurred for violent movies, war movies, and sexual scenes. There is no consistency in the decisions. We watch movies that have some violent scenes, war scenes, or sexual scenes. I don't select movies if any of those categories is prominent. To eliminate these altogether would narrow our choices considerably. I eliminate all movies without captions because it is difficult for Jane to follow without them. Jane's decision to reject movies often appears to relate to her mood and the kind of day she had.

In the movie last evening there were no exposed breasts, buttocks, or pelvic areas. There was suggestive dress with exposed cleavage and short skirts. The story clearly implied sexual liaisons. I thought it was an interesting story of complications in several intertwined relationships. I said to Jane a couple of times, "Are you okay with this movie?" She said she was. After 40 minutes passed, she said angrily, "I don't want to see any more breasts of women all over my television. This is disgusting. Do you enjoy this kind of movie? You can see where it is headed. Pretty soon they'll all be naked." I said I thought it was an interesting story about relationships but I would gladly turn it off.

Jane continued with a variety of similar comments. I kept reassuring her I was in agreement to discontinue the movie and was sorry I had ordered it. We talked for two hours. She was fully placated by the time we finished and said she made a fool of herself. I insisted that was not so. She didn't like the movie, the scanty clothing upset her, and she was right to let me know how she felt. She was concerned about me seeing some unscarred arms and legs and thighs and breasts in the movie.

At times Jane takes a rather puritanical position about these issues. It is related to how she sees her own body. She is concerned about the veins on her feet and hands. "My body is rotting. The Alzheimer's is going up my legs and will eventually kill me." She examines carefully the veins on her forehead and expresses concern about them. "Soon my whole face will be scarred like this. I won't be able to leave the house." It seems she has just discovered the changes produced by aging. She continues to mention her larger and harder left breast. "I want something done about my breast. I can't stand it anymore." I remind her that the plastic surgeon did not recommend surgery because it would not resolve the capsular scarring. I reassure her, telling her quite honestly she is still beautiful, I love to see her body, and hers is the only body I care about.

(Laura, Kathie, Bonnie, Paul, Bob 3/11/11)
Just had long talk with Mom about phone calls from "the kids." She is now totally opposed to the idea I sent you about phone calls. She agreed before and seemed relieved as a result of the plan. In retrospect I was being too protective of her and was trying to avoid the kind of confusion and anxiety

that sometimes results when she talks on the phone. This evening she said, "I don't want to think I can never talk to one of my children again on the telephone."

It might have felt like I was trying to "shut you out" when I wrote before. It might be sad for you to feel you could no longer talk to your Mom on the phone. Each of you is sensitive enough not to say things that would upset her, and I'm sure you can decipher her comments and figure out whether or not they are accurate. If you are giving her some information I should know, then please tell me directly, because Mom is almost certain to get it confused or forget it.

(Laura 3/14/11)
Mom has been doing quite well with her mood. She repeats some of her old stories a good deal and will tell strangers about her mother, grandmother, etc. Yesterday I was surprised when she asked me if I was married before. She knew I had children but never wondered who their mother was. She said she felt jealous when I told her I was married before. Life comes to her in pieces, not in stories, snapshots not running film.

We are looking forward to your visit. Mom said she hopes she behaves well when you are here and that she remembers what she needs to remember. I tell her you and the girls are very aware of her illness and know how difficult things are for her and there isn't anything she can do that would be wrong.

3/17/11
These have been good days. Jane is doing remarkably well. She talks about her memory deficit and says she can live with it because we are together and that is what life is all about. We speak frequently of our love for each other and how special it is and seemingly so rare. I volunteer comments often during the day about how precious she is to me and how she has made my life worthwhile and beautiful for the past fifty years.

We met fifty years ago this year. Most of the time she doesn't remember much about how or where we met, but when I remind her it comes back to her. I remind her I loved her the first time I saw her and she felt the same way. It was a story book beginning but very real. We have had a good life together and

I thank God every day for her and for our Laura. We still treasure our days and often say we live together, eat together, sleep together, talk together, love together, pray together. What could be more wonderful!

We returned to our parish church two days ago. It was the first time we saw the new pastor who was installed the previous week. We are delighted with Father Gerry, the new pastor. He is genuine, gracious, pleasant, and obviously very capable. What a relief to know we have a pastor whom we can understand and who has a good heart and mind. It brings peace to know our wonderful pastor has been replaced with a good man.

Recent emails to Laura show how "lost" some things are for Jane. She met Marguerite, my first wife, several times during the years, and of course was very aware of my legal issues with Marguerite which went on for years into our marriage.

Jane seems to be losing some of the more distasteful memories of her childhood. She rarely mentions her stepfather who "threw my dolls into the trash can." She never mentions her first husband.

One advantage of her memory loss occurs in our daily trips to the Mall. The store windows always seem to be freshly stocked because she does not remember them from the day before. "They must work every night to change the windows so often."

Yesterday Jane had a brief episode of anger over something I said. I was patient, apologized repeatedly, sat with her and told her how much I love her. After the episode she said she remembers "how I used to give you such a bad time. I was mean and horrible to you." I said my memories of difficult times are gone as soon as we are on good terms. I mentioned that Alzheimer's causes persons to behave like that sometimes.

I missed exercise after the episode yesterday because Jane was too tired to go with me. I would not leave her alone because I wanted to be present to assure her anger was resolved. When we came home from the Mall today, Jane said, "I'd like to lie down for awhile." When she mentions it, there is never any doubt in my mind it is needed. I will wake her in an hour to get ready for dinner. I will miss exercise again. I don't like to leave her sleeping because she may wake, become disoriented and frightened. I don't like to miss the exercise but first things first, and her well-being is always first.

3/20/11

We spent over an hour last night talking about what will happen to our "things" when one of us dies. Jane fears, "You might die suddenly and I won't know what to do." I told her to call the front desk and say she needed help immediately. She said, "They won't know what to do. They don't know anything about me. They don't even know who I am." I explained they have procedures to take care of emergencies and do this regularly.

Jane worries about the furniture and pictures and statues and jugs we have accumulated through the years. She agrees most of these will not be precious to the three children for whom they are designated. She acknowledges most objects will be sold—books, pictures, lamps, furniture, mirrors, etc. I said we bought things for our pleasure and happiness. We enjoyed them and still do. What happens to them after our death is relatively unimportant. She understood and accepted that as reasonable. She was grateful I took the time to explain it all.

I don't know how many times we have had this same discussion, regularly reaching the same conclusion. I'm sure we will have it again. If it gives Jane some temporary peace of mind, the time is well spent.

3/22/11

Yesterday was a horrible day. All was well in the morning. Jane's hair is almost to her waist. After it is washed, she puts it in a bun and tries to preserve the result for a week. She uses hair clips and hair nets at night. Each morning she adds spray. By washing time her hair appears matted because of the spray.

After washing her hair, I gently suggested she take it down every few days and brush out the dried hair spray. By afternoon the story was: "You don't like the way my hair looks. You don't want to take me out because it's ugly, and you want me to get it cut. You made fun of me because of the way it looks. You said it was all standing up on my head. You don't like the style." It was so ridiculous it could have been humorous, only it was sad and wasteful of our day.

I tried to explain what I said and, of course, only made things worse. I apologized for the comment and tried to sooth her. Every response increased the distortion. We would reach a more peaceful level but not for long because the hair issue would come up again. It seemed endless. It was endless.

Finally in the evening after we talked for two hours, Jane understood my comment and agreed her hair looked bad with the spray. She blamed herself for the bad day. I said I was sorry I made the remark. Her comment was, "If you apologized a little sooner, it would have made a big difference." My thought was, "sometimes nothing makes a difference."

I don't know whether I get angry at Jane or just want to turn her off. It is so unceasing, so bizarre, so sick, so sad. It wears me out. I know it is hard on her and for her. She is unable to leave it alone. Would she behave the same way if someone else was taking care of her? I doubt she would. Her expectations of me are unreal. They are fantasy.

A few days ago I commented about her posture. She occasionally tips the upper part of her body to the left and walks that way. She was angry at my comment. "I'm alive. Isn't that enough?" Perhaps I should make that the standard. She is alive. Why worry about her posture, her gait, her matted hair?

3/24/11

An event last night demonstrates how easily and how quickly everything goes to hell. We had a good day, shopped at Home Depot, went to the Mall for lunch, came home and exercised. I bought fluorescent bulbs and explained several times why I was doing so.

Prior to dinner I installed the bulbs in a few lamps. One lamp had a daylight bulb rather than soft white. Leaving for dinner, Jane saw the lamp in our hall showing stark white light. She attacked me. "What have you done? Why did you buy something without discussing it with me? Never do that again. I will never enter this apartment again with that kind of light. Does this mean we are breaking up that you should do such a thing?" I said I bought the wrong bulb by mistake and would exchange it.

Her comments continued during dinner. She wanted to leave the table. She wasn't going to eat. At one point she said clearly and coldly, "I **will** kill myself. You don't know I think about it all the time but I do." After dinner she wanted me to go and replace the bulbs while she waited at the table. I left her alone there.

When I returned, a dining room staff member had taken Jane into an office and was talking to her. When they came out, before Jane would separate from the staff member she insisted I promise not to be mad at her and not to punish her for what she did.

On returning to our apartment, we talked two hours and later in bed another hour. Nothing gets resolved by these lengthy discussions. We just go over and over the same material. She describes the terrible wrong I have done. I apologize. We talk about it, and she becomes calm and reasonable. Then she describes the event again. In no time, the calm is gone and the anger is back. The pattern repeats and repeats. Eventually she was either satisfied or exhausted and we got to sleep.

This morning was fragile. I did our ritual of greetings and hugs and kisses. After breakfast I took a shower. After the shower I dressed and went to my desk to complete some things I was doing. Jane was angry. "You are ignoring me. You are leaving me all alone. This is what you always do. You always call to me after you finish your shower. You don't love me anymore."

We spent an hour going over my unforgivable behavior. At some magical moment I say, "I'm sorry I didn't come in to see you," and she hears me. It doesn't matter how many times I said it before, now she hears it and insists I never said it before.

3/25/11
Last night we were talking about how our evenings have changed. A few months ago, we ate dinner in our apartment about 7:00p.m. Now we go to the dining room at 4:30 and are back by 6:00p.m.

Jane asked how we could spend this evening time. At one point, unrelated to anything being said, she asked, "When are we going to have sex again?" I replied we don't have sex as often because my age slows me down a bit. Our sexual patterns were not the focus of our conversation so I continued talking about what we might do in the evening. We discussed playing cards, reading, walking in nice weather, and going to some of the evening programs.

In bed Jane said, "I want to talk to you about something." She spoke in a loud, pressured manner and appeared distraught. "Why did you say we'll never have sex again? What's the matter with you? If there is a good reason, it will be all right with me but why did you tell me tonight? Why did you go on with those stupid things we could do instead of having sex? You just made it worse to come up with all those things."

I decided it would be better to approach this sitting up and with the lights on. We got out of bed and sat on the sofa. She insisted she was correct. I became irritated and told her how wrong she was. She finally accepted what I was saying. Then in her usual fashion she went over it again and got back to the same emotional place. After several rounds we went to bed about midnight.

This morning Jane remembers little or none of the evening conversation. She said what a wonderful day and evening we had yesterday. When I mentioned "the girls" (Casey and Tara) would be here tomorrow, she had forgotten they were coming. She asked, "Who do the girls belong to?" I said, "They are our grandchildren, Laura's daughters."

Life is full of surprises. Everything in life is a surprise for Jane but not pleasantly so.

3/27/11

Laura and the girls came yesterday. It was a difficult day for Jane. In a way she dreaded their coming. She saw it as a test of how much worse she is since the last time they were here. If it were such a test, sadly she failed it.

She had difficulty entering into exchanges with the girls and was awkward in exchanges with Laura. Last evening we had a nice conversation with Laura about her work. Jane was at ease but participated little. She complained of a roaring in her head most of the evening. After Laura and the girls went to their room Jane insisted on talking for two hours before she would even try to go to sleep. It was after one when she slept.

231

Today she is confused and remembers little about yesterday. Paul joined us for brunch. It went well, although Jane participated minimally and had difficulty following the conversation. After Paul left Jane agreed to take a nap, to my surprise. Laura and the girls are at the Mall. I sit here wondering what the next visit will be like. Will she know the girls? Will she be talking?

This visit compares poorly to past ones. Jane is not with us as she used to be. I see myself more as a caregiver than a companion. After they go she will mourn their going and her lack of interaction with them. She will be aware of the shortcomings for a day or two and then she will be saying, "When did Laura and the girls last visit?"

This visit made me more aware of the truth in what Jane says. "Don't you know how bad I'm getting? I'm going over the edge. Soon it will be over." I know it is not over but we are on a downhill slope. How steep? How fast? What's at the bottom?

3/31/11

I sometimes think Jane looks for things to be mad about but I know that's not being fair to her. It just feels that way to me.

Last night preparing for bed she started. "You never talk to me about my illness or how I feel or about the things that go through my head and can be there all day. I have no one else to talk to. I'm not going to see that therapist again. It doesn't help to talk to her. I'm going crazy and you don't want to talk about it. No one ever told me what it would be like to have Alzheimer's. Those little comments you make that 'things will be okay' don't help at all. You say those things just to pacify me like you would a patient." I said we often talk about her thoughts and about Alzheimer's. Such a comment only intensifies her insistence she is lonely with no one to talk to. These bedtime conversations are not unusual. It reminds me of an anxious child trying to postpone the loneliness and fear that invade the privacy of sleep.

We sat down to talk. She was concerned because I told her a while ago we would never have sex again. She insisted she remembered the conversation exactly. The subject has been on her mind but I was never willing to talk about it. She elaborated. "You told me the doctor said you could never have

232

sex again. I know you have some horrible illness and will die soon. I've thought of nothing else the past two or three weeks."

When I told her the only doctor I've seen this past year was our internist in her presence, she seemed to recognize things were not as she remembered them. When this happens, she acknowledges how wrong her judgment was. I think it is remarkable she has this much insight.

Today we had an opportunity to prove her fears to be false.

4/4/11
During the last several days, Jane is dealing better with her memory loss and times of confusion. Her greater acceptance makes all the difference in the world.

I felt lonely after Laura and the girls left. I felt homesick, the way I felt when I was a child at boarding school. I did well there and had friends and was compliant but deep down I always yearned to be back at the ranch. I did what needed to be done, but happiness was "back at the ranch." It seems farfetched but the recent bout of homesickness had that same feel. I need to do what I am doing but peace will come "back at the ranch" in heaven. Heaven seems more real and I look forward to being there.

After Laura's visit, I realized I don't have the usual sense of involvement and pleasure in exchanges with others. The visitor is not a primary connection, because my principal concern is how the visit is going for Jane. This is an observation not a complaint.

(Email to Laura 4/5/11)
Thanks for the email of yesterday. Mom got her card and was very pleased with it. She really responds to support and praise. I tell her several times a day how well she is doing, how brave she is, how proud I am of her, and how much I love her. It does seem to be a boost for her. I realize how much she forgets of everything I say, so I repeat it. Mom says she is determined to do as well as she can with the illness. She does have a remarkable spirit and I truly admire her courage.

Having you here was having another adult to talk to. I can talk pretty freely to Mom most of the time but her understanding is limited and her range of interest is too. I've stopped watching much of the news because there's no place to go with it.

4/7/11

Jane became quite paranoid last evening. She was convinced our new neighbor (Mary) is telling tales about her. Mary asked us to visit her and have dinner together. I told her we always eat alone. When we saw her later she seemed rather curt when we spoke.

Last evening Jane said she thought about Mary all day and can't get it out of her mind. Mary ate with five other residents a few nights ago and Jane insists she was talking to everyone about us. "I hate her and everyone else here." I sat with Jane and said, "Sweetheart, you are mixed up. We have lots of good friends here who love us. Mary was not talking about you and would have nothing negative to say about you. People on staff and other residents love you very much." That seemed to placate her.

4/9/11

I finally insisted on taking Jane to the bathroom during the night. When she goes alone she is confused and spends 30 to 60 minutes in her rituals, no matter how much preparation she makes before going to bed. On return to bed she is frustrated and angry. "I can't go on like this. This is too hard. I can't live this way. I wish I were dead." These episodes disturb our nights.

She is opposed to me getting up with her. I reminded her she has fallen three or four times during the night. I said I must make decisions I think are best. She reluctantly agreed. It works well. I turn on lights, steady her on her way, help get what she needs, and take her back to bed. The episode takes about five minutes. She gets back to sleep quickly. She got up twice last night and agreed it went fine. She was comfortable and slept well. I slept much better too. I trust this will be a regular plan.

(Email to Laura 4/12/11)

Mom has been doing remarkably well the past week or so. We follow a daily routine pretty closely and it seems to suit her. After breakfast, get ready to go to the Mall or to Mass and then the Mall. Lunch and home about 2:30. Get ready and go to exercise. She is going with me every day lately. After exercise, get ready for dinner. Later a movie and then to bed. Not very exciting but who needs excitement.

4/15/11

Jane was disturbed last evening after the movie. I stopped it several times to "catch her up" and thought she followed it fairly well. She said, "I'm so stupid. I didn't understand it. You understood it and I saw the same things you saw. I didn't know what any of it was about." I suspect she can't remember the beginning by the time we reach the end. She says she enjoys the scenery, the rooms, and the clothing even if she loses the story.

She sees the psychiatric nurse today. She was angry. "I'm not going to make another appointment. She isn't going to make me better so why should I see her." I agreed the therapist won't make her better and no one else will either but it may help her continue to do as well as she can. She said nothing more about stopping. What a fragmented, chaotic, frightening world my Jane lives in! I cannot appreciate how difficult her life must be.

4/18/11

Last evening Laura called. Jane did not want to talk to her. I told Laura, "It's not a good time for Mom to talk on the phone." Laura and I talked about fifteen minutes.

After the call Jane was furious. We spent the next three hours talking about it. Times like this expose the turmoil in her mind. She was furious with Laura and me. "It's always the two of you. I hate you both." Later she stumbled onto some reality. "I think I'm jealous when you and Laura talk on the phone. When she talks to me I don't have anything to say and she has told you everything already. But there is no reason I should be unhappy when she talks to you." I said I think Laura talks more freely to me and rattles on about things. That was not helpful. Jane decided Laura was telling me things she didn't want her mother to know. "Why would the two of you keep secrets from me? Are there things you don't want me to know? I don't want to hear what she said."

It's a merry-go-round nightmare. I try not to be quiet because that angers her. I choose my words carefully, but whatever they are, they are more likely to be irritating than helpful. I try to avoid disagreeing. If I correct something Jane said, she responds, "I know what I said and what you said. I'm right. Why do you always disagree with me and try to correct me? Are you trying to make me feel stupid? Well I'm not stupid, so don't try that." And then she tells me how stupid she thinks she is.

I want so badly to help her find some road to peace and calm. There seems to be nothing I can do. Then suddenly she is in tears and begging forgiveness for being so cruel to me, for hurting me so badly, for becoming such a monster. The aftermath of guilt is as relentless as the torrent of anger that came before. I explain again these are Alzheimer's storms; they come and they go. There is no damage to our relationship. No one is hurt. No one is injured. Our love remains intact and always will.

After a day or so she has forgotten the whole episode, and so have I. I don't feel hurt by these tirades. I am frustrated because I can't find a path to calm her but I am aware it is a period of emotional incontinence over which she has no control. I am sad for what it does to her. I am glad for the cleansing process of her forgetting.

(Email to Laura 4/18/11)
Mom fluctuates between listless and edgy. It is difficult to talk with her these days. She is not interested in most things and forgets things that interested her. If I comment about anything she does, it sounds like criticism to her. She is irritated easily but it goes away quickly. We talk sometimes about her empty head and how difficult it is for her to make sense out of everything.

The last several nights Mom complained of pain in her legs keeping her awake, usually after she returns from the bathroom during the night. Sometimes I think she isn't fully awake and imagining it. It is always "the worst pain I ever had in my life." Her legs are fine in the day time. She walks more slowly, sometimes so slowly it is difficult to walk with her. Her gait probably causes some of her leg pain because she takes such small steps.

4/24/11

Easter day! Jane is lost to the world and in the world. I have mentioned three times it is Easter and each time it is a surprise.

Jane continues to say she wants to do her best with the Alzheimer's so it won't be so hard for me. I think that is a principal motive for her courage and stamina. It is another way she loves me. I tell her I have new ways of loving her now.

We had a long talk about Jane's fear of dying. I talked about death as "going home," which is how I think of it. I suggested it will be more like "going to Aunt Edith's" for her since that was always the house she looked forward to visiting. I said I am not afraid of dying and don't think she should be. I reminded her she is a good woman, a wonderful spouse, a kind and loving person, someone who clung to her faith through difficult times, and she has no reason to fear death because she will be with God. A fitting topic for the season! She seemed reassured at the time but will she remember? No!

4/27/11

Last night after a bathroom trip Jane said her right hip was terribly painful and she could not sleep. While I went for Tylenol she got up. I got our robes and we sat in the living room. I prepared a hot pack in the microwave oven. It didn't help.

After fifteen minutes I suggested we return to bed. I put the hot pack on her hip. Within five minutes she was sound asleep. This morning her hip was fine and she did not recall the incident. When I mentioned how painful her hip was, she was defensive. "You don't think I made it up, do you?" I said, "Of course not," but I feel she exaggerates things like this. What need drives this behavior? Is it fear of dying, of my abandoning her, of being alone? When her physical condition seems not as terrible as she reports, I believe her complaints help her bridge the distance between us and between her and reality.

4/30/11

Jane bought a new lipstick two days ago. The clerk demonstrated several colors on her own hand for Jane to pick one. Last night Jane said she was unable to remove her lipstick. She forgot she removed it the previous evening with no problem.

She was frantic and talked about it for an hour, continuing after we got in bed. "I'll never be able to get it off. We have to take it back. I don't know if they will take lipstick back, but they will have to take it back. I can't afford lipstick in the first place. I shouldn't have bought it. It was a terrible mistake. I am so sorry. It must have cost three times as much as other lipstick. Don't tell me what it cost. I don't want to know." When I said we'll take care of it and please don't worry about it, she was irritated. "You have to say you will take it back." I said it and did not challenge any of her statements.

The next morning she brought up the subject. I carefully said I couldn't see lipstick on her lips and reminded her that her lips are normally quite red. I said the store would hardly sell lipstick that would not come off and we saw the clerk take the lipstick marks off her hand.

Jane agreed she was wrong. It seemed too easy. She was self-critical about how wrong she was and how strongly she had carried on about it. That knowledge will not benefit her because it will not remain with her. We talked about Alzheimer's and how it affects her in a variety of ways.

(Email to Paul 5/1/11)
Mom has just had a couple of remarkably good days. It truly amazes me she does so well. She clings to her faith these days and it is very meaningful for her (as it is for me during these times). She has a determination and spirit that are remarkable. I'm convinced she gets determined to do as well as she can so I won't suffer from her decline.

Last week there were a couple of days we went to the Mall and it seemed she could hardly walk. I even suggested it might be better to quit going so often if it was too much for her. She would sleep for about an hour when we got home. I think it was the result of her feeling depressed, frightened about the future, and overwhelmed. The last two days we went to the Mall she walked fine and we exercised for 30 minutes after we got home.

(Email to Laura 5/2/11)
Mom got your card on Saturday and was very pleased. Cards seem to be very meaningful for her, probably because she can see them, hold them, read and reread them. You write such loving comments. She will cherish them for a long time.

Last night Mom went to the bathroom without waking me. I remind her every night to wake me. I heard her fall. I got up and helped her back to bed. I told her this morning if I am to take care of her she will have to abide by some rules and not get up during the night without waking me. Well, that was too much. I never spoke to her so cruelly in all her life; I had no right to set up rules; she could do what she wanted, etc., etc. She finally settled down and agreed she was wrong, but she hates to wake me. I said I'd rather you wake me than to be awake two hours worrying about you after you fall. Fortunately she didn't hurt herself, just a bruised bottom.

5/09/11

Jane is doing remarkably well, considering how poor her memory is and how unfathomable the world must be for her. We had a pleasant visit with Paul two days ago. Jane is at her best when he visits. He makes it easy for her to stay with the conversation. She remembers little of what was said.

Jane had a session today with the Fitness Coordinator in the exercise room. She gave Jane three exercises to do. Additional appointments are scheduled. I enjoy seeing her work with someone she admires and appreciates. Jane is cooperative, warm and friendly, and quite humorous in their exchanges. I admire her for her spirit and her willingness to try something new. She is a remarkable woman who in some almost unbelievable fashion can find a way of being comfortable in a shattered, scattered world. What an inspiration!

(Letter sent to two of Jane's physicians 5/5/11)

Dear Doctor* * * * *

As you can imagine I worry sometimes I may predecease Jane, so I want to make as many preparations for that eventuality as I can. We have all the legal papers prepared except we do not have papers indicating Jane's incapacity. I am enclosing a document which I hope you will sign based on her last appointment with you this year. Then if you would please have it notarized, I would ask you to mail it back to me.

After I get this document and a similar one by another physician, they will avoid the possible necessity of a court proceeding, which would be emotionally distressing for Jane and cumbersome for Jane's daughter, who has power of attorney. I prefer this matter not be discussed with Jane because it would be emotionally traumatic for her and needlessly disruptive of our life.

If you need another appointment in order to sign this Statement of Incapacity, please ask your office to call me and I will arrange the appointment within a short time.

We appreciate the care you have provided both of us these past few years. I do not have any new concern about my health at this time but it would greatly relieve my mind to have this matter settled as quickly as possible.

Thank you for your cooperation.

5/11/11

Last night Jane went to the bathroom without me. She was immediately defensive when I mentioned it this morning. I said I cannot trust her. She promises and then does it her way. This is not how it should be. I reminded her she fell at least four times in the bathroom at night. She knew I was angry but I needed her to get the message.

Throughout the day she fluctuated between apologies and accusations I was being distant with her. I denied I was but in reality I wasn't really myself. I fear she will do the same thing again some night, guided by her immediate concern about waking me. I'm quite sure she doesn't forget to wake me but decides not to for my sake. I told her I'll be angry if she does it again and explained why I am concerned.

5/14/11

At lunch yesterday we talked about Alzheimer's. Jane gets frustrated each time she can't find something. Forgetting things does not have as strong an impact as losing things, because her "things" are more precious, more personal than "experiences" she has. As we talked I came onto a new thought about the disease. Jane does not accept that she will not be able to find things or remember things. Patients with Alzheimer's do not have a clear and present consciousness of their limitations.

Persons who are blind do not expect to see when they get up in the morning. Persons who can't walk have no reason to think they can walk the next time they get up from a chair. Persons with Parkinsonism do not anticipate the tremors will be gone after a nap. Most people with serious illnesses have shortness of breath or pain or physical limitation which reminds them of things they cannot do. But even though Alzheimer's patients constantly confront their inability to find things and to remember things, that inability does not remain constantly and clearly present to them. They begin to look for something with the expectation they will remember where they put it. Simply put, they don't remember they forget.

The unremitting pain of Alzheimer patients: to search for something and expect to be able to find it, to try to recall something as if they have access to it in their memory bank, to meet over and over again the harshness, the loneliness, the desperation, the frustration of separation from things, from thoughts, from experiences that have disappeared. And they are shocked each time it happens because nothing in their body or in their mind tells them this is going to happen over and over again—even after it happens over and over again. Yes, they know it but they can't remember it. And what good is "know" if you can't remember the "know."

5/22/11

Last night Jane wondered how long she will live "with the cancer in my breast? I know I am dying of cancer but the doctors won't give me any information on how long I have. They won't tell me because they don't want to alarm me. There is a hard lump in my left breast that is getting bigger every day and it is going to kill me." No matter how many times we have discussed this, I cannot convince her she does not have breast cancer. Her mind tells her, "A woman who does nothing about a hard mass in her breast will die of cancer."

Even after I tell her what the doctors said, she still wants the breast taken off. "My breasts are noticeably not the same and I can't wear any of my summer clothes because it will show." In fact she wears the same clothes in the summer she wears in the winter. "I won't be able to wear a bathing suit." She hasn't been in a bathing suit in ten years.

For several weeks Jane has been concerned about needing a refill for a cosmetic pencil she uses. Each time she mentions it I remind her I have refills. Her brain seems unable to exchange her fixed idea for what I tell her. At lunch today I mentioned the difficulty her brain has assimilating information when she already has her own belief about the matter. I thought it would help her know how aware I am of her difficulty.

She seemed to understand what I told her and I emphasized I was not being critical of her. At home she became hostile. She could not remember what I did to irritate her. Taking a guess, I asked if it was about the refills. Yes, it was and "how cruel you were to criticize me and tell me I always do that same thing. This is just an example of how bad and stupid I really am."

I finally convinced her I was not calling her stupid and did not mean to offend her. I was letting her know I have some appreciation of how difficult the world is for her.

5/25/11

My schedule has changed considerably from what it was six months ago. Then I got up at 6a.m. and had three hours before Jane got up. I exercised and read or worked on the computer. Now we get up together about 8:30a.m.

We go to the Mall every day for lunch now. Previously we went four or five times a week. Six months ago Jane often slept in the afternoon for a couple of hours after we returned from the Mall. I had that time to myself. Now she rarely sleeps in the afternoon and at most for 30 to 60 minutes. Most days I exercise 20 minutes about 3:30p.m. and Jane goes with me if she doesn't nap.

We go to the dining room for dinner at 4:30 so we can get a table for two. We used to pick up our dinner and eat about 7p.m. Now we finish dinner by 6:00 at the latest.

Advantages: I get more sleep, Jane gets more exercise, and we have more time together which seems to improve her functioning.
Disadvantages: I have little time alone. I have no time to read. I started a book of Sudoku puzzles my granddaughter gave me but I don't have enough time to follow through. I occasionally play a few quick games of solitaire on

the computer. I miss the hours alone but it is not a burden and seems not to affect my mood or state of mind negatively. And it affects Jane positively, so any loss for me is worth it.

Most evenings go well. We get Netflix movies. I sometimes read to her in the evening. She follows the reading well. A few months ago I stopped reading to her in the mornings when she does her hair and make-up. It distracted her from her preparations.

Jane continues to spend considerable time in her bathroom in the mornings and the evenings. She resents it if I don't come in regularly to see "how things are going." She accuses me of being at my desk all the time and ignoring her. Actually that is the only place I have to sit to be anywhere near where she is. I consciously try to be more attentive and pay her a visit more often. It is worth my time to do so.

5/28/11

During the night Jane went to the bathroom and didn't wake me. She had, of course, promised faithfully she would always wake me. I was awake two hours sorting it out in my mind and wondering how to deal with it. I was angry but tried to reason it through. Maybe she forgets her promise to wake me. I can't tell her how she must behave. She can show her independence if she chooses to do so. I decided not to mention it further because it would only cause irritation, defensiveness, guilt, escalating anger, fear of punishment from me, fear I would leave her, and all the other disorganized and disturbing thoughts of which she is victim.

PART 10 (JUN 11—NOV 11)

(Email to Laura 6/7/11)

Forgot to tell you—we had contact from a social worker at Arizona State University requesting permission to reprint part of Mom's book in an anthology they are doing. Their book will contain writings by individuals who have a cognitive illness. The book is designed to be used by students in psychology, social work, nurse counseling fields. We have agreed to participate. Mom is pleased, as am I. It is sort of a professional recognition of the value of the work.

6/24/11

For the past few weeks I have been reading these pages and removing extraneous and redundant material. I got a little obsessive about the whole project and although I thought about writing from time to time, I kept putting it off.

When I read the material I wonder what I can write that is new. Jane's memory is worse. Jane gets more confused. Jane has problems with irritability, sadness, fear. Jane has thoughts about dying. Jane worries how I will be when she is gone. All these things have been said many times.

But there are changes going on and exchanges which I want to note. Last evening she said she can't remember what the dining room looks like until we get there. We have eaten there every evening for over six months. When I say let's go to the exercise room, she doesn't know what we do there until I tell her. She has no recollection of the trainer who worked with her two or three days a week for several weeks. We leave the apartment to "go to the Mall for lunch" and in the car she asks where we are going. I am becoming more conscious of how lost she is and how easy it is for me to overlook it.

We talked last evening about her thinking process. Lately she focuses on how much worse she is. She agrees everything gets bleak and frightening when she does that. She feels better when her attitude is to accept how things are and try to live as peacefully as she can. That is a philosophy of life we could all use to our advantage.

The last few weeks have been as varied as our life has been these past several years. Jane is easily irritated at times. If I don't get defensive or critical, it is soon over. I think I have come to terms with the ongoing deterioration. I know there is an increasing need for me to be attentive to her, spend more time with her, and be more alert to her loss of contact with the immediate. I need to remind her frequently where we are going, why we are going, why we are where we are, what we are doing and why we are doing it.

She is interested in details we would never have discussed before. I recently discontinued a service we had from Comcast Cable. I had to return a converter box to stop the service. When I mentioned it to Jane she wanted to know all about it. I am quite inept in the electronic field, so I try to explain something to her I don't really understand. This happens with telephones, the computer and our digital camera. She asks questions I can only answer in vague terms and my answers are often not sufficient to satisfy her curiosity. It irritates her that I can't clarify. She erroneously assumes I am knowledgeable in a field foreign to me. I wonder why things like this now interest her so much.

We watch a Netflix movie almost every evening. Invariably at some point during or after the movie, she decides we saw it before, although she can't remember much about it. I suspect some scene finds a brain cell where a similar scene resides. The light for "familiar" goes on, so her assumption is we saw the movie before.

(Email to Laura 6/24/11)
Thought about writing several times this week but never got around to it. I am spending a good deal more time with Mom even if it is just to go in her bathroom and check on how she is doing. Keep in pretty close touch with her these days. Yesterday she went to get ready to exercise (I had just made the suggestion) and she came out dressed for dinner. Of course that is more upsetting for her than for me.
* * * * * *

Every day I keep learning more clearly how little she understands about everything we do and every place we go. That's why the Mall by the same route is so important. A couple of weeks ago we went in through Nordstrom and stayed on the first level to take her shoes to the cobbler. When we left the eatery I asked if she would like to go back on the top level since we came in below. We went up the escalator by the eatery and came back on that level. She was furious. Why did I change something we always do? Didn't I know it would mix her up? I could never convince her we came in on the ground floor, so I just let it go. The routine is: we go up in Nordstrom and the length of the Mall upstairs, then come back on the ground floor and out through Nordstrom.

Mom has her ups and downs and brief episodes of irritation but all in all things are going well. I think about the wild times of last summer and am ever grateful we are here and not back there.

6/27/11

Jane woke me at 3a.m. this morning, Saturday. Her left eye had been blinking for some time and she didn't know what to do. I turned on the light. Both eyes were blinking about twice every second. I was at a loss as to what to do. We've had some placebo effect from Tylenol so I gave her one, suggesting it might help stop the blinking. We sat together for about fifteen minutes talking about it. It didn't hurt but she could not stop it.

She wondered if she was going blind or if she was dying. I reassured her but I mentioned the emergency room to test how serious her concern was. She didn't think that was necessary. I said we would contact her ophthalmologist on Monday if it did not improve. I tied a small scarf over her eyes and suggested we go back to bed. She was asleep in a short time.

She took the scarf off in the morning. There was no blinking. The eye continued to water intermittently but we went to the Mall for lunch and exercised when we got home. Once or twice she said it was a little painful but after dinner it was "much better." After the movie she complained of pain in her eye. Before long she was accusing me of ignoring her all day and having no concern about her eye or the pain she suffered throughout the day.

I mentioned the emergency room again. "You don't care how much pain I have. I'm going blind and you don't pay any attention. You didn't suggest the emergency room during the day. I would have gone then. I don't want to go now. It's probably too late to get any help anyway." Her unleashed fury continued. I finally said, "We are not going to the emergency room now or any time for this. It is not an emergency. I have looked under the upper and lower lid and at your eye; there is no bleeding, no sign of infection or inflammation. You are not losing your eyesight. We'll call the ophthalmologist on Monday if it isn't better."

We slept well. Sunday morning Jane asked about fillers for her cosmetic pencil. I told her again we had the fillers. Within two minutes she said we needed to visit the surgeon to see what he was going to do about her swollen left breast. I again went through the explanation. There is no cancer. The doctor did not recommend surgery when he saw her last December. The hard lumps are due to radiation treatment after the cancer was removed from her breast. The eye is not a worry this morning, the fillers were, and then the breast was. Her brain has a box of worries and Jane keeps finding one.

She never mentioned her eye until I asked about it in the evening. I hesitate to ask about issues that may have slipped from her attention. She said, "My eye was fine today. I should have told you earlier." She said she thought the problem may have been caused by eyeliner she got in her eye last Friday.

7/1/11

We watched a movie last night. The main character, a woman named Percy, was washed downstream in a river. Although she was face down in the water when she was rescued, it did not seem certain she was dead. The next scene was a funeral. I said, "Percy must be dead." Her name was mentioned several times in the eulogy.

Jane completely lost contact with the movie after the scene of the girl in the water. Later we discovered the answer. The name "Percy" meant nothing. Jane has no box for names. If I had said "the dark haired girl who was in the river is dead," Jane would have followed the story. As it was, the remainder of the show became incomprehensible.

I should have realized this. Jane doesn't remember the name Marilyn but she knows "the woman in the wheel chair you always talk to." She doesn't know the name Ruth but she knows "the woman who lives with her husband in an apartment just like ours." She doesn't know the name Syd but she knows "the woman who gave us the parking place." She doesn't know the name Ruby but she knows "the woman who stops and talks to you in the dining room." She has known Marilyn and Ruth and Syd and Ruby since we moved here. She knows them now only by description, not by name.

(Email to Paul 7/5/11)
Wanted to let you know I mailed the certificates of incapacity to you this morning. * * * * * * And I'll give a copy to administration at Vantage House. Hope there won't be a need for them because I expect to be around.

(Email to Kathie 7/7/11)
Thought I would let you know I have two "certificates of incapacity" from two of your mom's doctors. I have given Paul copies of them and there will be copies in Mom's medical chart in the clinic here. * * * * * *

Mom is unaware of these and would be very angry if she found out about them. If something happened to me and these were not available, it might be necessary to go through a court proceeding to establish incapacity and that would be horrible.

7/10/11
I'm not sure I want to write this but I'll see what it looks like and then decide what to do with it. Jane and I had a bitter evening yesterday. She would call it a terrible fight. I would call it a miserable time. The cause of her anger was relatively insignificant.

We visited Kathie in her new apartment yesterday. When we got home Jane felt tired. I encouraged her to lie down and she accepted. I turned the covers down and was waiting to tuck her in. She came out dressed to exercise. I had decided not to exercise because I didn't want to leave her alone after a rather bad day. She was irritated and didn't nap.

During dinner she said she thought Kathie made a bad choice of apartments. I said Kathie looked at a lot of places and probably liked the size of this one and maybe the quiet location. "Why do you always have to disagree with me? Why do you always have to take the other side? You want to show me how stupid I am."

I responded, "I'm sorry I said anything." She glared at me across the table and said rather loudly, "If you make any more remarks like that, you'll be sorry. I'll make a scene you will regret forever." We finished dinner and returned to the apartment.

My response about Kathie was an attempt to soften things for Jane and help her see them in a brighter vein. I often respond in this manner. She can't tolerate it if I don't agree but in addition I apparently must say I do agree. Any other view of the subject is forbidden.

On returning to the apartment I suggested we sit and talk. Jane lectured me for two hours about not talking to her. "This has been a problem all our married life. You don't talk to me and you do it deliberately to hurt me. I don't know how many times through the years you have done the same thing. It is how you have always punished me. And I have always been afraid of you because of it. I never knew when it would happen. You did it over and over again. And you do it now and it's going to kill me. Will you do the same thing when I'm dying? Will you not talk to me then and let me die with you mad at me?"

In bed we achieved some semblance of peace and Jane went to sleep. I was awake a couple of hours and woke early this morning. I'm trying to piece it all together. I always thought Jane was as happy with me as I am with her. I don't think it any more. I know she loves me but I believe she has always had a fear of me and consequently a doubt as to my—my what—my integrity, my loyalty, my fidelity—I don't know just what to call it. Perhaps my dependability. No wonder she gets afraid I'll leave her. No wonder she feels alone and uncertain.

No wonder she gets as angry at me as she does and as quickly as she does. I thought these anger storms were so violent because they were fueled by memories of anger she felt toward her mother and her first husband. Now I see they are fueled by the anger and resentment she carries toward me. She doesn't forget being hurt by others. It is one of her unsavory traits. She remembers the mean things her mother and her first husband did. And about me she remembers "you would always not talk to me because you wanted to hurt me and you know it hurts me more than anything else anyone can do."

I've thought a lot about my not talking when she is angry. I've written about it often. I truly don't know what to say to her that is of any value. She feels miserable and wants me to say something so she won't feel so badly. She is not interested in my thoughts about the subject of her anger. She is not interested in any of my feelings or ideas about what is going on. She just wants me to say something that will make her life rosy again. And I don't know what that is!

If I hadn't kept quiet through the years, we may not have stayed together. If I had said some of the things I used to think when she was furious and unreasonable and unreachable, she would have considered me abusive and placed me in the box with her mother and her first husband. I'm not sure our love would have survived it. I rarely get angry, but when I do I can be pretty critical and sarcastic.

So here we are. I needed Jane in my life. I still do and I guess she needed me. She certainly does now. But I wish she could look back and see it as happy a life as it was for me. I come away feeling self centered and selfish. I was happy and felt I was always a good husband, a very good husband. This morning I don't feel that way any more. Could I have done better? Probably, but I'm not sure how. I'm not trying to justify my behavior. Maybe Jane was looking for something I couldn't give her.

When she is angry, I close down. To openly quarrel with her would be a disaster now and I believe always would have turned out badly. To be able to talk to her when she is angry and help her out of it may be a possibility but I have never discovered the secret. Responding never works because whatever I say is fuel, and so is silence. Now with Alzheimer's complicating the picture I worry about the future and at the same time regret the hurts of the past, apparently still fresh for her and to remain so.

It makes me sad when I realize a few quarrels of the past remain the basis of and fuel for present fires of anger sounding like hate. Why can't she forget past times? I suppose she can't because I keep doing the same thing, viz. "not talking in order to make me angry." I don't remember quarrels of the past because I wasn't destroyed by them as she was. I wasn't frightened afterwards as she was. My attitude is more directed toward "forgive and forget," because incidents and events get pushed out by other interests and activities in my life. Jane's disposition has been to harbor grievances. She is forgetting most of the old ones about mother and classmates and first husband and the women from the pool. But her old grievance with me is kept fresh by regular renewal.

7/17/11
When I wrote a week ago, I was depressed after a difficult time with Jane and I perhaps took something she said too seriously. I think we have both been happy in our marriage and know no one else could have made either of us any happier.

Things have been going well the past several days. I feel differently about our situation. I am more aware of the deficits in Jane's thinking, responding, and feeling. Although she is still the love of my life, I begin to see her as the patient she has become. In the past her good days encouraged me to minimize the terrible toll the illness is taking and hold onto the belief she could on occasion respond at her normal level. I must now accept her "normal level" is abysmally low compared to what it was before. I tried to believe there were days when she responded "just as she always was." How many times have I written that phrase? How many times have I said it to myself or to others? Not any more! "As she always was" is gone, gone, gone.

I must see her in the full light of her illness. She has no concept of time. She cannot remember what we just talked about. She is never immediately sure who her children and grandchildren are. She recognizes faces but persons are a mystery. When I talk to her she understands some of what I say and the rest is meaningless. What we are doing may be understood but it has no connection to what we just did or plan on doing next. Her concerns about her body need to be considered with sensitivity and patience even though they tend to be exaggerated. She often does not hear because her attention is not in proper focus. She often does not understand because she does not hear, can't grasp the meaning, or has lost the first words concentrating on the last. Joking must be simple and non-threatening. A different opinion than hers must be avoided or spoken carefully with assurance hers is certainly valid. Topics of conversation must be simple and kept at an easy level to follow. Explanations of who, what, why or how should be readily available and given in simple, easy to follow sentences.

There are some additional limitations to accept. The paper doilies under ice cream dishes in the dining room are "collector's items." Empty tissue boxes

251

in the lounge area are fair game. Discarded ends cut off 8.5 by 11in. pieces of paper are valued strips from someone's waste basket. Careful adjustment of the sofa pillows after every sitting is a necessity. The line up of matching hair pins is a daily ritual. None of these are insignificant or minor items from Jane's point of view. I have come to accept these more gracefully as part of Jane's current adjustment to her narrowing and harrowing life.

With these realities of Jane's "normal life," she remains a kind, thoughtful, caring woman who is warm in her exchanges with others and as loving toward me as she has always been. I'm learning to adapt to this new partner. I know the other one is gone and will not return. But I find a glimpse of her in the smile Jane gives me when I tell her how much I love her, in the joy of lying close to her in bed, in looking across the table at dinner and seeing the most beautiful woman in the room, in the prayers we say that have been an integral part of our day for many years, in the satisfaction I have holding her hand when we walk together.

A certain pleasant banter takes place between us **when the mood is right**. Jane, "I don't know how you put up with me." Response, "Gladly." Jane, "You are an angel." Response, "I live with one." Jane, "I'm really stupid." Response, "Stop picking on my wife." Jane, "You're a sweetheart." Response, "You have to have one to be one." Jane, "I know I'm crazy." Response, "Crazy in love?"

7/20/11

An example of Jane's difficulties: she was getting ready to go to the Mall. I helped her pick out a pair of white pants and a pink cotton shirt. She put them on and we agreed they looked good. Ten minutes later she had on a different pair of white pants and a checkered black and white shirt. Five minutes later she had on a pair of tan pants and a striped shirt. She said we could not go to the Mall because she could not get ready. When I mentioned lunch here, she wanted to go to the Mall but didn't know what to wear. I said, "Why don't you put on the black pants you always wear?" Now she is dressed like she is every other day, apparently more at ease and ready for the Mall.

Jane complains she has no summer clothes. In fact, she has many that look good. I believe her mind cannot make the switch from winter to summer. When she tries them on, she doesn't look like she expects to look. She can't remember what she looked like in summer clothes. She wants them off as soon as possible and she doesn't want to talk about it.

Since I wrote the above, Jane has been in a storm. On return from the Mall, a staff member stopped me and said my recent article in Vantage Views, a news leaflet done by the residents, was wonderful. She was full of praise and said she cried when she read it. The article has been on one of the bulletin boards for the past ten days. Jane had no idea what the woman was talking about.

She became very angry. "How could you write something for anyone without telling me about it? Why didn't you show me this on the bulletin board? It's here for everyone to read, you wrote it, and I know nothing about it. You have changed recently. What does this mean? What other secrets are there?"

In our apartment I asked her to sit and talk. I said I read the article to her before I submitted it, showed it to her when it was published, and showed it to her on the bulletin board. As I explained this she became increasingly distraught to know her memory was so bad. "I knew I forget things but I never realized I was losing my memory." We talked about other examples of her memory loss. "I can't live this way. I won't live this way. I'll kill myself."

She was unreasonable and unreachable for almost an hour. She described herself as a cripple. I said we both need to be grateful we are not crippled. We see people here every day that can't walk, can't see, can't hear. We walk and go to the Mall. We talk and enjoy being together. We enjoy seeing our beautiful apartment, the trees and sky from our windows, the shops at the Mall. Many people here are alone. We have each other.

I continued. "Alzheimer's is a terrible illness, a tragic handicap. It destroys your memory and causes you to have periods of confusion. It allows your emotions to run away with you at times and drag you around. But it isn't the worst illness in the world. We still do things together and we still enjoy our life. We have to live with it and make the best of it. This is much harder for you than for me. You carry the real burden. I will help you in every way I can. I do not intend to 'put you away somewhere.' I want you to stay here with me and I will get help if I need it to take care of you. But we will be together until one of us dies."

Jane was calmer after we talked and was at ease getting ready for dinner. She was quiet during dinner and seemed preoccupied but we often don't talk much because it is noisy and hard to hear.

On returning to the apartment she came and sat near me. She calmly asked what disease was going to kill her and what did the woman say to me today about when she would die. I was dumbfounded. Where did this come from? I could not have imagined such thoughts were going through her mind during dinner. She believed we "spoke to a small woman" in the Mall or in this building who referred to an illness Jane has that will soon kill her. She believes one of our doctors told me she was dying and I decided not to tell her. "What is the name of my other disease?"

I spent an hour trying to clarify for her. We did not talk to any small woman today about her. We did not talk to anyone who made any reference to death. I have not talked to any doctor without her present. I have no information she is dying. We are not aware of any disease other than Alzheimer's. We are both in good physical health. Alzheimer's is not an illness that will kill her and it is not causing the redness or blotching of her skin nor is it creeping up her legs as she believes it is.

As she began to understand how far afield her worries had taken her, she criticized herself for being stupid. I said her lack of memory, her confusion, and her exaggerated worries took her to where she was. I think she put bits and pieces of the past together in some frightening combination that fits her worry about dying. Worry's emotional components get fired up with no damping influence from reason, and take her off into a dark forest of fear.

When she relaxed and accepted what happened, I encouraged her to tell me when thoughts like these are in her head. "Do not wait until after dinner! Dinner can wait!" As I look back on this day I am relieved the fires were put out, at least temporarily. I think I handled it calmly and I hope wisely. I wonder what happens to an Alzheimer's patient who has no opportunity to talk about distorted thoughts like these.

A note about my comment to Jane that "Alzheimer's is not an illness that will kill you." The Alzheimer's Association would probably take major issue with that statement. The Association states Alzheimer's is the 5th leading cause of death in older age groups. The data I could find indicate the commonest causes of death in these patients are infections from pressure ulcers, urinary tract infections, or pneumonia. These are common causes of death in many old people. Alzheimer's could be considered a contributory cause.

(Article mentioned above from Vantage Views July 2011)

THE DEDICATED

The months of May and June commemorate people in our lives who in some way provided care for us. Mothers are honored in May, fathers in June, and veterans on Memorial Day. It seems appropriate to give thought and honor to other people who now have that role in our lives.

Residents of Vantage House are surrounded by caregivers day after day, week after week. Often when one compliments or expresses gratitude to a staff member, the response is, "But we are family." What a loving expression of their view! "We are family!"

Families typically have disparate members and certainly all of us compose a rather hodgepodge group. But these caregivers in our family manage not just to "put up with us" but to show us kindness to the point of tenderness, responses that go far beyond our spoken need, thoughtful awareness of our limitations, and a keen sense of the pain and sadness we often try to hide from others.

These women and men of Vantage House Staff bring more than just services to this house. They bring consolation to calm our distress, gentleness to soothe our discomfort, patience to restore our strength, faith in us to help us continue to have faith in ourselves. They often reach out to us before we know to ask for help. And when we do ask for help they respond with a grace and generosity that preserves our sense of dignity and leaves intact our faltering pride.

These "employees" are not just employees! They are more than "caregivers!" They are friends! They are not here just for a salary. They could find the same kind of work with persons who are more independently mobile, persons who can hear what is said the first time it is said, persons who recognize them because they can see them, persons who are always in a pleasant mood because they have no pains, no handicaps, no daily fear of what tomorrow will bring. They choose to work with us.

This is a good time to step back a bit from our personal and private anxieties and consider the significance these "friends," these "family members" have in our lives. When I pause to do that, names come flooding into my mind: Travis, Lisa, Karen, Amy, Harold, Chris, Vivian, Musa, Katie, Beulah, Dontre, Ken, Mike, Meriann, Karpo, Marvin, Shirley, Gloria; and the list goes on and on through another fifteen or twenty names. These names have become more important to me than the names of past co-workers, long ago college friends, recent neighbors, and most family members. These are our present, and they have become more important than most people are from out our past.

We are important to them. We are why they are here. However, we must realize those who work here have their own lives, their own cares, and their own feelings. We do not participate directly in their lives as they do in ours. But we are in their feelings and in their thoughts and undoubtedly some of us go home with them at times. We may go home with them because they were touched that day by some exchange we had. We may go home with them one day because they feel uneasy for being unable to comfort and console one of us as they wished they could. We may go home with them a day when they feel satisfied because they were able to make someone here a bit happier, a bit more responsive, a bit more peaceful. And there are times when many go home sad because someone who was here is no longer here. The most difficult task for a caregiver is to face the loss of one to whom they gave care.

Our caregivers face that loss over and over again at Vantage House, and they are unable to share their grief with us as we share our grief with them.

Our caregivers leave behind their worries, their troubles, their bad times and their good times and meet us daily with their gentle, thoughtful presence. They listen to our concerns, our complaints, our conflicts. They accept us on our good days and our bad days and our terrible days. Their being with us somehow lifts our spirits and makes the pain a little less and makes the loneliness not as frightening.

We should think about them often, be grateful for their presence, and honor them for all they do to make our world not just a more livable place but a better place to live.

(Email to Laura 7/24/11)
Mom gets more often and more easily confused. She always interprets it as going crazy. I've been praying she will have peace of mind and heart during these remaining months or years. Then I realized about a week ago that God probably is depending on me to help her achieve the peace I'm praying for. I begin to see her more in the "patient" role and it makes it easier to dedicate my time and my energy to her care. It is strange to feel I'm talking to her as I would if I were her doctor but it does give me a much more objective attitude and makes me realize things she says and does are not directed at me but just a result of her confusion and sadness and fear. Our relationship has changed a little but she is grateful for my added attention. The change helps me realize she is not really able to interact the way we used to and I need to accept that.

(Email to Laura 8/3/11)
Looking forward to seeing you in a few days. Mom has had a couple of pretty bad days. Just seems to get into another world of worry and fear. That usually doesn't last more than a day or two. So I hope she'll be chipper for the visit.

8/11/11

Laura and the girls came Monday evening and left Wednesday after lunch. When we were sitting together Monday evening, I brought them up to date on Jane's present condition. I wanted to summarize the situation for their sake and for Jane's because she was concerned she would do or say something "wrong" or "crazy" while they were here.

I explained with a few examples how poor Jane's memory is. I said when a person can't remember what they just did or what they plan to do next, the person is certain to get terribly confused. "So Gram gets confused and sometimes thinks she is going crazy when that happens. Or she thinks she is being stupid." I explained one area of the brain that deals with feelings is usually controlled by another area of our brain, so feelings don't get out of hand. But those connections in Jane's brain are not working the way they should, "so Gram can have very strong feelings over little things that happen. She can suddenly be very sad or very frightened or very angry. She doesn't want to be that way but the feelings just run away with her and drag her along. Gram worries you may be frightened or not understand if something like that occurs. You don't need to worry. She will be calm again in a short time." I explained Jane worries about doing the wrong thing or saying the wrong thing and others will think she is stupid. "Gram may make mistakes but it is because she gets confused. So they are not really mistakes, she just can't help things like that."

Laura and the girls were attentive but there was little discussion. I don't think there was much new in what I said. Jane was pleased with my comments and added a few of her own. I believe it set a comfortable tone for her during the visit.

We went to the car with them to say our goodbyes and waited to wave as we watched them drive away. Today we talked several times about how wonderful the visit was.

8/13/11

Today is my 92nd birthday and not a terribly happy occasion. Jane had a hard time yesterday. We went to the grocery store, then to Mass and had lunch at the Mall. After we got home Jane asked when the girls would be coming to the apartment. It was difficult to convince her Laura and the girls were gone.

She remained confused throughout the evening. She had a bout of sudden diarrhea after dinner which I was able to tidy up for her. It was a disturbing and embarrassing incident which added to the confusion and sadness she was already experiencing. By bedtime she focused on the tragedy of her illness and the impending doom of her death. We were awake until midnight talking about her fears and her belief she will die within the next few days if not that night.

Things are somewhat tense today. Jane slept until almost eleven. I gave her toast and tea for breakfast. We will maintain a light diet for two or three days to clear up the diarrhea which actually began on 8/11.

(Laura 8/17/11)
The visit was really grand. It worked out as perfectly as anyone could wish. Mom went through a time when she thought you were still here, but she has it pretty straight now. Your last email helped revive some of the details and she and I talk about them.

Mom had a messy bowel problem over the weekend but I kept her on tea and toast for over 48 hrs. and it has cleared up now. Anything like that frightens her because she is convinced it will go right to death. She is doing well these days. She flares up briefly on occasion but if I stay calm and reassuring it goes away quickly

8/30/11
Confusion abounds. There seem to be fewer periods of real clarity for Jane, although she puts up her usual good front. On occasion, she says, "If you knew all the thoughts that go through my head, you would be worried to death." At other times, "My head is empty." She insists she is going crazy. "I've always been a candidate for it." I tell her someone who lived life as fully and as well as she has does not go crazy in their 80's. I also insist people with Alzheimer's do not go crazy. To get confused, to get lost, to not remember, to not know people—yes, but to go crazy—no.

We bought a jigsaw puzzle a few days ago. Jane was in full agreement and enthusiastic about it. We spent a few hours on it. She picks up pieces and looks at them. She often recognizes where they go in the picture but makes no attempt to find related pieces to put together. When she said she could not do it, I did not encourage her to continue. I said I would put the puzzle away because I didn't want to work on it alone. Her reply, "I have lots of projects to do, sewing, and other things, so I'll sit here with you and do them." Of course there are no other projects. The puzzle is back in the box.

8/31/11

Jane's annual visit to the oncologist was today. She was uneasy in the examining room. "They are not going to lock me up, are they? I couldn't live without you. I'm afraid they will see I'm crazy and lock me up. I won't know how to answer their questions." What torture she must go through inside her head! I assured her why we were there and no one was ever going to lock her up and she is not crazy.

The doctor found no indication of cancer but the left breast was enlarged since his exam a year ago. I mentioned our visit to the plastic surgeon last December. The oncologist spoke about the possibility of surgery and likely benefits. He recommended we see the plastic surgeon again, saying her breast might continue to enlarge and be more painful.

Jane was relieved by the visit but understood little of the content. She said she was relieved he did not recommend surgery. My impression was he felt it might be the best course of action but was leaving it up to the plastic surgeon to decide. I told Jane but I doubt she understood. I think she would be fearful of surgery.

At dinner this evening as we sat across from each other, I looked in Jane's eyes. They look the same but I can see she is not there like she used to be. On our usual day I tend to ignore or overlook the devastation her illness has wrought. But every once in a while it comes at me with startling clarity—my Jane is no longer with me—not the Jane I lived with and loved all these years. This is Jane, the handicapped, the Alzheimer's patient, the one I take care of and watch carefully and whose hand I hold so she won't fall. This is Jane whose judgment I cannot trust, whose propriety I cannot depend on, whose dependability I cannot expect, whose companionship I cannot fully find.

9/1/11

In bed last night I spent an hour trying to help Jane understand what the doctor said yesterday. No matter what I said or how often I said it, her final summation was, "If I don't have surgery to remove my breast, I will die of cancer."

Today nothing was mentioned about yesterday. It is as if it never happened. Or is Jane just avoiding the topic because she doesn't want to think about it? What an alternative—topics she doesn't want to think about or topics she can't remember.

I failed to mention how disorienting last week was for Jane. The dining room was closed for new carpeting. We ate buffet meals in the auditorium and the lounge outside the dining room. We did get a table for two. Every meal was anxiety provoking and disorganizing for Jane. The people seemed different, the food seemed different, the environment was markedly different. It was a trying week and left its mark on Jane's shaky sense of stability.

9/7/11

Jane is calmer this week. We have returned to the reassuring regularity of the dining room. I got salad for Jane from the salad bar one evening during the prior week. Now she seems pleased if I get her salad every evening. It is less stressful for her since the many choices at the salad bar only confuse her. She was a bit like the kid in the candy store—get some of everything even though you're not sure what it is. I know what she likes, so getting her salad has become a relief to both of us.

Jane was less irritable the past week. When she does "snap" at me I usually hold her and talk to her a while or I just say I'm sorry and walk away. She soon gets over the irritation and often apologizes for it. I don't get angry but I have a hard time convincing her I'm not. I believe she thinks I should be.

There is a support group for dementia caregivers starting here in October. I doubt I will go. First, it would be difficult for Jane if I was gone for that amount of time. She would be uncomfortable and possibly paranoid if someone stayed with her. Secondly, I don't feel the need for that support. I'm more comfortable with our situation than I was sometime ago. I think I have come to terms with what is happening to Jane and I believe I am becoming more of an "instrument of peace" for her, which brings peace to me.

9/10/11

Lately when we return from our Mall lunch, Jane is often tired and ready to lie down for 30 to 60 minutes of sleep. She is more easily fatigued these days. Is it possibly due to the change of season or to the several gray days we recently had? Or is it just the inevitable progression of the illness? Before getting in bed today she said, "I think it is moving up my spine these days. I get so tired." She continues to believe Alzheimer's is moving up her legs and will eventually immobilize her. On most days we do leg exercises the physical therapist recommended. These and the daily walk from our car through the Mall to the eatery and back should maintain her mobility.

I begin to realize how easily one day blends into the next. There is almost no variation in our schedule. I feel like I have a part in a play with each day demanding a repeat performance. At the same time, each day is a completely new show for Jane.

Yesterday we looked at pictures from our many visits to the Montana ranch to see my brother, Don, and his wife, Helen. Jane was deeply impressed by the pictures of the sky, the mountains, the sunrises and sunsets. I have asked our kids to combine our ashes and send them to my nephew in Montana to be buried near my parents and Don and Helen. I have not discussed this recently with Jane. Nor will I. Death is not a topic for discussion any more. She would never have wanted to live in Montana but I know our ashes will be at peace with my family and with the beauty and peace of the landscape.

9/19/11

Conversation with Jane becomes increasingly difficult. Two or three hour talks at lunch or sitting at home are less frequent, unless we are talking about her symptoms. The change is difficult for Jane because "words" are a mainstay of her life. Small talk is quickly exhausted . . . . the weather, the leaves turning colors, the number of baby carriages in the Mall, their great variety, and on and on. The repetition of topics seems not to bother her. The silence is not difficult for me but I feel pressed to make conversation because of her need. Words are one of the few connections she has with the world around her. They are a form of touch for her . . . comforting, reassuring.

Jane rarely mentions the children. When Kathie called last evening to say she was coming, it took several prompts for Jane to realize who Kathie is. The fading of faces and of the persons they belong to is becoming more apparent. I know she is frightened by these changes because they warn her of "how things will be."

We just returned from the Mall. We must go 350 days of the year. What is monotony for me is stability for Jane. It is small sacrifice for me when it provides her with so much . . .fashions to see and comment on in stores and in windows, people of different races and ages and dress to observe, activity all around her that does not draw her in or make demands on her. Occasionally she says it must be a sacrifice for me and it is good of me to take her so often. That's a bit of insight too, but I tell her I enjoy going to the Mall with her. I do! What is good for her is good for me!

9/20/11

For the second night in a row, Jane began getting out of bed to go to the bathroom without waking me. I woke and accompanied her with her objection. "I can do this on my own." I worry and wonder how to manage this. Before going to sleep Jane promises to wake me. During the night she is obviously reluctant to do so.

We talked about it at lunch today. She insists she doesn't remember getting up and has a hard time believing she goes to the bathroom each night. She doesn't accept that she has been doing it for years. I am convinced her night time lethargy prevents these forays from being captured in her memory. In spite of the lethargy I believe there is a cell in her brain with a big sign, a night light, saying, "Don't wake Robbie. He needs his sleep." It is difficult to deal with this when Jane cannot understand the reason for my concern.

9/23/11

A few days ago we had the worst clash-period we have had in a long time. I took some summer clothes out of Jane's closet to make room for winter clothes from storage. I offered to place the clothes on the bed for her to see them before I put them away but she was uncooperative. I proceeded without her acceptance and said it had to be done.

She mentioned the incident several times. The other evening she brought it up and would not let it go. She became increasingly irritated and agitated. It went on for three hours. She was loud and threatened to leave the apartment but made no move to do so. I kept "defending myself," as she called it, by telling her summer was over and we needed to have the winter clothes available. I must have said a dozen times, "Summer is over."

She took the summer clothes I had boxed up and put them back in the closet. She was "going to iron the shirts to wear them for the summer." She was furious, in tears, attacking everything I said, hating me for "being so cruel." At some point, I said again, "Summer is over." This time she heard it.

She was shattered. "I was so stupid to go on and on the way I did. I can't believe I could be so wrong. Why didn't you tell me that before?" The whole scene was different when the seasonal change became real. It was tragic to spend three hours in bitterness and hostility only because her brain did not compute those simple words I repeatedly said, "Summer is over." How many more times will we clash because her brain does not recognize the meaning of words I say or words others say? How much sadness, fear, and anger will result from this deficiency? I must be attentive and, if I can, avoid this problem at all costs for her sake and my own. On the other hand, how can it be avoided?

9/28/11

"It's terrible to go for so long without knowing anything. I think there should at least be an intermission sometimes. I feel like an empty shell. Do you think a person can die from not knowing?" Remarks Jane made as we were getting ready for bed. To some of her comments, I often say, "I know. I know." Tonight I said, "I don't know. I can't begin to know. I can't imagine what it is like for you." She said, "I know I am such a burden for you." I took her in my arms and said, "You are not a burden and you never will be a burden for me. You are the one who carries the burden. I'm privileged to be with you. My faint idea of how difficult life is for you makes me sad. Your thinking is not like it used to be but your love is the same and that will never change."

We saw Jane's plastic surgeon today, the one who did breast implants after her cancer surgery in September 1999. He noted the enlargement of her left breast and suggested the option of surgery to remove the implant and traumatized tissue. Without surgery the breast will continue to enlarge and could be life threatening. Surgery is scheduled next Tuesday.

Jane was relieved by the decision and I believe it was clearly the right decision. She had repeated questions throughout the afternoon. She thought I might get weary of answering the same questions over and over. I assured her she can ask any question as often as she wants, and since she may not remember what I tell her, ask again and again and again.

"I feel lost. I don't know what I'm doing. I was accepting the 'forgetting,' but then I pick up something in my hand and when I look at it I don't know why I picked it up. I don't know what to do with it or what it is for." A comment Jane made before getting in bed. We spent thirty minutes talking about her memory loss and how difficult it makes life for her. She said she appreciates being able to talk to me about it. It becomes less frightening for her. I told her how remarkably well she is managing her life considering how fragmented and uncertain every moment must be. She said during the day everything comes to her in separate little pieces. Life is not a continuum for her. It is not a running film but a series of separate, often blurred or incomplete snapshots she has to try to put together in the right sequence if possible.

10/2/11

Jane continues to do well in anticipation of surgery. Talking to Laura on the phone yesterday she got confused and thought one of the girls was having surgery. Laura told me about the confusion. After the call, I talked with Jane. "I'm so stupid. I can't understand how I could get so confused." I held her and said how confusing all of life must be at times and it is amazing she is able to keep anything straight. She relaxed and that seemed to end it.

I enjoyed Jane's reaction at the lab when the phlebotomist prepared to draw her blood. The woman looked at Jane's arm where there is no indication of available blood vessels. She said, "You don't have much by way of veins." Jane answered, "Well, the ones I have are certainly willing." It is the kind of humor she exhibits with medical personnel when they are about to cause some pain or discomfort.

She deals well with the pain medical procedures cause but she readily complains about some minor ache or irritation. Her legs hurt when she walks; her teeth hurt when she brushes them; her back hurts when she gets up from a chair. These are all "sometimes" complaints. I believe any unusual sensation in her body alerts her to Alzheimer's and becomes a warning signal of an unknown but frightening future. With medical procedures she knows the source of the pain and tolerates it well. Pain without her knowing the cause is threatening and easily exaggerated.

(Email to Laura 10/04/11)
Just a quick note to let you know how mom is doing. She got rather frantic last evening and was very concerned about the surgery. I think most of it was related to what she should take with her—and that's always a problem. The solution was simple, but not for Mom. No jewelry, no make-up, and loose clothing. But for Mom it was much more complex.* * * * * *

Home from the hospital, Mom agreed to lie down and sleep. Once she saw the drain with blood in it she started complaining about pain. I think that was the cause of increased pain. More fear than physical pain. She went to sleep quickly.

10/05/11
Surgery went well yesterday with two hours of anesthesia. Recovery room took about three hours and I was with her when she woke. The surgeon said there was a large hematoma in her breast, probably from an injury a year or more ago. She had no injuries I was aware of, so it must have occurred during a fall in the bathroom. She had a couple of bad falls with a skinned knee once and a bump on the back of her head another time.

Today she mentions pain at the surgical site but declines pain medicine. She remembers little of yesterday. At one point she became very talkative and went on for almost an hour telling about dreams she had. Some of it was bizarre. "I walked through the Mall with a head hanging from a string. We invited a lot of people to our apartment, and because it was so crowded we hung pieces of furniture from the ceiling. My grandmother came to visit us. My mother came to visit." She enjoyed telling the stories and sounded intoxicated.

Today has been much different. Jane had a difficult time walking this morning. She stumbled and nearly fell repeatedly. I kept a hand on her most of the time.

After breakfast she seemed surer of herself. We planned to go to the Mall but we could not because she was too unsteady. We had dinner delivered.

(Email to Laura 10/07/11)
Mom is having a bad week. Easily confused. Awake a couple of hours last night while I tried to convince her surgery is over and she still has both breasts. She is wearing a surgical bra and won't have it off until she sees the doc next Tuesday. So she has not had a view of the result.

Walking is difficult and talking is very slurred. She gets angry if I ask what she said. She is back to my needing hearing aids. We haven't been to the Mall since surgery because her walking is so bad. When we talked about it yesterday she seemed to agree it's all in her head. Some of this may result from the anesthesia but I think most of it is just the stress of the week—nothing has been regular or routine. We got down to dinner for the first time last night. May go to Mall today if she is walking better. That might be an incentive for her to put more effort into it. But I don't want to get her over there and have difficulty getting her back home.

10/08/11
The past few days were difficult. Nothing pleased Jane. Everything displeased her. She was irritable, accusing me of being angry. "You look angry. I know you are angry. I can see it on your face." There was a point when I showed some irritation over her incessant comments about me being angry. I worry about her, her slurred speech, her unsteady gait, her uncooperative and hostile manner. She certainly sees that on my face.

By bed time last night I was very worried because of her deterioration. Her speech was garbled and slurred. She put no effort into being understood and became irritated when I asked her to repeat. Her gait was worse than unsteady. She looked like she was about to fall. She had difficulty putting clothes on or getting them off. She couldn't find anything but would not ask for help. She resented my intrusion if I tried to help.

Throughout the day she complained of pain in her legs when she moved, about the drain in her breast, about her loss of memory, about the things she can no longer do, about the television, about my anger, about not being able to hear me. Whenever my voice is low, she doesn't just ask me to repeat; she

267

gets very angry. "I can never hear you. Don't you know that? I have to ask you 'what, what, what' all day long."

Before I went to sleep last night I felt very sad. My thought was, "I wish we could both die soon and have all this over." I was lonely. Jane slept almost three hours during the day. I felt very alone during that time, abandoned, perhaps a bit resentful of the situation, and blaming her, I suppose, for my misery.

Today was a much better day. I made a conscious shift in attitude. I had forgotten my attitude of seeing Jane as a patient I am caring for. I slipped back to the expectation she should be my companion, my partner, my close ally, friend, and confidant. In this latter role she is, sadly enough, a failure, because Alzheimer's has taken those qualities away from her and from me. She is my patient again, as she was 50 years ago when I first met her in my psychiatric practice. Now she is part of me, of my life, my well being. At times I try to see her in a patient role so I can keep a clearer and healthier perspective for myself and more realistic expectations for her.

We had an excellent day today. We went to the Mall for lunch, the first time in five days. This time the store windows had really changed. Her walking was never mentioned. She walked more naturally, more freely than she has in weeks. Her speech was clearer and she seemed to put more effort into talking clearly. Her thinking was clearer. She had no significant complaints. After we got home, she readily accepted my invitation to exercise. That's the first time she has been in the exercise room in three weeks.

Last night I checked the calendar to see when our appointment is with the neurologist. I was concerned about her gait and repeated complaints about her legs. For months she has talked about "it" coming up her legs. In the beginning "it" was in her ankle, then "it" was in her knees, then her thighs, and yesterday "it" was in her waist area. In an attempt to allay her fears I suggest it may be rheumatism and mention Tylenol as a possible aid. She never asks to take any. The other day during a rather candid talk about "it," she said it may all be in her head and therefore a sure sign "I'm going crazy." There have been times when she acknowledged that "it" was Alzheimer's. Today I became less anxious to see the neurologist.

I'm not sure what "it" is but I know it was not prominent in her mind or in her legs today. Now that the last few days are over I feel light and free, relieved and happy. It was a good day. I know bad days will come and I will again be staring at the bleakness of yesterday. I must remember Jane's instability of mood, activity, and responsiveness. And I must remember all that she has been and find it again in this woman I cherish.

(Laura 10/09/11)
Another quick note. Wanted you to know that yesterday and today have been much better for Mom. We went to the Mall for lunch yesterday and today. Just got home. Mom is walking better than she has been in some time. Speech is clearer. Mood is improved. We had a long talk at lunch about her Alzheimer's and the confusion she has. I try to convince her she is not going insane; she is confused. Went over what will happen to her "things" when either of us dies. Explained all of what I have sent to you before. She understood and seemed greatly relieved. But of course she will forget and wonder again.

But she is back to where she was before the surgery so I couldn't ask for anything better than that. We went down to exercise yesterday and going again today. That was the first time she has been down to the exercise room in two or three weeks.

10/12/11
We had the follow-up visit to the plastic surgeon yesterday. He removed the drain from Jane's breast and said everything looks fine. We return next week for a repeat check of the site. Jane was greatly relieved and the rest of the day went well.

This morning we rose at seven so I could go to the barber early. Jane stays alone. I leave a large note saying where I am, the time I will be back, and my cell phone number. I turn on all the lights and make the coffee before I go. Each time we do this, she assures me it will be fine. And each time when I return, she is edgy, a bit confused and disappointed she "didn't get a lot done." Soon after I was home she complained of severe pain at the surgical site. I gave her a Tylenol and said if it did not give her relief I would give her a pain pill. The pain was never mentioned again.

She planned on taking a shower and washing her hair but was reluctant to do so because of the surgery. I encouraged her to go ahead with the plan. I have no doubt apprehension and anxiety were the cause of the "pain" she had this morning. She feels unsure of herself today. During the past two weeks, the preparation, the surgery, and the follow-up markedly increased the uncertainty in her life. She has done well to maintain the fragile stability she has.

Two nights ago we attended one of the music programs which Vantage House regularly provides. Dale Jarrett played the piano and sang. We have attended several of his performances. On several occasions I requested he sing "What Now My Love." He was prepared this time and did a beautiful rendition of the song. It is a very special song for us. Jane was delighted and for her it brought back feelings of our past but without the attached memories. We decided to send Dale a copy of Jane's book. I enclosed the following letter to him.

Dear Dale,   10/11/11
After your concert last evening Jane was delighted to send you a copy of her book. We wanted some way to acknowledge your gift in bringing "What Now My Love" back into our lives.

We first heard it when we danced to the music in the Sheppard Room of the Drake Hotel in New York City in our courting days. The words were in French but we fell in love with the melody which seemed to express the powerful, dramatic affection we feel for each other. Sometime later when we heard the words in English, they only confirmed the depth and permanence of our bond because the words told us what we both knew, without our love there would be nothing else. They were not sad then.

Jane was ecstatic hearing the song last night. It did not bring back memories to her because she has almost no memories of our 50 years together. But the music brought back the feelings of those years for her. It was beautiful. I never felt sad before when I heard the song because it confirmed our dedication to each other. Last night the words put me where I am going; they helped me face the loss that is already there and becoming greater as the weeks go on.

Please, continue to play "our song." The music will bring Jane the feelings of commitment and union we have shared through the years. The words will help me work through the grieving that is with me daily.

Jane never wants to play any of our CD's. The music by itself disturbs her in some way—like she doesn't know how to feel about it or what to think about it. I don't know where her mind goes when she hears a CD. They trouble her. Your music is different for her. You are there. She can see the person doing it. She can identify with it all. Others in the room give it a background so it makes sense for her to be there and hear you. She stays with it, and somehow it is right.

10/13/11

We rarely have long talks these days but yesterday we talked two hours at our Mall lunch. It was about Alzheimer's and Jane's mental processes. She said she is sorry for all the mistakes she makes and wants to do better. She also sees herself as stupid when it takes her so long to get ready to go anywhere or do anything.

I took the position that she does not make mistakes. She does as well as she is able to do. She said the outcome is still the same because it turns out not to be right and she is to blame. I took a rather far fetched example for my argument. As a result of a stroke, a man at Vantage House uses a wheel chair. I said, "Do you think Ed is wrong when he sits in the wheel chair because he should get up and walk to dinner? Is he making a mistake? Is he to blame for not walking to dinner?" Jane said it was not the same. I commented, "You have a lame brain. It is not a blame brain. You function as well as you can. When you can't do something because of your illness, there is no mistake, no stupidity, and no blame." I think she understood my point and accepted it.

She said she sometimes makes up things in her head and thinks they really happened. I said I noted that. I started thinking about how my mind works in contrast to hers. In my thinking I am constantly referring to the past, a few minutes ago, earlier today, yesterday, or perhaps some time ago. There is always that reference point in my thoughts. Jane does not have that base. Her mind is working; she is awake, alert. So what goes on? Is it only what is in front of her now that gets taken in—all by itself? What can she do with it? What does it mean to her? It has no background, no depth, no fullness. Does her mind try to give it depth and meaning by grabbing onto bits and pieces of her world lying around in the corners of her mind? Thus, the stories. I discussed the idea with her and she seemed to understand and agree.

Jane feels she is doing much worse than she did a few weeks ago. I agreed she is having a difficult time but I pointed out important background for it. The past two weeks were very busy, very focused on arrangements, very anxiety and fear provoking. We saw the surgeon and decided to have the surgery. There was the physical exam, the EKG, the lab work, the anticipation of the surgery, the surgery, the aftermath with the drain and the suction bulb pinned to her bra for a week, and finally the return visit to the surgeon. Busy times, scary times for her. Our routines were disrupted. We missed going to Mass for two weeks; we missed going to the Mall for five days; we missed going down to dinner two evenings. She accepted what I was saying and seemed to relax a little.

At one point Jane mentioned getting another lipstick. "The one I have won't come off." We have been over this many times. I said calmly, "Sweetheart, the lipstick does come off. I showed you on your hand and on mine it comes off easily with a tissue. We have been over this many times, and that's ok. It seems an idea gets stuck somewhere in your brain like a bug hiding out for winter in some cozy spot. No matter how many times we go over it, the idea remains and pops out when lipstick comes to your mind. My love, we can go over this as many times as it happens. It doesn't upset me and I hope it won't upset you. We can also get you a new lipstick anytime you want." The remarks seemed to impress her but only the future will tell.

Jane again mentioned how "it" is moving up her legs. She acknowledged she thinks "it" is going to kill her and she does associate it with Alzheimer's. I again told her people do not die of Alzheimer's. They may die of problems related to having Alzheimer's. That is not the same as directly dying of cancer or a stroke. I don't know what "it" is but there is no reason to see it related to death.

As our talk ended Jane said how good it was to be able to talk about things she has in her head. Her remark reminded me we had close friends who met the problem of Alzheimer's quite differently. The husband told me they never used the "A" word in front of his wife. Alzheimer's was never mentioned to or discussed with her. I can't imagine what it would be like for someone with the illness not to have an opportunity to talk about it. Our frequent discussions of what goes on in Jane's mind must be of benefit to her in dealing with the disease. It also benefits me because it increases my awareness and understanding of her experience and helps me accommodate better to her needs.

Jane asks what I think the future will be like for her. I say I truly don't know, but I expect she will be less able to identify people she knows or even know she knows them. I expect she will be more confused at times. I think she will always know me and she may continue to know the children who visit often. I think we will continue going to the Mall for a long time so it is important to continue our exercises. We have no reason to think she will become difficult or "a monster" as time goes on. She is a loving, gentle woman. That is who she is. Her brain may deteriorate but her heart will always be full of the love that has always been there. She may become bedridden at some time. If that happens I will get an aide to help with anything I am unable to do for her. She was reassured by my comments.

(Email to Paul 10/13/11)
As always your visit was most welcome. It is always great to see you, and Mom gets a great deal of satisfaction from your visits. * * * * * *
I wanted to tell you about a remarkable conversation we had during lunch today. It was a total surprise to me. Mom's thoughts were as follows: she made a fool of herself when you left last night because you were ready to go and she brought up something that delayed you. She worried I was mad at her over what she said and over delaying your departure. She was afraid to talk to me about it, because she thought I was angry. She went to bed sad, cried in bed and had a difficult time going to sleep. This morning she worried I would be angry and was relieved when I was not. She never intended to talk about this to me.

As you may recall, she mentioned her surgery when you were ready to leave. She felt stupid for doing so and was embarrassed. She remembered my saying, "We already talked about your surgery." She felt like a little girl being told, "Be quiet now Jane. You're talking too much." She decided, as you left, you were thinking, "What a stupid, mixed up person." I said I thought you may have been thinking the same thing I was, "How sad Mom forgets so quickly what we talked about."

It seemed so sad Mom would go through 16 hours of worrying I was angry, and that you wouldn't want to come back, and that she had been stupid, etc, etc. She said it was a wonderful visit and she ruined it all. I told her I was going to drop you an email and tell you about her thoughts.

This sort of thing happens sometimes and she doesn't tell me about it until much later. I tell her over and over she should mention things like this to me so we can get them straight in her head. She eventually tells me when something like this happens. Of course, there may be times she never mentions and they end up with all the other forgotten memories. But what a horrible life it would be for her if she kept all of it bottled up inside. Sixteen hours was bad enough.

Just thought I'd pass this on so you are aware of her thinking. I talked about her Alzheimer's when you were here and I do that with you and Kathie and Laura. I want her to feel it is an open subject with all of us and I think she feels that way and is comfortable with it. Your visits are always welcome and are a tremendous support for both of us.

10/20/11
The above email was sent to Paul the day after the event in question. I think we finally cleared it up today, one week later. I don't usually include email others write to us but I'm going to include most of the email Paul wrote to Jane.

(Paul to Jane 10/13/11)
* * * * * *

I am heartbroken to think you felt burdened with thoughts you could have possibly done anything to keep me away. I treasure the bond you and I have. It is so helpful and meaningful in my life that I feel your love with me everyday. There is NOTHING you can say or do that can stop me from loving you. I hope you won't ever have that thought again. One of the things I hate most about the Alzheimer's disease is that it allows you to think about things in a way that can make you feel so isolated from the people that love you. The forgetfulness is certainly a difficult part of the

disease but it never stands between us in any way. I don't care if you tell me something you've already told me before, or if you get some details mixed up about something that happened, because I always know I have YOU with us. I never have any thoughts you are 'mixed up' or doing anything 'foolish'. I know Alzheimer's is taking away some of your memories and you may not have all the details of everything that happens but it never occurs to me it keeps you and I from having our special 'connection'.
* * * * * *

I thought the letter spoke clearly and lovingly to Jane's concern. I copied it and read it to her the evening it came. She was relieved and accepted gladly what Paul wrote.

Two days later, she spoke about ruining the evening when Paul visited and making a fool of herself. I reminded her of Paul's letter and that Paul and I both knew she forgot we talked about her surgery soon after Paul arrived. Since we knew she did not remember, there was nothing wrong with her mentioning it before Paul left. I apologized for my comment to her and said I should have been gentler, reached out and touched her, perhaps put my arm around her and said, "Sweetheart, you forgot we spoke about this when Paul first came."

She was not satisfied that everything was really all right. She said, "I think Paul's letter did not respond to my concerns. I think he is still angry and may not ever come again to visit." I could not change her thinking.

Last evening she exploded at me over some unimportant little thing. I apologized and left the room as I often do now. Then I heard her crying and asking me to come back. I went back and put my arms around her and talked to her. Before long it became obvious the evening of Paul's visit was still the major issue. I again read his letter slowly to her emphasizing his expressed feelings.

She listened attentively. "I find it hard to believe this is the same letter you read to me the other day. It sounds entirely different. I was so wrong not to be satisfied when you first read it." We talked about how things get stuck in her head and how difficult it can be to dislodge them no matter how wrong they are.

Today during lunch Jane mentioned again how she ruined the evening of Paul's visit. She said she broke into his conversation and took over so she could tell her story about her surgery. We went over the entire matter one more time. It was not a mistake. Nothing was ruined. No one was angry. Paul left in good spirits. They kissed and hugged goodbye in the usual way. All was well. I mentioned Paul's email. We again spoke of things sticking in her head. She agreed and my impression was the entire event was now in a more accurate perspective and will remain there.

It is recommended caregivers avoid arguing with Alzheimer's patients because it is a losing situation. I agree whole heartedly. But it suggests Alzheimer's patients can't acknowledge they are wrong. At this point in time, nine or ten years into her illness, there are times of such clarity for Jane she can recognize and acknowledge situations when she was not only wrong but was adamant and hostile about it.

I say "nine or ten years into her illness," when I previously dated it as beginning eight years ago. I've done a lot of thinking about a number of events in the two years before we moved here, events that suggest Alzheimer's was under way. She would become unreasonable about something or take a position on something quite out of character. There were two or three occasions when she was with one or two of our children and later reported to me behaviors on their part that seemed very unlikely to have occurred. There were times when she was very forgetful and would jokingly comment, "Must be my Alzheimer's." Now, I believe it was.

Jane sometimes tells one or another of the women residents she would like to get together and visit. She has tried such visits but the result is not good. On her own, Jane is unable to maintain a conversation. She doesn't remember what she wants to say and can't expand even on a simple subject. Later she can't remember what she said or what they talked about. She decides she behaved in a stupid manner and is embarrassed. Jane only talks about "getting together" but never refers to it again when we are alone.

10/24/11
The days go by and each one is much like the last. I think of the stability, the relatively slow progression of Jane's illness. From what I have read and heard it strikes me this course is rather unusual. I wonder what accounts for her

current functioning after these past eight or nine years. I mention things I believe contribute to her present state.

1) Her medicines must be a factor in slowing her decline. She takes two medicines for memory loss: Galantamine 24mg daily and Namenda 10mg twice daily. She takes two antidepressants: Venlafaxine 225mg and Fluoxetine 20mg daily. She takes Risperidone 0.25mg twice daily, and Alprazolam 1.5mg nightly for sleep. In addition she takes Pravachol 40mg daily for high cholesterol.

2) Staff members and other residents at Vantage House are a tremendous support to both of us. Many of them go out of their way to greet Jane, to say a cheerful word to her, to ask of her well being. Brief contacts are encouraging to Jane. We avoid lengthy interactions because these are typically stressful.

3) Avoiding stressful situations has helped Jane maintain a generally level mood in spite of occasional Alzheimer's storms. We have done this in a variety of ways which are mentioned in these notes.

4) Our religious beliefs and practices are helpful. Our faith not only maintains us but strengthens us in the face of the illness. We are aware of God's presence in our lives and frequently pray together. We each speak of talking to God during the day. We try to attend midday Mass twice each week. Together we say our morning prayers, a blessing before each meal, and night prayers. I recently began saying the Rosary daily. I have a list of about 170 saints (alphabetized) whom I petition during my exercises and getting to sleep at night. I don't get to them all each day if I don't exercise or if I fall asleep too quickly. I also identify and pray for about two hundred deceased relatives and friends, asking for their aid.

(As an aside, I should explain about the saints. About ten years ago, I began naming saints as a method of getting to sleep. I took them alphabetically, men and women. Initially I probably put together 30 or 40 as I went through the alphabet. Over the years the number increased until I have saints for every letter, some letters with ten or more. So I go from, "St. Albert, pray for us" to "Saint Zita, pray for us." I usually do about 75 while I exercise. I finish the others getting to sleep at night. They are great sleep aids.)

5) Going to the Mall almost every day is a positive experience for Jane and generally helps to clear negative thoughts and moods from her mind. I often mentioned this positive effect and the reasons for it. Routine brings calm and nourishment to her spirit.

6) Jane's attachment to the three children who put considerable effort into a continued close relationship is salutary. Laura's visits with her two daughters are the highlight of our life. They live in upper New Jersey so two or three visits a year is all they can do. Paul and Kathie are regular in their welcome visits. Paul and Jane are mother and son now, at Paul's request some time ago.

7) Our love for one another is, I believe, unusual. I have mentioned how often people, strangers and friends, speak to us about what a loving couple we are. People at Vantage House, strangers in the Mall, clerks in stores, people in church or on the street approach us and comment on our obvious attachment. It is a fairy tale relationship, only it is true. I tell Jane, "You fill me up." This relationship, deep, sensitive, and complete helps us through the turmoil of Alzheimer's as this writing shows.

8) Jane's deeply religious and strongly determined spirit is a key element in her adjustment to the illness. She survived a difficult childhood and a difficult first marriage. As she came to a time in life when she was free to be herself with the support and encouragement of one who loved her as I do, her inspiring strength blossomed. That spirit fed our years together and remains a key factor in her coping with Alzheimer's.

9) I learned some things and made some adjustments these years. I came to know more clearly my need for Jane, my need for her love, my need for her companionship. I have learned the pain of patience, the power of love, the value of another self.

10) We talk about the illness, about what goes on in Jane's mind, about our interactions with one another and the complications forced into our lives. These talks and our attitude about Alzheimer's keep the illness out of the shadows and help lessen the sadness and fear that must easily and quickly overwhelm Alzheimer's patients.

I would not try to prioritize these items. All are important. Would Jane's Alzheimer's be worse today if anyone of these was not present? Who is to say? In spite of all these factors I know the inexorable course of the disease will continue to make life more difficult for Jane and be with her until death.

(Email to Laura 10/24/11)
Sorry we missed your call yesterday. After lunch we drove out to the monastery where we had gone to Mass for a couple of years. They have a replica of the grotto of Lourdes and some beautiful outdoor Stations of the Cross. Occasionally on a nice day we drive out and sit on a bench by the grotto. It is peaceful and quiet. A nice place to chat about things different than what we think of in the Mall. The other day Mom said if she dies before I do, she will meet me there.

10/30/11
Had a return bout of jealousy last evening. A woman we both know stopped at our table in the dining room, greeted Jane with a kiss, asked how she was, and said she was happy to see her. When she spoke to me, I mentioned something about the parish we both belong to. She is a devout Catholic. She proceeded to tell me about different churches in the area and novenas, Masses and other services they have. We have known this woman for years because her mother was a resident here and the daughter visited her every day. Her husband greeted us as they went by. They were dinner guests of another resident.

After they passed Jane asked how we knew her and I explained the above. I mentioned the woman was a friend of a doctor whom I knew in my residency program. I said we see her occasionally at weekday Mass.

When we returned to our apartment I thought everything was fine. I asked Jane if she would like to watch a movie. "I will not do anything with you until we get this matter settled. I want to know what your relationship is with that woman. Why did she stop and talk to you and never say a word to me? Why was she flirting with you? Where have you seen her? How long have you known her? What were you talking about? Did you ever go out with her?"

I was totally surprised by the outburst. I put my arms around her and said, "My love, my love, you are very mixed up about this. We have known this woman several years because she came here often to care for her mother before the mother died. I never saw her when you were not present. I never knew her in the past. She is a friend of a doctor I knew in my residency. They are both from Cuba. She greeted you and kissed you when she passed our table. You heard what she was saying to me. She was telling me about religious services in this area. You are confused about all of this. You know you are my true love, my one and only love."

We sat together and talked for some time. Jane acknowledged how wrong she was and went on. "I have done this in the past and I was determined it wouldn't happen again. But I keep doing it and I'll always keep doing it. I know there was no reason for it." I said "This is another example of how a feeling runs away with you and sort of drags you where you don't want to go. It is because of the Alzheimer's but we don't need to worry about it. We always work it out. It never destroys or even weakens our love for each other, and it never will, no matter how often it happens. So don't be afraid it might happen again. If it does, we can deal with it as we did now. It is not going to lessen our love for each other or change our relationship in any way."

I am aware of the avalanche of Jane's jealousy and I am usually quite conscious of it in our contacts with younger women, especially if they are outgoing and friendly. I deliberately minimize my exchange with them to avoid these ideas on Jane's part. It is a reminder for me that Jane's life has mysterious byroads, perilous paths, hazardous turns leading to pain and unhappiness so easily. I am again reminded of the prayer of St. Francis: "Lord, make me an instrument of your peace."

10/31/11

I thought the matter of Paul's visit ten days ago was settled. Jane brought it up last evening and we talked about it for two hours. Jane continues to have hurt feelings about the incident but in her usual fashion blames herself for "jumping on both of you to tell my story. Who would be interested in my surgery anyway? Why should I intrude with such a story?" I explained the situation to her as I have before and again read Paul's email to her. It was obvious we still had not reached some hurtful piece of it. Then I finally discovered the real issue. The offensive element of the episode was my saying to Jane, "We already talked about your surgery."

That statement was a put-down. There is no way around it. I defended my statement each time we talked about the incident. "What else could I have done? I should have been more delicate in how I said it, but it needed to be said. It would have been embarrassing for you if you began telling Paul about your surgery when we had already talked about it." I finally got the picture. Jane was angry and hurt by what I said, not by anything else. There was no other abuse or assault, just that. But her angry feeling spread over the scene and she decided Paul was angry at her. And I was angry at her because she spoke out of turn and was to blame for it all. Of course she was also angry at herself because that's what her feelings do.

The reality of the incident became clear to me. Why should I stop her from telling something we already talked about? What harm was there in that? She often repeats things she told me before. I am patient and happy to hear the same thing as many times as she wants to mention it. I feel her spirit had been crying out for justice.

How long would it have taken her to retell her surgery story? She would have recounted a few items and let me fill in the rest. Five minutes! Ten minutes at most! Paul was not desperate to leave. He would have gladly waited and heard it all. How thoughtless of me! How shortsighted! I thought I was protecting Jane from herself. I need to protect her from me and the tight little world I try to make for her. If she retold the story would she be embarrassed if she realized we already talked about it? Maybe a little embarrassed but not hurt and criticized and humiliated by the comment I made.

I gained an important insight last evening. Why did it take me so long? If someone doesn't want to hear her repeat a story, they will deal with it in their own way. Everyone knows she has Alzheimer's. I'm sure they will be gentler than I was.

11/01/11

We went to noon Mass today. It is the Feast of All Saints, a holyday, so there was a Sunday crowd. After the service I noted Jane had more trouble walking.

During lunch I asked if the morning was difficult for her. She responded, "It took my strength away." Such a precise and accurate comment! That's exactly what stress does to her. The crowd, the music, different procedures and prayers were confusing and highly stressful. This is what happened in the past when we attended Sunday Mass. This is the kind of stress we should avoid when we can. It was a reminder of what not to do.

The stress causes anxiety; the anxiety causes tightness in her muscles; the tightness causes her to walk differently; the difficulty in walking causes her to be concerned she has a major debility in her legs. We talked about it. "The doctor told me the problem in my ankles would go up my legs to my waist and I would be unable to walk." I asked, "What doctor?" "The doctor that examined my breast and did the surgery." I said, "That doctor never examined your legs and never mentioned anything about them." "Do you think I made it all up?" I replied, "No, I think the muscles in your legs get tense when you are under stress and then you feel something is wrong with them. I don't think there is any disease in your legs, and I don't think Alzheimer's is causing what you feel." Coming back home, Jane walked considerably better.

It is possible Jane has increasing difficulty recognizing the relationship of her body to her immediate environment. One might question if her proprioceptive sensations (which respond to position and movement) are neurologically impaired from the Alzheimer's. In addition Alzheimer's destructive course may have an effect on voluntary movements. The marked variation in her gait does seem connected to her degree of distress, her mood, and her sense of emotional stability.

(Email to Laura 11/02/11)
* * * * * *

I have noticed my mood changes sometimes. I can be feeling very positive and then some little thing seems to bring a cloud over everything. Probably in the background of it all is concern about the future and, as Mom would say, how things are going to be. There is really nothing else to do but try to make the best of the day and see what happens down the road.

I decided the other day there have been three great women in my life. The first was my mother. She was a gentle, kind woman, probably the most charitable person I ever knew. Never a gossip, never critical of anyone, always a positive word for others. The second was Mom. She has been and still is the best possible companion I could ever have wished for. She has always been right there beside me, helping me, encouraging me, and showing a spirit that continues to be remarkable these days. The third is my daughter, Laura. She has the gift of enthusiasm which certainly has been tested at times and still is tested. She has her grandmother's and her mother's strength of character. She is bright like both of them, responsive to others, and has a sense of the true values in life. And she has a natural and profound sense of motherhood, as did her mother and grandmother.

11/05/11

We went to the Mall for lunch. Jane has increasing difficulty getting ready. I get her clothes out and put them on the bed. She manages better than one would expect based on her current limitations. She couldn't find her faux diamond ring. I took a quick look through her bathroom and various other places. It was not to be found. I was hoping she would forget the loss before we left because I anticipated she would not be able to go until the ring was found.

We were ready to go. "There is something I can't find but I can't remember what it is." I asked if it was the ring. "Yes, that's it." I told her I had looked but would look again. The first thing I did was take a clock off a shelf in her bathroom and there was the ring. We might have looked for days and never moved that clock. It was the most unlikely spot she could have used. It's actually hard for me not to believe St. Anthony (the finder of lost objects) or my mother (a regular petitioner of St. Anthony) was not involved.

Jane's comment, "I put it there so I would remember where it was." My response, "When you put something down, please put it where it can be seen because you will not remember where you put it." How many times have I said that same thing!

Before leaving Jane said she felt she was falling apart and feared she was going crazy. I held her in my arms and said, "Sweetheart, you get very anxious when you're getting ready in the mornings. It's hard for you to find things and hard for you to decide what to do. Let me hold you a couple of minutes. Take a deep breath and try to relax." For a brief time she was a sweet child cradled in my arms. Then we left.

I write about these things because they are the beautiful moments we share. They are not spectacular. They are not exciting. They are simple and passing but they remind us both of similar times woven through our fifty years of togetherness.

The Mall was crowded. We entered through Macy's instead of Nordstrom because we parked in a different area. Jane thought she had never been in the store before and repeatedly asked what store it was. I showed her the corridor to Nordstrom and explained where we were in relation to our usual path to the eatery.

The kiosks fascinate Jane. She likes to touch the handbags and the scarves and the stuffed animals. She is child-like as she admires things with interest and enthusiasm. As we leave the area she often says to the clerk, "I'll be back." Her merchandizing background wants to cheer the salesperson.

I am concerned I may become too conscious of what I write these days and be unable to keep the flow of words as free as in the past. I decided to ask one or two good friends to be readers of these pages, making corrections and suggestions. Will I become more aware of others reading what I write? Will it alter what I write and how I write? In a way I see these pages as a betrayal of Jane's simplicity and innocence. Am I breaking the trust we always maintained? We never kept anything from each other during these many years. Now I am keeping something important from Jane. Is there reason enough to do so? Will this writing be of value to others someday?

I have corresponded by email with Harriet Lerner for several years. I recently sent her part of this journal to read. She was encouraging and thought it should be published for its value to others. Her comments ease my conscience about deceiving Jane. I cannot share these pages with her because some of them would be devastating. If she could read them with the bright intellect and gentle compassion of her past, there would be no problem. But now because of her confused thinking and reinless emotions, they would destroy her peace and stability. If the pre-Alzheimer's Jane could have read them, she would know a great deal more about the illness that is taking over her life.

Friends who read this will have expectations of me, as our children have expectations, as Jane has expectations. I repeatedly pledge to Jane she will live in this apartment with me until she dies or until I die. What if I fail? What if we reach a point where I can't do it? Not that it can't be done but that **I can't do it?** I would lose Jane and my self-respect. I could only see my life as a failure. If things came to that point, I guess it wouldn't matter what anyone else thought. How could I live with what I would be thinking?

11/08/11

I write more frequently of late. Is it because I note more changes I want to record? Is it because I gain new insights or ideas about Jane's struggle? Or is it because I have more time or perhaps more need to talk to someone about it all?

Last evening after dinner Jane became irritable and hostile. I truly had no idea why. I embraced her and tried to talk to her but she was unresponsive. Sort of a "leave me alone attitude." I told her we could watch a movie when she was ready. We sat down about eight o'clock for the movie. Instead of turning it on we talked until after ten.

She didn't seem to know what was troubling her. "I feel like I'm losing it. I'm going crazy. I kept trying on hats so I wouldn't have to wash my hair before going to Mass tomorrow. I couldn't seem to stop. I don't know what I'm doing. Everything is strange. Nothing is familiar." She obviously felt bewildered and seemed to blame me for it but couldn't identify what I did to cause it. "It felt like everything was coming at me at one time." She acknowledged and apologized for her hostile behavior. "I feel like there is a black spider crawling around in my head making me say things I don't want to say and do things I don't want to do." I said we know Alzheimer's lets her emotional responses overpower her and cause behavior beyond her control.

As we talked it became clear that during the evening I had mentioned several items relating to that evening, the next morning, the next day and the day after that. Too many ideas, too many plans, too many comments, all crammed into a shrinking brain. My train of thought and conversation left Jane at the station, bewildered, lost, frightened, with no idea of what to do next. I was totally unaware of how overwhelming my comments were.

Talking together made it clear to both of us. I know most of "the plans" I spoke about included words and phrases like, "we might," "if we have time," "possibly," "maybe we will." Those words don't compute for Jane. "Might go" means go. "Possibly do" means do. "To have time" is without meaning and irrelevant. To measure time one needs a reference point. Jane has none. "Maybe we will" means this is what we will do. I must speak her language with care and recognize the lack of clarity in my own.

Toward the end of our conversation I said to Jane, "I want to write some of these things down so I will remember them. I write down things like this sometimes." She thought it was a good idea and said nothing further. Now I have told her I record some of what happens during the course of her illness. That eases my feelings about it all.

11/16/11

Things fell into a pit the last few days, days in which Jane became angry over nothing of significance. I ask her to repeat something she says and she is furious. "Why don't you get hearing aids? You're always asking me 'what, what, what.' I'm sick and tired of it. Everyone else hears me. Why can't you?" Her speech is slurred at times. Laura mentioned it two years ago when we were at her house so it has been going on for some time. She enunciates poorly and speaks with little mouth movement. At times she talks to me from the bedroom and assumes I will understand her in the next room. I am confronted with a dilemma. Do I ask "what" and risk her wrath? Or do I assume what she said was not important and reap her anger because I didn't answer her? I suspect the illness may cause some of the speech difficulty. In addition some of the medicines have this potential side effect.

There were other unprovoked tirades. In bed a few nights ago she began talking about Laura visiting. She was furious because I had not insisted Laura arrange her Christmas visit with me. It went on and on for over an hour. I was picking cautious responses not to fuel the flames. Laura said she and the girls will come at Christmas. Laura is very busy and will make those plans when she has the time and the information she needs to do so. The girls' father needs to be considered in the planning. I finally said, "If you want to continue to talk about this, let's get up, put our robes on, and go in the living room and talk." She didn't want to do that because she was finished talking about it. After another ten minutes of talking about it, she fell asleep.

The whole discussion was without reason or meaning. Facts are completely ignored and reality is a myth. It is sad to watch this flow of speech that seems to have no goal other than to make words which don't make sense. Experts say, "Don't argue with an Alzheimer's patient." Agreed, but to open your mouth is to argue, and to keep it closed is to risk more hostility. The trick seems to be to say words that sound like they mean something but which don't challenge the absence of meaning in the whole conversation.

Jane's confusion was apparent the last three evenings as we prepared for bed. Three nights ago, she asked, "Is Laura coming to visit tomorrow?" Two nights ago, she asked, "Is my mother going to be here in the morning?" I replied, "Sweetheart, your mother has been dead many years. You are an eighty year old woman now." She accepted it as gently as it was said. Last night, she asked, "Did you say you were going to call John tomorrow?" My son, John, has not been mentioned in weeks. I reflect, "What world, what scenes, what pieces of the past go through her mind during the silent times of her day? How does her world of wonder fit into the world of words we exchange?"

Several days ago we went through a number of photographs. I suspect that brought more clearly to mind people from the past, including Laura, Jane's mother, and John. Experts speak of going through pictures of previous times and events. My question is: "What does the patient do with the information? Does it confuse the present and the past? There are vague and fluid boundaries between the two."

Our most trying recent period began yesterday and continues even now. I took our car for oil and filter change. Jane accompanied me and while waiting we had coffee and a muffin at a near-by coffee shop. When we went back for the car, the service manager said we should consider repairs in both front axle assemblies. Jane was in the service area, although I had asked her to wait in the store section. The mechanic showed me where and what the problem was. I authorized the repairs and they loaned us a car.

Getting ready to leave, Jane wanted to get everything out of our car and take it home. I said there was no need to do so. That produced bitterness and endless hostility for two hours yesterday afternoon, four hours last evening, a short time this morning, and a renewed assault this afternoon.

Jane's version of the scene in the service department was rather simple. "You left my car with total strangers. You didn't ask any questions. You have no idea what they are going to do or if it needs to be done. How can you trust those people? You don't know anything about them. When that woman said it needed to be done, you were ready to let her do anything she wanted. That's my car too, you know. Why didn't you talk to me about it before you agreed to have it done?" It probably didn't help the situation that the service manager was a young, not unattractive woman. Jane did not remember the mechanic taking me under the car and showing me what needed to be done.

My first big mistake was not asking Jane if she agreed to get the repairs done. There was some foundation for her irritation because she felt demeaned by my not consulting her. I never discussed car repairs with her in the past and did not expect to do so on this occasion. But in her mind I was ignoring her and listening to a young woman tell me what I should do. Put that together and "voila."

My second big mistake was not agreeing to take everything out of the car, put it all in the loaner, and bring it home to our apartment. That was the unforgivable! Her things would be stolen! I said we left the car initially for over an hour and this would only be a few hours longer. I knew what everything was in the car, and I had confidence it would all be safe. I've dealt with these people for over twelve year and I trust them. Any reassuring words were only an insult to her intelligence. She knows what people are like. She would never trust those people with anything of hers.

Jane worries all the time about people stealing. She worries someone will steal from the apartment. We have our own lock on the studio door. I explain this to others by saying we have medical records there and it is for their security. She keeps a few things there because I carry the key. She worries about people stealing her coat or mine at the Mall so she ties the sleeves to the chair. In the eatery, she puts her foot through the shoulder strap of her handbag so no one can steal it. She was always concerned about people stealing but never to this rather bizarre extent.

Unfortunately the car repair has still not been completed. A needed part was not readily available but should be delivered this afternoon. A remarkable story has developed regarding objects in the car. Last night Jane said there are two pillows in the back seat which she covered with fabric years ago. They were there for the children when they sat in the back. She also said she left a pair of gloves and two books in the glove compartment. This afternoon out of nowhere—no, out of that mystery land inside her brain—appeared an addition to the above. Two black skirts she can't find are in the back seat of the car. In fact there are no pillows, no gloves, no books, and no skirts in the car.

Yesterday was a terrible day. We sat down about 7p.m. to watch a movie and talked for four hours. She was hostile, critical, unforgiving, merciless in her condemnation of my two grand mistakes. I was truly weary from it all. I think she could have continued several more hours had I not insisted we stop talking about it. My real mistake, by the way, was letting Jane get involved in the whole affair. She is unable to think clearly, much less wisely, in any situation requiring a decision.

She began talking about the car this morning. I told her I would not speak of it with her. She was angry about that but quieted in order to get ready for her appointment with the neurologist today. At his office she was well spirited and cooperative. They had an interesting exchange. Doctor: "Would you like to do a little arithmetic for me?" Jane: "No." Doctor: "Well, that's all right, but you did some for me before." Jane: "You asked if I would like to. I would not like to but I will." My sweetheart is still pretty sharp. The neurologist raised a question about the number of medicines she is taking. He suggested we talk to the psychiatrist about them when we see him next month.

Same date—four hours later.
The car was ready about 4p.m. Jane went with me to get it. On the way home she said there were two white skirts she couldn't find and thought she put them in the back seat of the car. I said there were no skirts in the back seat. She said nothing further about our belongings. Everything was intact as I expected it would be.

After dinner she mentioned the skirts. I said I didn't remember any white skirts. She said they were black and described them, saying she couldn't find them. I found them in her closet. She was pleased and said she was confused about them being in the car.

Perhaps all this sounds critical of Jane. It is not meant to be. It only describes her difficulty in dealing with things outside our daily routines. Between the anger sessions, she expressed remorse and promised "to do better." Even that can be irritating because she repeats her apology every five to ten minutes and continues for a couple of hours. I tell her there was no harm done, it was not her fault, it is a result of Alzheimer's, I am fine and not angry, and there is no need to apologize. She says she is afraid I will leave her forever because of these episodes. I respond, "My love, I will always stay with you. You need not worry. You are my life. Without you the world would be meaningless. Nothing will ever come between us."

This behavior shows a marked obsessive quality, a natural response to Jane's insecurity and fear. She finds herself unexpectedly and unwittingly in one of two roles. She has the role of "warrior woman," ready for the contest, plunging into the battle, determined to prove her side with whatever arguments she can muster. It is win or lose time. There can be no compromise, no middle ground. Her insecurity drives her into obsessive behavior: repeat the story over and over, give no ground, never give up, never concede, continue the struggle, go over it again and make it true even if all you have are the same word-weapons you used before.

Her other role is "fragile woman," an insecure, frightened little girl lost in a land of giants whom she does not understand, does not trust, and does not really know. Are they friendly? How would she know? What information does she have of their love or their behavior? None, because that information is lost. So she gathers paper doilies, leaves, tissue boxes, and keeps them for security, and she sorts her hair pins by size each night so she will sleep more safely. This is what remains of the sweet, loving, highly capable, accomplished woman she was before Alzheimer's began to steal her brain cells. But it can't take her heart!! She is fragile and frightened but she exudes love to all who come within the dawn of her smile or the tenderness of her words and her touch.

I cannot imagine how difficult it is for Jane to live in and be comfortable with her daily life. It is filled with uncertainties and insecurities. But the real tragedy is when the illness drags her by emotional bindings into the "combat life." Isolation, desperation, loss of personhood, and threat of losing her caregiver leave her battling blindly and without hope or future. It is an unthinkable time, a horrible time when she becomes, for a period, unreachable. How does she survive? How does her mind maintain sanity? No wonder she says she wants to die. No wonder she threatens suicide.

Jane often says she is insane or will be insane. It is her recurring comment and fear. Yesterday during our visit to the neurologist I mentioned her fear. He said to her, "As a professional, I can tell you that you are not insane and you are not going to become insane." He repeated it before we left the office. Jane expressed great relief from his words. If only she could remember them.

I mentioned Jane's two roles. I have somewhat the same experience. I have a "positive" life where I have confidence in the future, faith in the strength and permanence of our love, belief in divine providence and recognition of the blessings in our lives. There is also the "negative" life that was prominent the last few days. There come doubts about the future, about my ability to care for Jane, about my stability to deal with the onslaughts of her anger, about my faith in divine aid. At these times, all I can do is rely on my determination, continue the same prayers, and not get angry or vengeful.

11/17/11

Today was a better day than we've had in a long time. Jane was warm and interactive throughout the day. It was one of those days when we exchanged various phrases of love. It is ritualistic, but it is also valid and supportive of our presence to each other. Jane thrives on these words of affection, and once spoken I know they are soon forgotten. Repetition is as necessary as her next heart beat.

Washing her hair took us most of the morning. I mentioned it during dinner. She forgot we washed it today. For a few moments, the awareness of the lost memory hung between us and then was gone. The stark reality of how lost she is in our world stays with me.

At the Mall today Jane said how happy she was to be there and how much there is to see. She looks at items in windows, in stores, and on the kiosks with associated observations. These outings expand our world. Jane looks forward to them and never suggests we go anywhere else, even though I've mentioned other Malls and other stores. Sameness of the frame makes her comfortable with slight but continuous modification in the picture.

The Mall also provides part of our "socialization" program. Experts recommend continuing social contacts. Jane can't maintain lengthy conversations except with three of our children and even those can be difficult for her. Brief encounters with people we know at the Mall and at church and brief contacts with staff and residents here provide all the social interactions her limited repertoire can tolerate.

11/19/11
Lately we have talked more as Jane has shared more of what's in her head. Yesterday she felt she was "in a pit." She didn't recognize friends in the dining room. She described periods of not knowing what was going on or where she was.

My sense tells me Jane's head must be a haunted place. Surroundings become shadowy and strange. Nothing is familiar. Ghosts of the past, faces and scenes come out of nowhere. Are they from before or are they now? She is unsure. There are unexpected events that startle her, make her want to run away. But no place feels safe. All is fearful and sinister. There are dark empty spaces where evil and death hide. The past and present intermingle in mysterious and troubling stories, the product of reality and fantasy. Only one thing is certain in this place of torment. She will not get back to sanity! She cannot tell anyone about it because there is no one there. Although I am with her in body she cannot tell me because I am in a plane her spirit cannot reach with words.

Several times recently Jane said she did not want to tell me what happens in her head because it is too terrible for her to talk about and too terrible for me to hear. Of late, while embracing her and telling her of my devotion, I try to help her find words to bridge the space between us. I help her express her thoughts by saying what I imagine must be in her mind. The above paragraph is a distillate of our talk and thoughts and love.

In the midst of all this she fears she is a burden to me and I am suffering because of her. "I am always asking you something you already told me. How can you put up with someone who is so helpless and useless? What good am I to you? I never do anything for you, but you are always doing things for me. I'm just dragging you down. You must get tired of taking care of me."

My responses are along the following lines. "I don't care what questions you ask me or how many times you ask them. I will never tire of telling you things or answering questions over and over again. You are as good for me as you have ever been and your presence in my life since the day I met you has been the richest of blessings. It will always be so. You never drag me down. You lift my spirit every day as I see how brave and determined and good you are. You do for me what you have always done for me. You share my life, my world, and your presence, your sweet tender love make it a better life and better world every day we are together. My only sadness is to know how difficult life is for you with the illness you have. I am grateful to God I am with you and have you in my life each day we are together. I don't feel I am taking care of you. I am living with you and loving you as I always have. We will continue to take care of each other. That's what we do."

11/21/11

This is Monday. Laura called on Saturday, talked to her mother for a while, and then she and I had a long talk. We exchanged ideas about Christmas. She had some thought about coming by herself. I encouraged her to bring the girls.

I told Jane they would come the week after New Year's. To my surprise Jane thought it would be better if the girls did not come. She said she would not do well with them and didn't want them to see "their crazy grandmother." We talked about her decision for a while. She was calm and composed and continued to say it would be better if Laura came by herself. Actually I think it is the right decision. We will have a better visit with Laura and it will be less trying for Jane not to have to fuss about the girls.

I called Laura and we agreed she would plan to come down the weekend after New Year's. I mentioned the plan several times to Jane and her opinion remained unchanged. She says, "I will never see the girls again." When I tell her they may come next summer, she responds, "I will be dead before then." She is very focused on death these days. This plan is a major change for us. We have been with Laura during the Christmas season every year since Laura returned from London.

293

This morning Jane said, "All our friends were eating dinner together last evening. We have obviously been dropped from the group. I think they may be afraid of me and what I might do." She was disturbed because a group of seven or eight did not ask us to join them.

I told her we have invitations to dine with different people but I decline because we agreed we are more comfortable eating by ourselves. It is less stressful for her. She decided, "You are ashamed of me and worry I will do something to embarrass you." I said, "I will never be embarrassed by you or how you behave. I am proud of you. You are a good, loving woman and many people here care very much about you. Many of them go out of their way to speak to you in the dining room and in other places where we see them." I told her others know she has Alzheimer's and that we prefer to eat alone.

I feel very strongly we are coming to a downturn in the road. I anticipate the holidays will be a difficult time for us both.

11/25/11

We spent Thanksgiving quietly and calmly and managed to get through the brunch experience without difficulty. Brunch is usually unsettling for Jane because we do not have our usual table, there are a number of strangers in the room, the menu is different, and "all is not in order."

We spent a special love time in the late afternoon, a time which brings us more closely to who we were and what our life was before Alzheimer's took away our easy togetherness. Our love time requires no memories because it is a lived memory. It requires no history because it breathes history. It has no space for doubts or fears because it is filled with oneness. And there are words that cover all the aches and sorrows of other times, words beyond the mundane and trivia, words that take us beyond the boundaries of ourselves.

As nature would have it, this time is reassuring to Jane in a way no other time can be. It is a renewed pledge of commitment; it emboldens her faith in our bond; it instills a reality without need of memory-life. This time immerses me in the depth and breadth of her being; it renews my life that first dawned in her eyes; it tells me again the value of vow.

Bonnie is visiting from Iowa and will come this afternoon. She called yesterday and made the arrangement. I mentioned it to Jane several times today and each time it was news. Information rarely stays in her mind long. Words go in, are understood, and then are gone. Their meaning goes with them. We are at a new point of forgetfulness.

We go for Jane's annual mammogram this afternoon. Each time I mention it I remind her it is routine for a woman her age to have the test each year. That is the only reason she is going. It does not suggest in any way she has breast cancer.

Her mind makes strange and sometimes wild associations. During lunch today I was talking about the past and mentioned a psychiatrist friend whom Jane knew quite well. He worked for the CIA. Several years ago he asked me if I knew a priest who was a good theologian with whom he might talk. I gave him a priest's name. I said I wondered if his concern related to the program of prisoner torture.

Later in the same conversation Jane said, "Did you want to see someone to talk to about us?" What got her there? What dendrite caused that twisted outcome? Did the words "priest," "talk," and "torture" come together and suggest to her that I wanted to talk to a priest about "torture?" "Torture" she might see herself as causing? Conversation is not only limited by Jane's narrowed experience and interest but also by the safety and propriety of subjects. I can't guess what her brain might do even with innocuous topics. This one was a poor choice on my part.

11/27/11

The night before last was difficult. When we finished the movie Jane said she didn't understand any of it. I said the plot was rather intricate and hard to follow. I asked if we should stop watching movies. She denied she ever had difficulty before. This was the first time, and "you could certainly have been more understanding and sympathetic. I thought you would cry when I told you about this major change in my condition. I don't know why you can't be more helpful when I'm falling apart. What's the matter with you?"

We spent two hours talking about it without getting anywhere, another hour in bed doing the same. We both woke early yesterday after about five hours sleep. The day went poorly. When we returned from the Mall she said she had not been comfortable there. "I felt out of place and not myself."

The movie last night was an American film set in Tokyo. All the characters were Americans except for waiters, hotel clerks, etc. The latter spoke Japanese. About half way through the movie I asked Jane for the second time if the movie was all right. She said she couldn't understand it and didn't see any reason to watch it. I said we need not finish it and suggested we go to bed.

She said she hated the movie from the beginning but was afraid to tell me. She couldn't understand why I got a foreign movie. I said it was an American movie set in Tokyo. She insisted all the characters were speaking Japanese. When I said they were speaking English, she became irate.

I believe she is embarrassed when she realizes she is wrong, and anger is her natural defense. Or maybe she still believed she was right. She asked how I picked the movies. The whole process of choosing movies and the queue at Netflix has been mentioned many times. How the movie gets here and the fact it is not a TV show never stays in her head.

In bed she continued to talk randomly and irrationally about the movie, about her failing memory, about her fear of dying, about "things in my head I never tell you because it would make you sad." I suggested it might be helpful if she did tell me those thoughts.

This morning during breakfast she said what a good day we had yesterday. Actually she remembers little of yesterday. That is the sunshine of Alzheimer's land.

When we left the Mall today I suggested we drive to the monastery, which she likes to do. She said she was tired and would like to go home. She is napping now. I massage her feet when she lies down for a nap. It is a good time for me to say a decade of the rosary, ten toes—ten Aves. Is she tired because the last three days were different than our usual schedule and thus more difficult for her? Or is this additional evidence that the slope downward is suddenly much steeper?

Jane often says she doesn't want to tell me things because it will make me sad. I respond, "You don't make me sad. Life is sad. It is sad for both of us but especially sad for you because you have Alzheimer's and it is a sad illness." This afternoon I am sad because I realize I need to make a special effort to remember the Jane who was my bright, beautiful, energetic, enthusiastic, gifted companion. I no longer look at her and remember. I only see her sad smile, her empty eyes, her fatigued body, her listless demeanor. To remember her from the past, I have to recall some scene: walking on the beach or in the streets of Spokane, talking over dinner in a favorite restaurant, enjoying a show in Reno or Vegas, visiting on the ranch with my brother and his wife. I can't believe, I can't accept I have to consciously and deliberately look in some distant place and some past time to find her. It is painful to do so. It does not seem fair. Life is sad!

11/29/11

How easily Jane's world becomes a dreadful experience! How easily she absorbs and misinterprets the feelings of others! Last Friday we went for a mammogram. It became an ordeal. The tech doing the mammogram made three trips to the radiologist while we waited with apprehension and a sense of mystery. Then the radiologist ordered a sonogram. It seemed like we should do it right then, not just that we could do it then. Apprehension and mystery and urgency!

The tech doing the sonogram made three trips to the radiologist and finally returned with the doctor herself. The doctor did not instill confidence or calm in either of us. She spoke about possible problems in Jane's breast and talked about additional tests without explaining anything. Apprehension, mystery, urgency, uncertainty! I did not challenge her because I lacked confidence in and patience with her and I wanted to get Jane out of the situation as soon as possible without making a fuss.

We came away with a sheet saying "not malignant" and "repeat ultrasound in 6 months" or "3 months" if you read another place on the page. I explained the results simply to Jane and put the matter behind us.

The last three days at the Mall were different. Jane was uneasy. Yesterday she became irritable and fearful. As she talked about it she said, "I'm going to die in a week. The doctor told me that." I couldn't believe what she apparently believed for several days. I told her forcefully, "No doctor ever said that to you. That is absolutely wrong. It is not true. I don't know where that idea ever came from but it is not true, not true."

In bed Jane again mentioned her belief and wondered how it got into her head. I mentioned the doctor she saw for the mammogram. That was the origin for her "death in a week." The emotional atmosphere of that afternoon contained a sense of urgency, a feeling of uncertainty, a note of warning. None of that was spoken. It was in the air. The doctor seemed full of doubt and apprehension. In retrospect, I think it was more about herself than about her patient. The death sentence came out of the unspoken threats hidden in the scene. I cannot guess where Jane got the time frame "one week." A news show, a TV ad, a chance remark of mine or someone else—who can tell?

The Alzheimer's mind not only gets confused about what happens but fills in the blanks with pieces of unknown origin. As Jane and I agreed in a later discussion, the facts disappear but the feelings remain and build a picture to fit the fear.

PART 11 (DEC 11—MAY 12)

12/06/11

What I would call "an Alzheimer's story" developed over the past several days. On Sunday we went to the Mall. Christmas decorations are everywhere of course. We walked by a shiny new store highlighting new purses. We also walked past the Build–A-Bear store.

During lunch Jane suddenly said, "I want to know who is going to get 'Puppy.' I want to give him to someone now. If I give him to one of Laura's daughters I need another stuffed animal to give the other girl. Is there a store here that might have one?" "Puppy" is a small stuffed dog we bought for Jane about five years ago at IKEA. He has become our household pet. He sits in an arm chair looking at us as we sit on the sofa. We talk to him on occasion to make him think he is real.

Jane was clearly and strongly invested in this need to have a second stuffed animal as soon as possible. I said we could look in the Build-A-Bear store but we would have to go back on the upstairs level. She was agreeable to the change of route.

We looked at the animals in the store window and Jane thought one might be a suitable mate for "Puppy." The clerk took it down and held it for us to see. We agreed it was not acceptable. Jane was disappointed. I suggested we could bring "Puppy" with us someday and see if there was a better match. Or we could go to IKEA after the holidays to see if we could find a similar puppy. (I thought "after the holidays" would give Jane time either to forget the idea or decide it wasn't necessary.)

Christmas is part of this story because Jane can't resist wanting to get the girls something for Christmas. We gave them money last year and agreed to do the same this year. But that little feeling sneaks back into her head and her heart, "we need a Christmas present for the girls." Death is also in the story because it is ever-present for Jane. "I will be gone and what will happen to 'Puppy'."

Emotional catalysts included concern for "Puppy" and wanting to know where he would go when she dies, love for the grandchildren and the need to gift them, and love for me so I wouldn't have to dispose of "our pet" after her death. This sounds a little overstated, but Jane's emotions are always overwhelming, over-expressed, over-lived.

The Alzheimer's story continues. Before leaving the apartment the next day to go to the Mall, Jane said there was something in the Mall she wanted to buy but couldn't remember what it was. During lunch she continued to mention a planned but forgotten purchase. "I saw it yesterday. The clerk was holding it. She said it was for sale. I decided I would buy it today." "No, it wasn't clothing. No, it wasn't at a kiosk. It was in a store. The clerk was very nice."

I asked, already knowing the answer, "Was it the stuffed animal in the Build-A-Bear store?" "Yes, of course." I went over the details of the Sunday scene with her. Her reaction was a surprise to me. "How could I be so far off the track? The idea of giving 'Puppy' away now doesn't make sense. It wouldn't be a good time to give stuffed animals to the girls anyway."

Later in the afternoon Jane had an appointment with her audiologist. As we sat in his waiting room she said, "I don't know where I got the idea I wanted to buy that purse the woman was holding to show me. It was pretty but I certainly don't need a new purse." The new purses were in the store near the Build-A-Bear store. We were never in it.

A person has to stay alert to keep up with the workings of Jane's mind. At lunch today she said, "There are different sizes of panic." I said that was an astute statement. She replied, "I'm better than you think I am. I just act like I do to get attention." What a remarkably playful comment for her to make when she is fully aware her life is filled with confusion and loss.

I went into Jane's bathroom this evening to see how she was doing. She said, "I have my face washed and my hair net on. Isn't that great?" I took her in my arms and said, "Do you know what's great? That we are here together, that's great! That we have the life we have in spite of your illness, that's great! That we can still do the things we do, that's great! I know life is hard for you. The world falls apart around you. But you take hold of the pieces and somehow make them into something good and beautiful. You hold them together and you hold yourself together and you hold me together. I have always seen you as a gift from God and every day I am grateful for this wonderful gift you are." At times like this Jane is real, complete, full of the life and the love we have shared. For the moment we travel together through the years past and bravely into the future.

12/08/11

Some people worry about how Jane's illness affects me. I've been thinking about what it has done for me. Alzheimer's has certainly not brought positive changes in Jane's life but it has brought positive changes in mine. We don't fully know how certain events change our lives but we can search for an understanding of their influence.

My life is richer and certainly more dear as a result of Jane's illness. It is richer because I now have the opportunity to fill my days and nights with an unselfish love for and attention to the person I most treasure. It is dearer because I am sharply aware of the importance and meaning of my presence in the world.

I'm not sure how I might have accommodated to a usual retirement. I would have avoided it for a few more years by continuing the practice of psychiatry and teaching. When those necessarily ended I might well have been at loose ends. This small apartment would have closed us in too tightly, if our usual energy and interests had been maintained. We would have gone to Montana sometimes, to Rehoboth more often, to art galleries more often, to Laura's more often. But all those enjoyable possibilities would still only be time-fillers. I would have needed "something to do." Through our years Jane and I worked together on the houses we lived in, painting walls, tiling floors and cabinets, building shelves and closets, altering rooms, collecting antiques and decorating. These were our hobbies. Now we live in a five room apartment. We've finished the changes we wanted to make here. There is nothing left to do.

Jane has always been a blessing in my life and she remains that now in a new and special way. Her presence fills me with tenderness not just for her but for all the people I see who are ill or handicapped in some way. There have been no tragedies in my life or in the lives of those close to me. I haven't known what it is to take care of a handicapped child or an invalid parent. I've never been present day after day even to observe, much less care for, someone who is mentally, emotionally or physically losing ground each passing day. Jane's daily deterioration is immeasurable and almost unobservable because it is so slight, yet I know it is happening because each day it fills the space that separates us.

I just tucked Jane in bed for an afternoon nap. Massaging her feet I am a father encouraging sleep in a small, troubled child; I am a lover looking at the beautiful woman who graces my life and shares my bed; I am a husband returning in some small way years of devotion from a dedicated wife.

I get tired; I get impatient; I get edgy sometimes. These last nine years I have learned much about myself and about life. I believe I am a better person as a result of this time with Jane. I have learned the demands love can make and know they are not really demands but opportunities for love to be expressed in new ways and with new meaning.

As I look at years past I realize I was the center of our lives. My work took us to Reno, Nevada where I was Superintendent of the State Hospital and Director of the Department of Mental Hygiene. My decision and my job took us to Grants Pass, Oregon. Moving to Spokane, Washington, then to Baltimore, Maryland, then to Georgetown, Maine, and finally back to Maryland were all related to **me, my** work, **my** practice of psychiatry.

Life is different now. It is no longer "all about me." It is "all about Jane." And something deep inside me is grateful and says, "Now, you are the kind of person you should be. Now you can give to someone else all you have to give. And the only rewards you will have, the only rewards you will need are her sweet smile, her flash of humor, her warm hand in yours, her gentle face across the table, her loving caress at bedtime."

Jane's determination, her quiet dignity, her gentle demeanor inspire me and give me strength and courage to face each day. I know I have written about her anger, her recounting of ills, her suspicion of others, her doubts about me. That is her Alzheimer's life, without faith, without friend, without "us." But she has another life never to be extinguished: her spirit, her gentle self, and the world of faith and love matured within her. We shared that life, and now I share as fully as I can her Alzheimer's life.

When I was the center of our world it was a bright, cheerful, encouraging world. There were restaurant dinners, theater, museums, movies, close friends, intimate family ties, delightful visits, trips to the beach, to various cities and abroad. We traveled to annual professional meetings, to various educational seminars, to lectures and workshops I gave throughout the States. It was an energetic, active, enticing and entertaining world. We enjoyed it together and it filled us with happy memories of wonderful times.

Now Jane is the center of our world but it is a drab, constricted, flat world. There are Subway sandwiches at the Mall, home movies from Netflix, gin rummy, friendly faces without names, uncertain visits from our children, pictures of people and places no longer real. It is a world that meets Jane's current needs and so mine. It is alive and active. It is safe and secure. It is a world where we live as fully as we can and love as fully as we ever did. Our world is between us and in us. It does not change.

12/18/11
It has been hard to write recently. I'm not sure why. Everything seems unsteady, uncertain. Jane is showing additional deterioration. She has such a difficult time getting ready in the mornings. She "can't find things" that are right in front of her. She can't decide what to wear. She is easily irritated if I intervene. All of this has been said before but that is the land of Alzheimer's: repetition, repetition and uncertainty, uncertainty.

I've again started reading to her as she does her make-up and hair. I don't know if she understands much of it but my presence is a benefit. She often says, "I don't want to be alone." Her bathroom is the loneliest place because it is the most removed from the rest of the apartment. She won't consider changing to the bathroom both of us use, which is directly across a hall from the studio. I read to her mostly because it gives me an opportunity to be with her during a lonely time. If I don't read she thinks I should talk to her and talk is hard to come by these days. Small talk is quickly exhausted.

There is not only the loss of immediate memory but more is being lost from the store room of the past. Places we lived, people we knew, trips we made are no longer recalled even with prompts. Jane's comments: "I don't know who I am any more," "My head is empty these days," "I don't know what I'm thinking sometimes," "Things in my head just melt away," "I have fumble in my head." In contrast to those dismal statements she recently said, "I want to do some sewing after the holidays. I want to go through everything in my closet and decide what I want to keep for the future. I'm going to write a Christmas card to each of my three daughters." None of these statements gives an accurate picture of where she is or what she does but they tell where she used to be.

One minor struggle has faded from the scene. The use of the lipstick is no longer an issue or even noted. The whole episode has disappeared.

I recently mentioned to Jane that our friend, Harriet Lerner, has encouraged me to write about our experience with Alzheimer's. Harriet's name and reputation is familiar to Jane. She responded, "I think it would be a great idea. You should do it." So I covered an issue that troubled me. Jane is aware of this writing. I doubt she will show an interest in reading it, which indicates clearly how great a change has occurred. Nor will I encourage any further discussion of it or reference to it.

Jane is increasingly less able to confront each day as she did in the past. Much of life seems to be "too much." I can't think of a better way of putting it. Many events just pass her by. It's like she sees them but does not observe them. Things she hears seem not to register. She seems less aware of how unaware she is. And that may be the phase of Alzheimer's haunting us now. All of it "seems."

An older couple (99 qualifies for older here) used to pass our dining room table every evening and stop to talk to Jane. Ten days ago they told us they moved to the nursing unit. Jane created a picture of their move out of her own fears. She decided someone came to their apartment and made them move. I explained they moved of their own volition and probably because they were both using walkers and were becoming unable to care for themselves. No matter how many times I explained the move, her version remained dominant in her thinking.

Jane asked about the couple this evening. I went through the details and said we talked about it several times. "When you tell me that, I feel so stupid. I never know what's going on. I don't know how you put up with me and my stupidity. I always thought I was stupid as a child and no one ever told me otherwise."

I said the reason I mentioned telling her before is because I want her to know I am trying to keep her informed of things that happen to our friends. I said, "I have known you 50 years and I know you are not stupid. If I had Alzheimer's it would affect me the same way it is affecting you. You were always bright and participated in every decision we made. Your opinion was always important and many times more correct than mine. You have Alzheimer's, my love, and it has taken your memory. That is not your fault and it is not something we can change."

Later when we sat together in the apartment Jane said, "I don't know how you put up with me. It must be difficult for you to be with me. You got stuck with me. I'm afraid I'm changing into someone else. I want to do better. I know I can do better." I took her in my arms and said, "Sweetheart, I don't put up with you. I love you and I will always love you. You're the one with the tough road to travel. I have you and that makes everything right for me. I didn't get stuck with you. I have been blessed with your presence in my life. You won't change into someone else. You will always be you, my sweet loving companion. And you don't need to do better. Please, try to be satisfied with how you are doing because I think you're doing great right now."

Jane frequently says how difficult things are for me, how good and patient I am with her, and how much work I do for her. I tell her my responses are my way of loving her and the "work" I do in a day could easily be done in thirty minutes and I have nothing else to do. Her sensitivity to the situation is remarkable.

12/26/11

Christmas was a very good day. Brunch went well. Staff saved the two-table we like when things are set up for the buffet. In the afternoon we drove out to the monastery and visited the Christmas crib in the chapel there. After an evening snack we watched a movie and went to bed.

A few days ago we visited the older couple in their current setting. They are in a room with two single beds, a small wardrobe, two chairs and a TV on the wall. There is a dayroom and a dining room down the hall. Jane keeps the scene in her mind and is terrified it will be where we or she ends up. "I will kill myself before they put me there. I won't go there. It was terrible. I won't be locked up there. I can't stand to think about it." I remind her they are almost one hundred and are both quite incapacitated. They may welcome the relief of not trying to maintain themselves independently in their apartment.

In bed last night Jane was full of thoughts about the older couple and how sad their life is. She was full of fear the same arrangement will be her fate. "I couldn't live like that. They don't have any of their furniture. What did they do with their things? Why would they give up their apartment? I won't go to that place. I'll kill myself before I go there." I tried to reassure her. "We will stay in this apartment. You will not have to go anywhere. My health is good and I pray every day I will live to take care of you. If I need help I will hire someone to help us. Their move has not changed anything in our lives. Several people we knew moved there during the years. Several people we knew died during the years. None of that affects our lives directly or changes anything about our plans for the future. I am sad for that couple but their being where they are changes nothing for us."

We talked for over an hour. After making a comment I realized Jane was not answering. I was lying on my side facing her with my arm around her and my legs by hers trying to comfort her. I lay very still and waited. Her breathing became heavier and I continued to wait for her to reach a deeper sleep. It is amazing how many spots on my body burned or itched or hurt or tickled during the fifteen or twenty minutes I did not move. Then very slowly I removed my arm and turned on my back to sleep. All the itching and hurting was gone but I was wide awake due to my vigilance. It took a few more saints than usual to put me to sleep.

I recently realized Jane speaks a language of superlatives because superlatives express strong feelings. Her comments to others and about others and about her environment expose the unsupervised and unmindful run of her emotional life. Background noise in the dining room varies from one night to another. Every night Jane says, "The noise is the loudest it has ever been." The same thing happens in the eatery. Every day, "This is the noisiest it has ever been here." No matter what the crowd is, "This is the biggest crowd we've seen here." Each scarf or purse she likes in a window is, "The nicest one I ever saw." Clothing she dislikes is, "The ugliest I ever saw."

When she is angry at me, "That is the cruelest thing you ever did," "The meanest thing you ever said," "The worst thing you could possibly do." There are no dividing marks on her scale. If it is at all, then it is all of what it is. When another resident or one of the staff stops to say hello, Jane's typical response in those few minutes includes at some point, "I love you." People often seem uncertain how to respond to such a statement. She compliments people (one might say indiscriminately). "Your hair is beautiful," or "That blouse is the prettiest one I've ever see," or "I love that necklace you are wearing."

Her comments are not to ingratiate. They express something she feels. And it is difficult for her not to express feelings because they are unrestrained, ungoverned. Jane lives in a world where thoughts are dried bones but feelings are warm flesh attached to what she sees and what she hears.

We returned from the Mall a short time ago. It was an adventure to brave the crowd the day after Christmas. During lunch Jane asked, "When is Christmas?" She was not shocked when I said it was yesterday. The blow of knowing how much she forgets is not as brutal as it was a few weeks ago.

12/31/11

New Year's Eve, a time to examine the past and wonder about the future. This past year was certainly easier than the preceding one. Jane is obviously more forgetful and much more confused but she is far less volatile and an easier companion.

We had an example of her confusion a few days ago. We came home from the Mall through Macy's. Jane saw a scarf she greatly admired. We looked at the price and I asked if she would like to buy it. Her response was, "No." As we walked away she added, "I don't need another scarf. I don't really need to buy anything."

On the way home we exchanged a few comments as we usually do. Shortly after we were home she began, "You never said a word to me all the way home. I wanted that scarf. I don't know why you didn't let me buy it. I thought I was

307

going to have an allowance. I need my own money so I can buy whatever I want. I always shopped on my own and I never spent too much." I reminded her of our exchange about the scarf. She said she told me she wanted it and I refused to buy it for her.

We sat down and talked about it. Initially she insisted we go back to the Mall and buy the scarf. The parking lot and Mall are very crowded these days. I told her I would not go back then but we could look at the scarf the next day. "I know it won't be there tomorrow. You should have let me buy it today."

Getting ready for bed Jane began talking about the robe she saw in Macy's which I refused to buy for her. "I've always been economical but you never tell me I am. I don't spend much money. I don't buy things. There is nothing I need but I would like to have that beautiful black robe I saw while you went to get the car. Later on I may be in bed more of the time and it would be nice to have a pretty robe."

The next day we went to the Mall. I took Jane directly to the scarf she wanted to buy. She decided it did not go with anything she wore and declined to buy it. Before we left the Mall she talked about the robe she saw the previous day and wanted to buy. I told her she must be thinking of the scarf, because she was not alone in the store, and we never looked at a robe.

At the Mall two days later she again mentioned getting the robe, only now it was a white robe. When I repeated what I told her about not seeing a robe, she was disturbed to realize how confused she was over the whole scarf-robe affair.

Today I asked if she would like a new robe. We discussed it. She definitely did not want to buy a robe and was sorry she was mixed up about it and caused so much trouble. I assured her there was no trouble and no reason for her to feel badly about it.

As we left the eatery today Jane said, "Are we going to buy that purse today or not?" When I asked what purse, she knew she was off the track again. "My head gets very confused these days. You can't really trust what I might do. I'm glad your head still works well. I don't know where we would be if it didn't."

Jane is accommodating better to her confusion than she was a few weeks ago. She is calmer and less irritable these days. If she has a flare up I either say I'm sorry for whatever caused it and walk away or I hold her in my arms and try to soothe her. I'm not sure what determines which course of action I choose. Perhaps I've learned to sense which is the better way to go.

Her confusion doesn't worry me as much as it did. Her flashes of anger don't unnerve me like they did before. It just seems to be another part of a day and not a prologue to disaster. The Christmas season is nearly over and was much less traumatic than I anticipated. We are expecting Laura next Saturday for an overnight stay.

There is no use speculating about the next year. Alzheimer's will continue its destructive course. Our love will continue intact and inviolate. The routines of today will be altered to accommodate the needs of tomorrow. We will continue our trust in God and meet as best we can the challenges of 2012.

1/4/12
"I'm a mess. You should get rid of me. I'm a burden to you. Why don't you lock me up somewhere? How can you put up with me? I'm going crazy. I don't feel well this evening. I think there is something seriously wrong." All comments Jane made this evening. As I took her in my arms I said, "You are not a mess and you are not going crazy now and you never will go crazy. You are not a burden to me and you never will be a burden. You will always be the treasure of my life. No one will ever lock you up. You had a difficult day. Your memory didn't work very well today and when that happens, you get frightened. We will sit for a while this evening and talk about how you feel and how things are working in your head. It doesn't matter how many times you ask me the same question. I know you forget. It doesn't matter how many times I find something for you. We can sit down anytime and talk about anything you want to talk about."

Laura is coming in three days. "How will I be when she is here? How will she understand me? What will she think? I'm afraid." "Sweetheart, Laura knows how poor your memory is. Everyone who loves you knows how poor your memory is. You don't have to worry. Everyone knows you get confused as a result of your poor memory. There is no reason to be afraid. I will be with you and there isn't anything the two of us can't deal with or work out."

At the Mall today Jane commented about feeling pressure to buy something the last few weeks. It suddenly became clear to me. During the Christmas shopping season Jane was caught up in the emotional tone of the Mall. It was shop, shop, shop and buy, buy, buy. No wonder she felt the need to buy something, anything, just go with the mood. There was a stuffed animal, a scarf, a purse, a bathrobe, another scarf, another purse. The contagion of emotion spread easily to her vulnerable mind. She could never settle within her mind what it was she wanted to buy but the feeling was there and was strong. Today seemed to be a relief to her to know she was not there to buy something.

Vantage House is a somber place to live. We see people we have known for several years growing feebler. Walkers, canes and wheel chairs seem to multiply. I've been thinking lately we have nothing to look forward to. During our years together there was always something waiting in the future: a vacation, a trip, a holiday, an outing of some kind, a special evening together, a change of some kind in our routine. We no longer go to Rehoboth. We no longer go out to dinner. Holidays are just like any other day.

We look forward to visits from the children but these are infrequent and short lived. Laura will be here soon. Jane said today, "Laura is coming to see me before I die. This will be our last visit." Even Laura's coming has a sour note for Jane.

The reality for us is the same for all the residents here. Somewhere in everyone's mind, not hidden away too well, is the realization we are waiting here to die. I spoke about the contagion of emotion. It is not surprising Jane has death on her mind so often. It inhabits the facility and every two or three weeks we see posted a name and date on a card with a black border. Jane resonates with atmospheric emotions others only sense dimly.

1/8/12

Laura just left for home. She arrived yesterday about 1p.m. It was a good visit but very limited for Jane. Paul joined us for dinner last evening.

Jane stayed with the conversation at dinner and throughout the time with Laura. She contributed a comment for time to time, some were on target and some not. Last evening Jane was very confused. Although we took Laura to her room when she arrived, Jane wondered where Laura was going to spend the night. She asked when the girls left and why they didn't stay. She decided they came with their mother the previous day but their father came and took them away. When I told her Laura came alone she was irritated and said, "No matter how wrong I am about things, I don't want you to correct me again tonight. I've had all I can take." She slept peacefully.

This morning she volunteered the comment, "I made up a whole afternoon for myself yesterday." An accurate description of what happens on occasion. We visited with Laura until afternoon and then walked with her to her car and waved goodbye as she left, a scene Jane usually does not remember. There are few she does remember these days.

Jane is presently napping prior to our going down to dinner. I just returned from exercise which I usually do during her afternoon nap. During exercise I began to realize how lonely I feel. For whom am I lonely? "Jane." Having a visitor for a lengthy time separates me from Jane. Even short visits seem to put her in a shadow, the dark of dimmed awareness. I missed going to the Mall with her today and having lunch there.

Others interfere with the pattern which is becoming as precious to me as it is to Jane. I am lonely for Jane now. But as I say that I also realize when I am with Jane, I am lonely for her, for the Jane that was, for the person who was close companion to me with or without visitors present. She is no longer a close companion and hardly a companion when one of the children is with us. I am aware my deepest loneliness has no cure. And I know visits from the children do not and will not lessen it. It is interminable.

Laura talked quite freely about her life, her work, her relationship with her two girls and their father. During our conversation I often thought, "We could come up and I could help you. I could paint that room. I could clear the dead branches out of your yard. I could fix the refrigerator grill. I could help you move that furniture. I could help you put together the IKEA furniture you plan to buy." I miss going there and participating at least a little in the care of her house. I miss seeing the children. But most of all, I miss Jane.

1/16/12
I have mentioned how the emotions of others or of a situation or place can have a marked effect on Jane and carry her into the same feeling field. How

come I never applied this directly to the two of us? Might it place too heavy a burden on me and my behavior? I have often said how she reads emotions on my face, maybe not always accurately, but certainly regularly.

Jane had three or four days last week that were very trying for both of us. She was irritable with herself, with others, with me. Nothing pleased her. Things I said to be supportive were attacked or flatly negated. I became increasingly aware that I was feeling "out of sorts."

The question is: was I feeling out of sorts because of Jane's mood or was she having a difficult time because I was not as chipper as I usually try to be. I don't suggest I'm always a bright spirited person but I usually am in a reasonably good mood and maintain a reasonably positive attitude about life. I think caring for Jane takes its toll, so something small may become more significant for me. I have times when things are not so good. It may be a problem with the computer, a Netflix movie broken on arrival, or forgetting something at the grocery store. In the past I would gripe and complain about it to Jane and then it would be over. I can't do that now. She would want me to get a new computer. She doesn't understand the Netflix stuff. She would want me to go back to the store. I am left with an irritation and no place to go with it. It stays with me longer than it should. Of late it doesn't take a calamity to dull my day.

The question is: what effect does some change in my mood have on Jane? I am often astonished by her awareness of what I am thinking as well as what I am feeling. If she picks up on my diminished mood, it is going to set off some feelings in her that will quickly grow disproportionate to any reality. Then it is difficult for me to respond in a supportive manner and that magnifies whatever is going on emotionally for her. Her mood continues downhill and mine follows along not as precipitously but nevertheless in the same direction.

It is clear this analysis of the situation is sometimes correct, perhaps more often than I care to believe. I've probably had a dim awareness of it for some time but avoided looking at it as honestly as I should have. It was so easy, so simple and I'm afraid so natural to blame the worsening of my "out of sorts" mood on Jane's bad mood. I need to take inventory of my storehouse of love for Jane and I need to give more freely and more frequently words of love, times of tenderness, expressions of praise and gratitude, moments of seeing her as the beautiful, sweet woman she has always been. "Out of sorts" is no excuse for being stingy with any of these love notes.

1/20/12
Sometime last fall I decided to do some different writing. I was always impressed by Jane's faith. It had a childlike simplicity, a directness, a sort of "first name basis with God" component that made me somewhat envious. Anyone who has read the last few pages of her book, "Before It's Too Late," will understand why I say that. I have been saying the rosary regularly and decided to try to look at the Sorrowful Mysteries from the perspective of Jane's illness and her unsophisticated, uncomplicated faith.

As a result I wrote several meditations on the Passion and Death of Our Lord, approaching the work, as much as I could, as Jane might converse with Jesus. In that sense it is Jane's voice that speaks.

An Alzheimer Patient's Lenten Meditation

When it grew dark he reclined at table with the Twelve. During the meal Jesus took bread, blessed it, broke it, and gave it to his disciples. "Take this and eat it," he said, "this is my body." Then, after singing songs of praise, they walked out to the Mount of Olives. (Matthew 26:20-30)

I know you enjoyed being with family and friends, Jesus. You had a triumphal entrance into Jerusalem and now you gather with your closest friends to celebrate the Passover. There is food and wine and conversation and singing. Your friends are unaware your ministry is coming to an end. They see just another Passover. The shadow cast by Judas is not obvious to them. There is a shadow in my life that is not always obvious to others. I want to tell you about it.

When you began your ministry did you have doubts about how successful it would be? Did you confide in your mother from time to time? How did you decide which person you wanted to walk with, to work with? You only had a few years of ministry. Did you ask your Father for more time? Dare I ask if you were satisfied with what you accomplished?

When I was young I had lots of doubts about my life. I didn't do much confiding in anyone. I made some mistakes back then. Big ones too, at least I thought they were big. When I was about thirty I seemed to find the right path, the path I think you wanted me to follow. That's interesting. You were thirty when you started out on the journey leading to your death.

How will I know when my work is finished? Will I be satisfied with it? The shadow in my life is Alzheimer's disease, so I no longer accomplish anything of value. I don't sew or wash clothes or iron or clean or even shop for things we need. What should I be doing with my life now? Even as I ask, my spirit tells me my work has not changed. It remains simple. It is to live each day as well as I can with the gifts and graces you grant me.

Were you sad that last evening with your friends? It was a going away party but they didn't know it. But it was not a sad ending. It was a glorious beginning. It was the moment your infinite love reached out not only to your gathered friends but across the ages to all who would come to know you. Your Body and Blood became food for our spirit and strength for our trials. Sad times can produce unbelievable benefits.

I'm leaving my friends, not really leaving them, forgetting them. Will they forget me too? Can I leave something of myself for them as you did for us in the Eucharist? I can leave them my love because loving will always be part of me. My caregiver tells me Alzheimer's can take my memories but it can't lessen my ability to love.

I'm over eighty now. I am grateful for all you have given me during this wonderful life I've had. I can't remember much about past years but my spirit tells me they were beautiful. One special gift you gave me is my husband who is now my caregiver. He has had that role for eight years now but he has given me his care and his love for fifty years.

By the way were you angry at Judas? His behavior must have stirred some deep human feelings. I have lots of strong feelings these days; anger is certainly one of them. Sometimes I say things I don't really mean to say. I also have strong feelings of love for my husband, my children and friends. I hasten to express that as often as I can.

Alzheimer's casts a long shadow over our lives. There have been times when I felt betrayed. By whom? Yes, by you. I'm a little afraid to say that but you know what's inside my head. I never expected anything like this would happen to me. I had breast cancer twelve years ago and survived. I had some difficult times during the first thirty years of my life and survived. I thought I "paid my dues," as they say. I held onto my faith by a thread during my early years. I trusted you when I had cancer. How come you let me down this time?

My thinking gets very mixed up these days. There is so much I don't remember, so much I don't understand anymore. Deep down I know you have not forgotten me and I know you will not abandon me. Your gifts surround and embrace me still. We get to Mass and receive the gift of Eucharist twice a week. My caregiver brings me love everyday, every moment. I feel your presence in him and I am comforted. No, I have not been betrayed!

At the end of supper you sang songs of praise. I enjoyed singing and used to sing in a choir. My voice is rather harsh these days. I say words of praise to you each day and someday I'll sing them when I come home to you.

Robert John McAllister, M.D., Ph.D.

They came to a place called Gethsemane, and He said to His disciples, "Sit here while I pray. My soul is sorrowful even to death." He prayed to His Father: "Take this cup away from Me, but not what I will but what You will." (Mark 14: 32-36)

Were you frightened in the garden, Jesus? Did you know what was going to happen? Did you know the details or just that something terrible was going to happen to you? I guess you knew they were coming to get you and take you away. But did you know what it would be like? No one told you what was going to happen. I guess you knew some of it because you knew the scriptures. But you didn't know how it would feel, how it would hurt, how degrading it would become, how lost you would feel, how alone you would be.

I'm frightened because I have Alzheimer's and I don't know what is going to happen to me. I don't know the details but I know it is a difficult disease. I don't know much about how it is going to be for me. No one tells me what is going to happen or what it will be like. I don't have any idea how I will feel when I can't remember anything and my thoughts are confused and my emotions are in turmoil.

Did you wonder what your friends and your family would do when your enemies took you away? Would they know how bad it was for you? How would they know? How would they feel and how would they react? Would they abandon you? Would they try to help and find they could do nothing to help you? Did they worry about you?

How will my husband and my children and my friends know what is happening to me when Alzheimer's takes me away from my present life and from them? Will they wonder what is happening to me? Will they worry? How can I tell them about it? How can I explain to them what is happening in my mind and my body if I can't understand it? What will I do? What will it be like?

Was it difficult to pray when you were so sorrowful? Why were you sorrowful? Were you sad because of what was going to happen to you? Or was it because of what happens to us, all of us with our sins and our sorrows? Were you sorrowful because your feelings just sort of took over and clouded your thinking?

My feelings take over sometimes and confuse my thinking and change my behavior. That makes it difficult for me to pray. I get awfully sad sometimes, thinking and wondering and worrying. You had a lot to think about and even though you were the Son of God, your human nature must have worried about what was happening and wondered what would become of your mother and your close friends. I wonder what will happen not just to me but to my husband, my children, my loved ones.

Your friends fell asleep and later ran away. They were afraid. I wonder if my husband and my children and my friends will be there for me. Or will they, one by one, eventually leave me. Will they leave because they are afraid of the person I become and of what I might do? Will I be so overwhelmed with negative thoughts and feelings it will drive them away? Will I be so different they won't know me? Or will they just say they don't know me like Peter did?

You asked, "Take this cup away." Was the anticipation of what would happen that frightening? Did you really want to be out from under it all? Well, I do. How many times I have asked to have it taken away! I have told God over and over I didn't do anything to deserve this punishment! But He doesn't listen to me and I guess he didn't listen to you. Or did He just give you strength to continue on the path in front of you?

I've not been perfect but I don't think I did anything bad enough to deserve this punishment. On the other hand you never did anything wrong. I guess bad things aren't always a punishment. You were truly and completely innocent. And in the end you accepted everything that was ahead! I guess that's what I need to do. Will God give me the strength to do it if I ask?

They bound Jesus, led Him away, and handed Him over to Pilate. Pilate, wishing to satisfy the crowd, released Barabbas to them and, after he had Jesus scourged, handed Him over to be crucified. (Mark 15:1-15)

What a painful and degrading time it was for you, Jesus! You gave your sacred body to the whips of the soldiers and the whips cut deep into your flesh and opened the first wounds. How desperate you must have felt! How long would they continue in this merciless scene? Did you cry out in pain? Did you think about your mother and your friends? Did you wish you could die then? Your human nature must have taken you through all sorts of thoughts? Did you feel angry at the soldiers for hurting you?

My body often hurts. I don't know why. I always think it must be because of the Alzheimer's. Sometimes my legs hurt when I walk and I imagine the disease is creeping up my legs to destroy my ability to walk. I see the veins in my hands and my feet and they look like recently wounded flesh. I hate the sight of them. They frighten me. They are disfiguring and I am ashamed when anyone sees them. Your bleeding flesh was shown to many when Pilate brought you out before the crowds. Was that to shame you?

I had surgery for cancer twelve years ago. I have hard lumps in my breast again and I believe I have cancer and will die of it. The doctors tell me it is not cancer but only scars from the radiation treatment. But I can't trust them. Pilate wanted to set you free but he could not be trusted. I can't trust the doctors. They tell me things to make me feel better. I see them wash their hands too. But they don't tell me what's going to happen because of Alzheimer's, so why should I trust them.

Sometimes I feel the doctors are my persecutors. They ask me questions I don't know the answers to. They say things to me that are unintelligible or that I can't remember. Later I think I know what they said but when I tell my husband he says I am wrong. They talk to my husband about me and I don't understand what they are saying. When you were questioned by Pilate and by Herod, did you know no matter what answers you gave, things would turn out the same? That's how I feel when I talk to the doctors. No matter what I say, I expect one day they will take me away and put me in a cage somewhere for the rest of my life. That will be the end. Then I will lose my spirit.

I talk to my husband about these things. He reassures me and explains what the doctors say. Then I forget what he told me. He knows I forget, so he tells me over and over so I won't start worrying again. But I do of course.

Every pain in my legs or my arms or my breast or even in my teeth or anywhere is a signal to me that death is near. The pain tells me I am going to die. And I am afraid. The fear sometimes casts me into a kind of despair. I want to die and be finished with all the suffering. Were you afraid when you were being whipped? I guess you knew you were going to die at their hands. Did you find any peace of mind during the ordeal? Did you despair even for a moment? Was all hope, all good, all faith dimmed by the pain throughout your body?

I call to you in those times that are the most difficult for me because deep in my heart I know you will not abandon me. Many times while I am still pleading with you, my husband steps into the room I'm in to ask, "How are things going, my love?" He knows how sad and frightened I can become. I don't have to answer his question. He takes me in his arms and holds me tight and pours soft loving words into my ear. "You are my precious love. I will always take care of you. We will do this together. God will be with us as he has always been through all our years. His providence brought us to this retirement home right before we found out you had Alzheimer's. We are in a safe, good place to be at this time in our life. We have each other. We have our faith. Please, don't worry. You know I will always love you." And for a time I am at peace.

> **The soldiers led Jesus away inside the palace and assembled the whole cohort. They clothed Jesus in purple and, weaving a crown of thorns, placed it on Him. They began to salute Him with, "Hail, King of the Jews!" and kept striking His head with a reed and spitting upon Him. (Mark 15: 16-19)**

Jesus, did you wonder "what will they do next?" Or did you know how the whole event would be played out? I often wonder "what will come next?" The crown of thorns seems so real when I think about it. I can almost see the sharp thorns piercing your scalp and entering some depth into the bone of your skull. It was such an exaggerated form of mockery! And the purple cloak was to mock you. (I never told you; purple was my favorite color when I was a child.)

Was there some special significance in that event? I often wonder if it was to atone for all the sins we commit inside our heads. If the scourging atoned for sins of the flesh, did this suffering atone for my sins of thought? I have lots of those. I have angry thoughts, hate-filled thoughts, and jealous thoughts—beyond control, beyond reason, beyond explanation. I never had such hostile thoughts. They enter uninvited and unwanted. My husband tells me they come as part of the illness. I believe that is true but they are still mine and I fear I may be punished for them. For a while they seem to take over my life. Do your thorns atone for these thoughts of mine?

Sometimes I think of killing myself because I don't like what I have become. I think I am stupid when I can't remember the simplest things and I lose each thing I put down. I can't find it because I can't remember what it looked like. I hate feeling stupid and mean and especially for being nasty to my husband. I can easily feel like I'm a failure. I know you never felt like a failure because you continued on, no matter how painful and severe the course. I often feel discouraged about my illness and there are moments when I feel like I hate everyone including you.

I know that is wrong and all my hates are wrong but the knowledge comes only after they are gone. After the storm of anger is over I feel remorseful and ashamed of how I felt, what I said and how I acted. My husband is always there ready to forgive; although he says there is no need of forgiveness because these are Alzheimer's storms over which I have little or no control. Then it comes to me, "I am not a failure."

My head is full of thorns. I see little bumps and indentations on my face and on my forehead and I am certain something serious is happening to my skull. I know something is affecting how I think and how I feel. Are those small surface changes the cause? The doctor tells me they are insignificant, "perhaps due to aging," but he can't see what they are causing on the inside. Although others minimize them, these thorns are real to me.

The thorns inside are painful and more frightening than those on the outside because I cannot see them and check on them. But they are there! They wake me at night with frightening dreams. They disturb me during peaceful times because they push and prick inside my brain and tell me, "you are getting worse," "you will be crazy someday," "you are turning into a daemon," "you will be locked up and alone," "you are stupid," "someday everyone will abandon you." They hurt. They disrupt my waking time like the dreams disrupt my sleep.

I am grateful for my ever-present caregiver who repeatedly assures me I am not crazy and not going to be crazy, not stupid and never going to be locked up and alone. Your gift comes through him, Jesus, and the painful, frightening things are gone for a time. I am comforted in his arms and by your continued love.

> **Then Pilate handed Jesus over to be crucified. So they took Jesus and, carrying the cross Himself, He went out to what is called the Place of the Skull, in Hebrew, Golgotha. (John 19: 16-17)**

The scriptural passage suggests to me you had an option. Did you? There is the tone of "volunteer." Would someone else have carried the cross for you? But we know God's way is to show us the way. A fundamental thing to learn as a Christian is that we must carry our own cross. How clearly the message comes down through the centuries! How clearly it confronts me these days!

I didn't volunteer and I still don't volunteer. But I am here and I am carrying the cross you gave me. I'm not happy about it. But how can I speak of happiness considering these horrible scenes of your life and death. Because life is often so sad I need to speak of happiness sometimes. I need to think about it, to be aware of it, to mention it. I need to remember that Golgotha was only a stopping off place, not an end place.

As I picture these continuing events in your trip to death, I feel exhausted. What strength kept you going? How could you go on? I guess the soldiers whipped you if you stopped or fell but how could you find strength to get up? The blood and sweat must have dripped from your body, drained your strength, and hampered your vision. Did you see your mother somewhere in the crowd? Did you catch sight of your friends? After Veronica reached out to you and wiped the blood and sweat from your face, you could more easily search the onlookers to catch sight of those especially dear to you.

The ninth Station of the Cross has always captured my imagination. It seems like such a pivotal moment, one of those "do or die" times. How could you get up after you fell that time? Where did you find the strength, the determination, the will to go on? After all, your humanity had been tried before the Sanhedrin and was now being tested to the limit. You lost a great deal of blood; you were severely dehydrated; your physical strength was depleted. Wasn't your spirit broken? As I ask the question, I respond to it, "Of course not, never, impossible!" Because you were God? No! Because you were the one with a love that surpassed all those limitations.

Simon of Cyrene was called to help you carry the cross. I have often wondered, "Was he a willing helper? Or did he help because he had to? Did you speak to him with words or only with the way you looked at him?" I'm sure he was blessed forevermore as a result of his service to you, whether forced or voluntary. My husband helps me carry my cross and does so most willingly. He calms the emotional storms that knock me down. He holds me and comforts me on my journey, as I'm sure your mother wanted to hold and comfort you as she saw you on your journey.

I fall a lot, you know. I intend to do better each day. I plan to be patient with myself and with others, especially my caregiver. I plan to remember things and to put things in a place so I will be able to find them later. I fail over and over and over again. I am defeated by my failures. It is so hard to get up again and go on, especially when I know I will continue to fail. But I forget I can't remember, so I get up and continue my journey with new resolve until I find myself flat on my face again. I get tired of getting up and worry someday I will stay down. I will just lie there, go to bed, and let everything go. But I think of you when you fell the third time. You got up and went on to meet the end you were destined for. And so must I!

I am sure Veronica and Simon received your blessings of gratitude throughout their lives. They were your caregivers on your journey to death. My caregiver does not always fare so well. Instead of gratitude and blessings he is too often met with anger and harsh words and bitter times. That is not what I mean to do but the storm clouds of Alzheimer's dull my judgment and somehow unleash the lightening of my hostility and the thunder of my angry words. There are many others who reach out to me and express their concern and willingness to help. The women of Jerusalem reached out to you. I always feel these friends have needs of their own to take care of but I am grateful for their presence and their kind words.

> **When they came to the place called the Skull, they crucified Jesus. Darkness came over the whole land until three in the afternoon. Jesus cried out in a loud voice, "Father, into Your hands I commend my spirit." And when He had said this, He breathed His last. (Luke 23: 33-46)**

This passage brings me to thoughts of death, my own and that of my spouse. You left the garden of your prayer and spent many hours helpless and alone throughout the suffering you endured. Even in your last agony you had concern for others. You left your mother in John's care. You prayed for those who treated you so horribly and forgave them. You responded generously to the man crucified beside you. And when all those matters were settled, you returned to your Father.

One could say, "You settled your affairs." I use that phrase because "my affairs" is a matter that disturbs me greatly and often. First of all, I worry most about what will happen to my husband. Who will take care of him when I die? Will you? The good thief went with you to paradise. My husband is a good man and I want so badly to take him with me when I die. I cannot leave him, though I know I must. I cannot bear the thought of it but "thy will be done."

You had no "belongings" to dispose of, to settle. They even had to borrow a tomb for your burial. My "things" are troubling to me. They are too much with me. They are too important to me I know. Now I cling to them even more desperately because in my increasing confusion I find them reassuring and consoling. They are always there. I need not know their names. I can talk to them or not and either way we have a closeness that is familiar and warming to me. We have no unfulfilled expectations of one another. Before I die I want to know where they will be after I am gone. I want to make decisions about their future. But it is my future I need to be concerned about, not the future of "things."

Maybe I focus on the future of my things to avoid thinking of what will happen to me. I fear I may not go to heaven. I am filled with thoughts of how unworthy I am. The intensity and depth of my anger seems wicked to me. I sometimes am angry at you, at your Father. I have always been ready to doubt the love of others, even my husband. Why should I not doubt your love? Still I dwell on the reality and the force of it as I contemplate your passion and death. Was it for me too or just for the chosen ones?

My husband says I should go straight to heaven because I have purgatory with me now. I wish I could believe what he says. I stole once or twice when I was little and again a few years ago. When I was young I didn't know how wrong it was. In recent years I was too confused to know I was stealing. If I'm a thief, can I be your good thief? Will you take me home? My husband says dying is like going to a happy home. I never knew what a happy home was until I married him. So I guess heaven will be something like our life now, only no fears, no sadness, no anger, no mistakes, no losses, no stupidity, no Alzheimer's.

I have forgiven all those toward whom I have harbored resentment. I have no others on my list to forgive. But I'm sure there are quite a number on the list from whom I would ask forgiveness—my husband for my lack of gentleness, my children for my lack of presence, my friends for my lack of the strength and wisdom to be the friend they needed, and my enemies who may have been made so by my shortcomings.

I wrote a little prayer several months ago. I keep it where I can say it every day. "God, how quickly comes your love to me. Can I join with your pain and suffering? Could I? I do not feel any words are needed to explain to you. You are with me. I know I must accept my condition. I want to carry it well for myself and my loved ones and for you. I pray to go to heaven to find the Creator of love, the Mother of peace."

Can I commend my spirit to you now and believe you will be there to receive me when I die? Can I ask that my husband be with me when that time comes and that I will recognize him and know he loves me? Do I ask too much? When I have fulfilled your plan for me, will you release me and return all my beautiful memories to me?

> **Two of them that same day were making their way to a village named Emmaus. In the course of their lively exchange, Jesus approached and began to walk with them. They said to one another, "Were not our hearts burning inside us as he talked to us on the road and explained the Scriptures to us?" (Luke 24:13-32)**

Of all the Easter stories, Jesus, this is my favorite. The scene is probably afternoon on the dusty road to Emmaus. There is no sunrise or morning dew or angel or earthquake or empty tomb. There is no running or shouting or weeping. There are just two men walking and talking. It is so simple and so beautiful,

Jesus, it almost takes my breath away. My imagination can witness the event and I am there.

I don't handle excitement well. It unnerves me. Or perhaps I should say it "nerves" me because any big "to do" stirs all kinds of emotions in me and you know I don't handle emotions well. With Alzheimer's my feelings just go charging off in any direction they please. Unusual and unexpected events can make me angry or anxious or sad or frightened or even "crazy" (as I call it). My responses are completely unpredictable.

The scene at the tomb is too much for me to grasp and to hold onto. It is too "busy," too hectic, too unreal. There are strong emotions everywhere and I want to run away. Someone in "dazzling garments" would frighten me. I have a hard time recognizing the people I know even when they are calm and relaxed and dressed in familiar clothing.

As always I have questions. Why these two men, only one of whom is named? What was special about them to have so much time in your presence? You seemed to think you needed to reveal yourself to them in a gentle and careful manner. Why was that? Maybe Cleopas or his companion had a weak heart or possibly an illness like mine. It was so thoughtful to make them feel at ease and then bring them so tenderly to an awareness of their risen Lord.

My Easter wish is to walk quietly down a path hand in hand with my husband and have you join us for a time. Or even better the three of us sit and just talk. It is difficult for me to converse with someone when I am walking. I understand another person better if we are face to face. It helps me focus on what is being said.

During the day I sometimes feel very comfortable talking to you as if you were in the room. If someone can hold a little gadget in their hand and talk to another person in Europe or anywhere else, it is not difficult for me to envision you hearing me wherever I am.

Words are a great consolation to me. They are another form of touch, only they reach more deeply into me. I wish I could learn to hear your voice as some holy people do. Talking with my husband is a great blessing in my life. We often talk for two or three hours. We used to have lengthy conversations about life, about religion, about philosophy, about world events. I don't know much about any of those topics now. Mostly we talk about my illness and how it affects our life. Talking helps me understand better what is happening to me. My husband is kind and loving. He encourages me and tells me how brave I am and how I inspire him. We agree our life continues to be a good life because it is filled with our love for each other and with the blessings of physical well being and our deep faith.

My greatest fear is dying and leaving him alone. He says if he dies first I will not remember him. But if I die first, I will live on in his memory and in his heart. Come to think of it, that's how you live with us now.

I submitted the piece, "An Alzheimer Patient's Lenten Meditation," to the National Catholic Reporter (NCR), a prominent and popular biweekly Catholic Newspaper. After several promptings by phone I finally reached someone who agreed to read "from the stack of papers on my desk" what I sent. The editor was interested in publishing the material. At his suggestion I expanded the meditations from five to seven.

1/30/12

I've written books and numerous articles during the past years. On each occasion I had both a purpose and a goal or endpoint. My purpose when I started writing these pages was not to publish. I wasn't writing for others to read. I think I started to keep myself company. It doesn't seem to be "the company" it used to be. Has the thought of publishing this material changed my focus and my freedom?

The endpoint is the real issue. When and how will this journal end? These uncomfortable questions confront me every day. No, the questions don't confront me, the answers do. I will stop writing if I become too ill to write or die. In that case the end would come abruptly, unexpectedly. The most likely answer, the one I don't want to face, is that I will stop writing when Jane dies. There would be no more reason to write, only to say she is gone.

The story will be over. Life will be over. I can't imagine living in the emptiness. Sometimes when we are at Mass I think about being there for Jane's Memorial Service. How will I be able to continue going to Mass without Jane? When we are in the Mall I think about never coming back once Jane is gone. When we are at dinner I wonder how I will be able to go to the dining room ever again without Jane. How will I go to bed without Jane? Or get up?

In the event I die or become too ill to write I should perhaps consider asking my son, Paul, to get these pages from my computer, add a brief note of his own and then send them somewhere for self-publication. Harriet Lerner has suggested that possibility based on her strong feeling they should be published.

There could be another endpoint, too painful for me even to consider, but I must be honest. As Jane's health fails I may reach a point where I cannot care for her in our apartment. I would find that very disturbing and I know I would feel a great deal of guilt if I needed to make such a decision. On the other hand, I would not condemn any caregiver for reaching a point where she or he could not continue in that role. Jane would want me to be equally gentle with myself.

Thoughts like these are with me lately. Maybe it's the winter weather. Maybe it's the cold I've had for about ten days. Maybe it's because I haven't exercised regularly of late. Maybe it's just me.

I often say to Jane, "You are my life." We talk about the two of us being one. I am confined to the life Jane has. This **is** our life. For me it does not have the "lost" feeling, the desperation, the emptiness it has for her. I am not lost but I am wandering. I am not empty but I am shriveled. I have memories but in some ways they only make it more desolate. Our life is not going anywhere, not doing anything except repeating the patterns and rituals we have created.

Sometimes it feels like it is over; and we just keep going, waiting for it to end. I don't feel depressed. I'm tired. I just want to go home.

I occasionally talk to another resident I see in the dining room. He is short of breath, has difficulty walking, and sees very poorly. His wife died some years ago. He often says, "I just wish this could be over and I could be out of here." I understand what he feels.

Even as I write this I feel selfish and ungrateful. This is not a bad life or a difficult life or an empty life. Perhaps what is bothering me is: I need to know now how it will end. I'm not good at the waiting, the uncertainty. We could go on as things are, perhaps worse, undoubtedly worse, for a long time. How long, oh Lord, how long?

2/2/12

Jane has been having a difficult time the past few days. She is often confused and easily irritable. She bought a scarf in the Mall yesterday. It was the "prettiest scarf I ever saw." Today she wanted to buy another so she could give this one to Kathie and another to Bonnie. I said she liked the scarf and should keep it. She couldn't remember what it looked like.

She wanted to buy greeting cards for Kathie and Bonnie "to take to them when we visit them." I said we don't visit them but "you should get the cards to send to them." Shortly after we got home, she wanted to send cards to her mother and her grandmother because "I'm not in touch with them very often." I replied, "Sweetheart, your mother and grandmother have been dead a long time." She accepted it without comment. I don't think it disturbed her to learn how far off the mark she was, because the words melted away as they went through the air between us.

Sometimes in the evening, usually at bed time, Jane seems to change into a different person. She becomes argumentative, very opinionated, and off on one or more tangents of confusion. It feels like she is prepared to turn on me over anything I say. It is difficult to comfort her, much less reassure her. Basically I try not to make matters worse. I am careful what I say and how I say it. I try to be present but not intrusive. I try to be gentle but not overly solicitous. If I become too involved she says I am trying to make her feel "stupid" or "crazy." It is one of those times that a year ago would have escalated to her leaving the apartment or threatening to kill herself. It has the same feel, the same tone, the same ingredients, the same direction. But these episodes play themselves out quickly or fade away as she falls asleep.

I mentioned how Jane absorbs feelings from others or from situations. My emotions certainly respond strongly to her mood. An evening like this leaves me disheartened and fearful about the future. I start thinking every day of our lives will become like this. It is a dismal picture, a depressing, hopeless future. The fears that dwell in my subconscious become real. This is our future, until death do us part!

Then the next morning after a good sleep Jane is back, pleasant, loving, looking forward to our day together. Sleep surely helps us both but it is loss of all memory of the night before that makes everything right for Jane. It is the smile on her face and the love in her embrace that makes it all right for me.

(Email to Paul 2/3/12)
Dear Paul,
You left just a short time ago. When we got to the apartment I asked Mom if she wanted to play cards a while and then take a nap before dinner. She opted for taking a nap. Visits are obviously tiring for her.

I wanted to tell you how remarkable Mom was during the visit. I have not seen her so bright and cheerful and sharp in many, many days. Last night she was terribly confused as she often is in the evenings now. She wanted to send a card to her mother and her grandmother. She felt desolate about her life and insisted a doctor recently told her she had six months to live. When I said I was with her every time any doctor talked to her, she initially seemed to accept what I said. But within a few minutes she was repeating the comment and said the doctor told her on the telephone. A clever maneuver! I just gave up and let it go.

Last night she was also caught up in our need to make plans for the future, meaning of course our deaths. She has "a lot of things I need to do while I still can. We have to make some decisions about all of this. You know I am dying." We have talked many times about this very thing. I encouraged her to postpone our discussion until tomorrow. Of course, she has forgotten all that today. Last night she was sad and frightened and unreachable to any reassurance I tried to give her.

(Paul 2/7/12)

Paul,

I seem to be inundating you with emails the last few days. This is one I have long deliberated about.

I have over 200 pages I have written since December 2006 about our life with Alzheimer's. I have called it "An Alzheimer's Love Affair." Harriet Lerner, the well know author of "Dance of Anger, of Intimacy, etc., etc." has encouraged me in this. * * * * * *

Now, the main reason for this email. If I become unable for any reason to complete the writing, I am asking you to work with Harriet so it can be submitted with her help for publication. She feels very strongly about this and I must admit I have become more invested in publication. Her email address is in my Gmail.

* * * * * *

The writing seems very personal and private to me, almost sacred, so I have hesitated to share it. In the past few months I have asked two close friends to proofread the material. In a week or so I'll send you a section of it. * * * * * *

2/11/12

A few nights ago Jane commented, "I'm going to quit going to those Thursday meetings. Nothing is being accomplished and I'm tired of going. I think I will just not go back." There are no Thursday meetings. Several years back Jane went to chorus on Thursdays but she stopped going long ago.

Last night apropos of nothing she said, "I'm not going to work with that committee any more. They just give me papers to write down names. Someone else can do that. It doesn't fit for me now." She and I were on the Marketing Committee here for several years. Is that the connection? Or is this related to a time when she worked as an assistant buyer nearly 50 years ago? To this comment and the previous one I just went along saying, "I don't think you need to continue that." I decided there was no reason to tell her how confused she was.

Jane's head works strangely these days. Her comments seem so reality based. Her mind is a playground for a never ending game of hide and seek. Some events and people from the past get in free, uninvited to the game, unexpected players. But there they are: a mother, a grandmother, a ring, a handbag, a scarf, fellow workers or participants in some long forgotten activity. Other events and people from a day ago or an hour ago stay in hiding and cannot be found no matter how many hints are given of their whereabouts. It is an uncomfortable game because there are no known rules, no limits on who or what gets in free, or on who or what might hide and never be found.

When we had arguments in the past Jane often referred to them in a demeaning way as a game and she felt she always lost. The hide and seek game goes on independently of her behavior, her intentions, or her moods. She is an unwilling player, a constant loser, a solitary figure. She is a child who doesn't want to play but has no choice, who knows something is unfair but cannot identify what it is, who is aware she is losing but has no way to measure how badly. I suspect this is reminiscent of childhood experiences. She was lonely and frightened as a child and participated poorly with other children. Her responses often seem primitive and pleading in the midst of her confusion.

Physical affection and calm conversation help us clear up much of the confusion that runs rampant and reckless in her head at these times. Even if it doesn't clear the confusion, it quells the accompanying fear.

We had a strange incident a few days ago. The supervisor at our Subway in the Mall has been a friend of ours for four or five years. He and his wife are the ones who brought a Nepalese lunch to the Mall for us about a year ago. They celebrated their 25th wedding anniversary this week. We were invited to the party on February 11th. I declined because it would be confusing for Jane and not a good evening for either of us. Jane and I bought a card for the occasion and earlier this week we picked out a picture album as a gift for them.

I wrapped the album and attached the card. I showed the package to Jane and explained what it was. Later that afternoon she took a nap and I went down to exercise. When I returned she was up and said, with some irritation, she was unable to sleep. When I asked if something was wrong, she said she couldn't sleep because she kept thinking about "the box of chocolates you are going to give some woman."

This obviously required some "sit down and talk time." I explained carefully and step by step what it was all about. Jane had no memory of Nandi and Binda, the couple, or of buying the card or the album. She accepted my explanation and apologized for "attacking" me. If this sort of thing is not dealt with as quickly and as directly as possible, it becomes an overpowering problem for her. Fortunately she was amenable to sitting down with me and discussing it. I have had at least two occasions to go over the details again to keep her mind on the facts and not go back to the "jealous player" in her head.

Later that same evening we had one of the best talks we've had in sometime. Jane brought up her concern about "how things are going to be soon." I reassured her I will take care of her. We talked about "our things" and what will happen to them. We talked about moves in the past in very general terms because Jane has no memory of specifics. We agreed each time we moved we were looking forward with anticipation to the place we were going. That always made moving easier. I said we are in the same kind of situation now. We are preparing to eventually move from here to another place, a place unknown and mysterious, but a real place we call heaven. We talked realistically about everyone here waiting to die. It was a very open conversation about the reality of our situation and the certainty of our death.

Jane said how good it was to talk about these things. It was remarkable how clear headed and logical she was, how cognizant of the realities of our life now, how accepting of the inevitable future. It was a comfortable, frank, and tender exchange between two loving partners looking at the "end time."

2/13/12

I want to give an example of something I consider important in interactions with Jane. We met Kathie at the Mall yesterday for about an hour. She has a bad cold, had not been sleeping well, and clearly was not in the best of spirits. The visit went well although it was a bit flat and slow. Jane was affectionate with Kathie and made many loving comments.

Last evening in bed Jane said, "I need to call Kathie in the morning. I don't want her to be angry at me because of the mean things I said to her today. I'm afraid she might never call again and I couldn't stand losing contact with her." This kind of thing occurs in Jane's head at times. She may have had some mild negative feelings during the visit because it was not bright and cheerful. Those feelings may then have become dominant in her mind in relation to the visit. Feelings trump facts every time.

I immediately responded, "My sweet love, you were gentle and loving with Kathie at the Mall. You were affectionate like you always are. You didn't say anything harsh or critical. There was nothing you said or did that could possibly make her think you don't love her. There is no reason to call her. Kathie knows you love her and she loves you."

Jane was relieved and acknowledged she would have had a difficult time getting to sleep if we had not talked. I said, "If you ever have thoughts that are disturbing you, please, talk to me about them. Wake me up if something is keeping you from sleeping. This is how we need to work together. We know your feelings drag you off into some strange thinking at times. Please, let me know about it. We need to talk about it. This is how we stay close together in our love."

What if she hadn't told me? What if we hadn't talked about it? What if we didn't have the kind of conversations we often have about Jane's thoughts and especially her feelings? We both slept well.

Two interesting incongruities: 1) Almost every movie we watch ends with Jane saying, "We saw this before but I didn't remember much about it." 2) Every lunch at the Mall has been a six inch sub with turkey, provolone cheese, lettuce, tomato, and honey mustard. Today after lunch Jane said, "We never had that before. It was good." Things she never saw she believes she saw. Things she has experienced repeatedly suddenly are new.

2/27/12

I last wrote two weeks ago. How much the world has changed in two weeks! My life has come undone! I've been avoiding coming back to write. I make lists of what to do because I can't remember things. I go from one thing to another in order not to come to this place and put something in words I do not want to write, to hear, to think about, to see. **Jane is dead. Yes, dead.** I don't want to write it. I don't want to say it. I don't want to hear it.

But I do say it so easily when I see people we know. I talk about it freely and tell them what happened. Somehow this is different. These words were my secret world where I lived with Jane and could say how things really were or at least how I saw them to be. Now to come back to this world and put this truth in these pages that contain our life, our love, our pain makes it more real, more cruel, more desolate.

I just realized I use these pages as a parallel world where I live not alone but privately. These pages gave me some distance from all that was happening. They were in some strange way a retreat, a refuge. In retrospect I believe they made things easier for me.

I sit here with an empty head and a heavy heart. I don't want to go over all the details but I must. On the other hand the thought occurs, if I just keep writing something then the story won't end. But the story has ended. I have to put it to rest, as she has gone to rest. Then I too will be at rest.

Last Tuesday, February 14th, we went to Mass followed by lunch at the Mall, our usual routine. We did our leg exercises in the morning before we left. They seemed more difficult for Jane but she completed them. Now I wonder if her goal has been to maintain her strength or to please me. I always praised her for exercising and said how important it was to remain ambulatory so we could continue our outings to the Mall. I think she pushed herself to the limit to keep our life going along as it was.

On the 14th we ate dinner in the dining room as usual. We went to a music program at 7:30 in the auditorium. We started a movie after we got home but Jane couldn't follow it. I do not recall bedtime being unusual. We slept well.

While fixing breakfast the following morning, I heard Jane call. She had fallen in the bathroom. She could not get up and was too weak to assist me in trying to help her up. I called the front desk and a nurse and the security man came to help her up. After an evaluation, the nurse recommended Jane go to the emergency room and she called an ambulance.

We spent the day in the ER at Howard County General Hospital. Jane had a urinary tract infection. They gave her an intravenous antibiotic and a prescription to pick up on the way home.

When we returned to Vantage House Jane walked in with me from the car. She fell on the first floor of our building. I took her upstairs in a wheelchair provided by staff. She was able to walk but unstable. I sat her in the living room. She was ill tempered and uncooperative. The emergency room had certainly been an ordeal for her.

I picked up two dinners from the dining room. Jane ate very little. We watched a bit of a movie but she was unable to follow any of it. We talked a little but she was quite confused. It had been a tense and tiring day.

I steadied her as she got ready for bed. She was extremely weak. Once we were in bed, she would not, probably could not, stop talking. I think she talked all night. I dozed for about half an hour a couple of times. She was angry, frightened, sad, tormented. There was nothing I could do to calm or console her. Most of her comments were directed toward me. She remembered every hurtful thing she thought I did over the past few years . . . all the things I didn't let her buy, not giving her money or an allowance or a credit card, not letting her shop on her own, bossing her, belittling her, ignoring her, smiling at all the women we knew and never at her, being friendly with the women on staff, in the Mall, at church. It was endless. It was merciless. It was Alzheimer's at its worst.

When we got up Thursday morning, I slid her from the bed to a chair with casters. I rolled her into the bathroom and slid her onto the toilet. Then I slid her back on the chair and rolled her into the living room. I slid her onto the sofa. She was weak and listless. I called the clinic nurse. After she did an evaluation and made a phone call to our internist, she recommended Jane return to Howard County General Hospital ER by ambulance.

We spent another day in the emergency room. I noticed Jane's left breast, the one that had surgery last October, was extremely swollen and very red. I had been putting cocoa butter on the scar every night, so I knew the swelling and the redness were very recent. It got the attention of the ER doctor and he called a plastic surgeon. (Our plastic surgeon was out of town.) After his examination and a review of the records, the surgeon told me they could do an MRI, which would be very difficult, and he felt certain he would have to operate on the breast. All of this, if I wanted Jane to be treated aggressively. He didn't say it but his tone seemed to suggest he was reluctant to proceed with what he proposed.

I chose not to have aggressive treatment. Palliative treatment was the alternative. That meant stopping the antibiotics and all medicines Jane had been taking. She would be continued on morphine as needed for pain and Ativan as needed for restlessness. She was admitted to Howard County General Hospital Thursday evening and remained there until Monday afternoon. Then she was transferred back to the nursing unit at Vantage House to await death. She died Thursday morning, February 23rd, about 5a.m.

There, it is all down on paper. It is done. It is fact. **Jane is dead. Yes, dead.** And I am still alive, and I cannot let her death leave me abandoned.

I chose not to have aggressive treatment. It didn't take thought to decide. It was in my mind waiting to be said. Did I expect the question? No. But a door opened and I was ready to let her go through. How could I say to the doctor and to Jane, "Keep her alive. Do whatever you need to do, but keep her here." If Jane had been conscious, and the question was asked of her, she would have said, "I can't leave Robbie alone. Do whatever you need to do, he needs me." She would not have said, "Do whatever you need to do. I want to go back to the life I've had for many years now. I want to go back to feeling stupid and crazy and being sad and frightened and angry and not knowing where I am or where I've been or where I'm going." As long as I live, no matter how miserable and lonely and lost I may be, I will never for one second think, "I should have requested aggressive treatment." Life had been aggressive toward my love long enough. No more, no more!

Paul and Kathie were with me last Thursday, and Laura came on Friday. The three of them spent most of the days and evenings in Jane's hospital room through Sunday. There was a sofa-bed so I stayed around the clock. Laura went home on Monday. Jane was transferred to the nursing unit at Vantage House on Monday. Paul and Kathie visited there Monday and Tuesday, and Bonnie came on Wednesday and spent some time with Jane the evening before she died. Kathie was also there. Jane was not awake then.

There were some jeweled moments during those days. Jane was awake enough to talk briefly to each of the three children and to me. She was for the most part her sweet, gentle self with them. On occasion she became agitated and tried to get out of bed or to pull out the oxygen, the intravenous, or the catheter. This happened more often during the night. She would call, "Robbie, Robbie." Her expectation was I would help her with what she was trying to do. She would become quite hostile and obstreperous when I thwarted her attempts to free herself from these limitations.

We had a special period Sunday evening. It was Jane, Laura and me, the three who spent so many years together from Laura's entry into the world to the time she went off to college. The three of us were reunited for a special, sacred time. I was leaning over Jane to do something . . . . she puckered up her lips and pointed to them with her finger. I kissed her and then she puckered again. I kissed her several times. Then she motioned for Laura to come and did the same thing with her. Jane was obviously aware of and united with us for that precious time. It was so right, so fulfilling, so blessed.

The following is a letter I wrote to the director of the nursing unit at Vantage House.

Barbara D'Anna   2/27/12
Director Health Services
Vantage House

Dear Barbara,

With a heart filled with sadness I write to tell you of my sincere gratitude and deep appreciation for the care the staff on the nursing unit provided to my wife during her short stay prior to her death. They provided excellent professional care and at the same time exhibited warmth and compassion to me and those who came to visit Jane.

There are names of several staff I would like to personally thank and commend but I'm not sure I have all the names and I would not want to miss anyone. Suffice it to say, everyone was kind, thoughtful and caring. I shall be ever grateful for their making these last days and nights as painless and as peaceful for Jane as they could possibly have been.

Gratefully,

Robert McAllister

2/28/12

I went to the mortuary the morning after her death. My friend, Dennis, called and insisted he take me. It was comforting to have him there. I picked out a cinerarium large enough for two. It has a solid cherry top and base, a birch body with oak stained veneer. Laura commented later, "Mom will really be happy with that box." Jane never saw a box she didn't love.

Her wedding ring was returned to me at the mortuary. Before I left there I put it on my little finger next to my ring and there it will remain for the rest of my life. The rings will be a symbol of our closeness. They will always be near each other, touch each other most of the time, but there will never be friction or hurt.

I got very tired yesterday afternoon and stopped writing. I wake rather early these mornings, although I sleep reasonably well. I returned to my pattern of exercising about 6a.m. Yesterday afternoon was warm so I walked to the lake on the path we so often used. We haven't walked it in several years. Jane always found hearts and faces and unique designs in tree trunks along the way. There were rocks and branches and leaves pleading to come home with us. I didn't discontinue the walk for fear of being weighed down with Jane's treasures; I feared I might be weighed down with Jane if she became too weak to get home.

Yesterday the walk was relaxing and reminiscent. What a weak word "reminiscent." I don't just remember Jane, I feel her inside me and I live in her presence. I don't just think about her, I talk to her. I don't like to walk without her hand in mine. I don't like to laugh without her knowing what's funny. I use her tooth brush and remind her it is hers. The quilt we folded across the bottom of the bed is now folded on her side of the bed so I bump against it when I sleep. I used to lie against her beautiful body.

When do I miss her most? All the time. I went to Mass today. I've gone two or three times since she died, and today someone came to sit with me. Today I sat alone and was more comfortable with that. The presence of others seems like an intrusion; they separate me from Jane.

I ate dinner this evening with two people I have known for years plus a relatively newcomer. As I looked around the dining room I felt more like an inmate and these were my fellow inmates. I know many people here and even though I speak to them in a friendly manner I seem not to have any genuine feelings for them. It's as if my feelings died.

At home I read the eulogy I am preparing and I am lost in my loss. I am tired and lonely and empty and no one fills any of the space. I seem not to care whether I hear from any of the kids or not. I drive an empty car. I reside in a vacant apartment. I live an absent life. It's a low point. I will feel better tomorrow.

Going to bed is so much easier since Jane died. What a horrible thing to say! Does Jane see what I write? What will she think when I write things like that? I should say going to bed is simpler now. She became so meticulous and so slow about brushing and flossing her teeth. I would wait until she was finished before giving her nighttime medicines. Then she would spend fifteen to thirty minutes in her bathroom before coming to bed. Several years ago I was impatient with her over this. How sorry I am for things like that when they come to mind. How I wish she were back to do it all again with as much time as she might want! How empty the world is without her!

2/29/12

I just go on from day to day, not even sure what's on my mind. It's difficult to pray. I know the words but my thoughts wander off. I keep rereading the eulogy and make changes every time and then print it again. I better get more ink for the printer. I want to get a few groceries tomorrow so Laura and the girls can have breakfast with me while they are here. They are coming on March 1st, the day of the evening visitation prior to the Memorial Mass on March 2nd.

Paul picked me up the morning of the 24th and took me to the Inner Harbor and the Aquarium. It was good to be somewhere else and to be with him. He and Jane were very close. He understood her well.

I've been going through pictures today for the Visitation and the Memorial Service. They seem not to have memories attached to them. I see the face I loved so long, the face I miss so much, the face that looked so tired, so worn, so empty the last few days of her life. She was comfortable those last days. She–she–she. Her name was Jane. It is still Jane. It will always be Jane. And Jane will always be with me.

There is so much I want to write but thoughts and words to match don't come easily. The thoughts come when I try to pray; then when I try to think, the words don't come.

Kathie and Bonnie are having dinner with me here this evening. Laura and the girls will be here tomorrow. We will go to the church in the afternoon to arrange the pictures I selected. The Visitation is tomorrow evening at the church from 7p.m. to 9p.m.

Jane was cremated. The ashes will be brought to the church tomorrow afternoon and left there until after the Memorial Mass on Friday. Then I will bring them home. The box has room for my ashes. There are two separate containers inside the larger box. I must get someone to take the walls out between the two after I am dead.

I realize I'm just writing a lot of words about things and not about Jane. Maybe I don't have those words yet. Or maybe I'm afraid I won't be able to stop if I start putting them down. I want it to be a time when I won't be interrupted, when I'm not expecting someone, when I don't have something else I have to plan or work on.

I notice the first of the meditations I sent last fall to the National Catholic Reporter is in the March 2-15, 2012 edition. This first one was over-edited by one of their people who had a need to use his words rather than Jane's. The original is the one that appears in the pages above.

3/2/12

The Visitation last evening was beautiful. Laura and the girls and I put the pictures up in the afternoon. They looked good. I included a book jacket from Jane's book, "Before It's Too Late," about her Alzheimer's. Our Maryknoll friend, Father Joe Heim, had dinner with us and then we went to the service.

Family and friends were there, the ones expected and some not expected. Mary, of the pool history, was there and spoke to me about her long friendship with Jane. Five or six people including the manager and his wife came from the Mall Subway shop. Three couples we knew casually from the Mall were there, and two of the women spoke to the group about the model of love Jane and I had been for them.

When Laura and the girls and I got home, we had some cheese cake Laura made and brought. I told them the story of Jane's death. I have not written about that but I need to now. No, I can't now. This is the morning of the Memorial Mass and we will be leaving soon. I have lots of thoughts but I don't have words. Later when I have solitude and can be alone with Jane then the words will come. Not now.

Later on 3/2/12

Four priests were present for the funeral Mass, a most unusual happening. During the homily Father Tillman talked about intellect, will and feelings with emphasis on the feelings. It set things up surprisingly well for the eulogy. Some people thought we planned it together. Father Tillman said to someone, "Jane arranged it."

This is the eulogy.

The pastor told me to take all the time I wanted. I have about 150 pages here. How does that fit your time schedule?

I thought that comment might make some of you smile. It made Jane smile. She is here you know . . . . watching all of this. It's probably one of the first requests she made after she got settled in up there. So don't think for a minute she would miss being here.

Others could have done this eulogy but I decided I needed to do it. Then when I went to my head to find the words I discovered they were all buried deep in my heart.

I want to welcome each of you to Jane's going away party. She asked me to tell you she had to leave a little early. I think what really happened she got the days mixed up. You know she had Alzheimer's. She couldn't remember the season or the month or the day of the week. I think she got Ash Wednesday and Easter mixed up. She got all caught up in Easter and the resurrection story and she just got carried away.

Jane grew up in Philadelphia. She lived with her mother and maternal grandparents. No one in the house practiced religion but her grandmother took Jane to Mass every Sunday and returned to get her. Her grandmother taught her the prayers and the two prayed together every night. Her godmother, Edith Ellis, was probably the motivator for all this.

Jane went to Sunday catechism taught by the nuns. Children who did not attend the Catholic school sat in the back of the church at Mass. At first communion time the veils and prayer books given to the "back of the bus" kids were not as elegant as those given to the Catholic school students. Jane never forgot that.

She didn't learn much about her religion during those classes and she always felt she was a second class Catholic. No more, sweetheart, no more.

I spent 25 years in Catholic institutions and learned that faith is built on reason, on dogma, on knowledge. But Jane's faith was not built on reason or knowledge. It was built on feelings . . . . and so was her life. Saying you loved Jane was never enough . . . . she had to feel your love. Knowing there was a God was not enough . . . . she had to feel God's presence . . . . and she did. She felt it in the churning of the ocean, in the latticed beauty of the stark winter trees and then their green summer dresses, in rocks shaped like hearts, in the wild beauty of evening skies, and the soft pillows of summer clouds.

She didn't live by doctrines or commandments or rules. She lived by her heart; it was her compass, her guide. I have a vague recollection that Thomistic philosophy said something about the natural law being written on our hearts. Jane read what was in her heart and she was a good woman. Let me read the closing lines from the book she wrote about her life and her Alzheimer's. "When my mind takes me to revisit a trip of long ago, do you go with me God? Do you hear me? Do you hear me when I rebel? When I am indescribably angry? What are you thinking? Do you know my pain? I want to see Mary. I want to be here for that so it will be right. God hold my face in your hands."

Did you ever pray like that? You don't get that out of a book or from some teaching. That comes from the heart. Jane's faith had a simple and primitive quality. Her prayer card has an Indian verse on one side and God's handiwork on the other.

Jane loved to tell the story of her grandfather's return to the church. He was home, seriously ill. Thirteen year old Jane asked him if he would like to see a priest. He said yes. The priest came and I assume heard his confession. After the priest left Paddy McQuade said, "If I had known how easy it was to get under the fence I'd have gone a long time ago."

Some years later Jane asked her grandmother if she would like to be a Catholic. She arranged for the priest to come and helped prepare her grandmother's entry into the church.

On completing high school Jane won a four year scholarship to the prestigious Moore Art Institute in Philadelphia. She married soon after completing art school and never had the opportunity to follow up on her training and her remarkable artistic gifts.

I met Jane 50 years ago. It felt like I was meeting someone I had always known somewhere deep inside me. We came to believe our meeting was truly providential. When people ask how long we've been married my usual answer is, "Not long enough." It could never have been long enough.

When we met Jane had three children and I had five. And we both had marriages on the way to bleak failure. Later we had the gift of our own child, Laura, here with our grandchildren Casey and Tara.

We lived in Nevada, Oregon, Washington State, Baltimore, Maryland, Maine, then Ellicott City. Every house we lived in became a showpiece, an artistic reflection of Jane's creative and beautiful mind. We worked side by side redoing every house to match her vision. She had a great eye for antiques and could also turn junk into works of art.

In the woods near Vantage House we found an old cedar fence post from pre-Columbia days. It now stands inside our front door, a remarkably decorative piece.

Jane's major in art school was fashion design. When we lived in Spokane she was a model for Nordstrom for several years. Fashion was her forte. She designed and made clothes for herself and for Laura. I still think that prom dress was a little too daring, Laura. I mentioned Jane is watching today to see who is here; she is also looking carefully at what everyone is wearing.

Just before her death Jane got a note from Tara, our 12 year old grandchild, which read in part: "You taught me to follow my dreams. I know that whatever dream I choose to pursue, you will be right next to me in spirit guiding me." Tara is quite an artist like her grandmother.

Eight years ago Divine Providence again entered our life in a major manner. A friend from this church invited us to dinner at Vantage House. We dined with four residents who spoke positively of their experience. We got details; we looked around. On the way home I said to Jane, "What do you think?" Her reply, "Let's do it."

We didn't know Jane had Alzheimer's when we moved. The radical change of environment suddenly made her memory loss more obvious. Over the past eight years our lifestyle has changed gradually but greatly. We stopped going to Rehoboth, stopped going out to dinner with friends, stopped going to plays or movies. Eventually we stopped going to Sunday Mass and substituted a week day Mass. Why did we stop? It became too confusing, too many unknowns, too many strangers or people who seemed like strangers.

Think about it. If you couldn't remember how you got here or why you're here or where you're going when you leave and you can't recognize anyone near you, you might decide you never want to come back again. That's why we narrowed our world to familiar, repetitive routine. It was calming, reassuring to go to the Mall for lunch, park outside Nordstrom, enter the store, up on the escalator, walk on the right side and down on the escalator to the eatery. We had the same subway sandwich every day. Back on the lower level, the right side, through Nordstrom to the car. To alter the path could cause confusion, frustration, and an emotional storm.

We followed this routine probably 350 days a year for the past two or three years. Jane was always happy to go. It was familiar enough not to be confusing, different enough to be interesting. Because of memory loss the store windows were always new for her.

There was a time when we talked about art, politics, religion, philosophy, everything. With memory gone conversation narrowed to the weather, the trees, the clouds, the traffic, the crowds, fashion.

One area we continued to talk about seven or eight hours a week, often two or three hours at a time. We talked openly, freely about her Alzheimer's. We talked about changes in her thinking, about her forgetting, her losing things, about things she could no longer do, things she wanted to do, about her fears, her sadness, her anger, about death, about our love, about God.

I always told her she might lose her ability to think but she would never lose her ability to love. Her loving heart was always open to others no matter how fearful or lost her day had been. Residents and staff at Vantage House tell me how they loved to see her, her beautiful smile, her warm greeting. She lived her feelings and others responded to them. The words were not important.

We often talked about death in recent months. Her greatest fear was she would die and I would be alone. I told her if I died first she would forget me because her memory was failing so badly. But if she died first I would always remember her and she would live on in my thoughts and in my heart, so we would continue to be together. My prayer is answered.

During the last week of her life I was with her almost constantly. When she was frightened or anxious or restless I tried to console her and would stroke her cheek or hold her face in my hands and say to her, "I'm here, love. I'm here. Everything is going to be all right. Everything is going to be just fine." She didn't realize the fine print said, "But you have to die first."

She wondered what I will do without her. I wonder too. On occasion I'm sure I'll hear her say, "I'm right here, love. I'm here. Everything is going to be all right. It's going to be just fine." But Jane was so honest and so exacting she will add, "Don't forget to read the fine print, Robbie." I know a generous God will share this gentle woman with me. After all, I always shared her with God.

A comment to our children and grandchildren. If you are wishing this bright star of our world to return, know this. She lived each day losing things, forgetting things, not knowing where she was, what was happening, or whom she was talking to. The result for this intelligent, creative, gentle woman was to feel stupid most of the time and crazy about half the time. Sometimes I would take her in my arms and say, "Love, you are not and never will be crazy. You are not stupid. You have Alzheimer's."

Now she can know she was a brilliant, capable, remarkable woman with passion for those she loved, for the beauty of God's creation, and for God. She lived the life her God-given feelings brought her. Don't wish her back.

Jane's book about her Alzheimer's, in which her granddaughter, Casey, wrote the epilogue, was published in 2009. Soon after that her writing began to fail miserably. She couldn't think of what she wanted to say and then when she knew what she wanted to say she couldn't find the words and when she found the words she couldn't spell them. This is the last coherent paragraph she wrote dated August 16, 2010. "God, how quickly comes your love to me. Can I join with your pain and suffering? Could I? I do not feel any words are needed to explain to you. You are with me. I know I must think and learn about my condition. I want to carry it well for myself and my loved ones and for you. I pray to go to heaven to find the Creator of love, the Mother of peace." Jane joined in Jesus' pain and suffering and now she joins in his resurrection.

My thanks to Father Tillman, our former pastor, who so generously returned from vacation to be here, thanks to our long time friend Father Joe Heim of Maryknoll, and thanks to Father Bowen for his careful attention during Jane's illness and for his generosity today. And thanks to Father Ferdinand for his presence.

And thanks to all of you for your love for Jane and your comforting presence today.

Instead of a going away party it turns out to be "a coming home party." Let's celebrate it. Come and have some lunch with us in the room next door and meet our wonderful children and grandchildren.

After the service, we had a catered light lunch which 75 people attended. There must have been well over 300 at the service. About 20 residents and a number of staff members came from Vantage House. The whole affair was a tribute to the warmth and charm and loveliness of my beautiful wife. Those who were there reflected back to me the love and goodness she had shown them. It was a grace filled, people filled, Jane filled occasion.

Father Tillman was our pastor for several years and has been mentioned in prior notes. It was very kind of him to return from vacation to say the Memorial Mass. I was very grateful. Attached is an email I sent him after the service.

Dear Dick,
I just had to drop you a note and again thank you for your generosity and graciousness in coming for Jane's Memorial Service. Considering where she is, if there is one thing that could have added to her happiness, you gave it to her. I shall be ever grateful for your shepherding the two of us and for giving Jane the special welcome she always felt with you . . . . and the special goodbye.

I'm doing well. I'm very sad at times but I don't deeply mourn a loss that was a gift to her and a blessing for me. I do not for a moment wish her back
Gratefully,
Bob

3/6/12
Laura, Casey, and Tara left yesterday after lunch. It was a grand and fulfilling visit for all of us. It was very different from any visits we had over the past six or seven years. Those visits always had the pall of Jane's Alzheimer's covering all that occurred. I believe we all forgot how visits used to be. It was refreshing, renewing.

I feel a tinge of guilt when I write that because it sounds like Jane is being blamed for times that were different or unpleasant. Not so! When I mentioned that kind of feeling yesterday, Laura reassured me her mother sees things much more clearly and more peacefully now. I know that is true.

After the Memorial Mass my daughter, Frances, invited the family to her house for dinner. Bob, my son from Seattle, and John, my son from Kentucky were here. John brought his thirteen year old daughter, Samantha, with him. It was a pleasant afternoon and evening.

I took the shard which Jane gave Fran at Fran's birthday party five years ago, the party that became a major issue for Jane. In fact that party was the last time we got together with Fran and her family. When I gave Fran the shard I told her Jane is in a place where all life's misunderstandings are no longer valid and I know Jane wanted her to have it five years ago, but her thinking became tainted with emotional reactions due to the Alzheimer's. Fran seemed understanding and pleased.

I have lots of "left over thoughts" from the past eleven days. If I count the days it is eleven days since Jane died. But I believe it is twelve days since she died. I believe she died the evening of February 22nd, which was Ash Wednesday, the beginning of Lent for Christians.

Bonnie arrived from Iowa that evening and got to Jane's room about 7p.m. Kathie was already there with me. Jane was unconscious, heavily sedated, breathing unevenly. Bonnie stroked her mother's face and spoke to her.

After Kathie and Bonnie left I was sitting near the bottom of the bed with my left hand gently rubbing Jane's feet and my right hand holding my rosary. There was no fan in the room and no air conditioner operating. No one entered the room or left it during this time. Suddenly I felt a cool, almost soothing puff of air on the back of my neck. I looked around because I thought someone had gone by, although there was little space for a person to get by without my moving. Within three or four seconds I felt the same thing again. It may seem farfetched, ridiculous fantasy, but I believe God's messenger came for Jane and took her spirit away at that moment. I think her soul left her body then. The physical machine was left behind to run down in due course, which it did about 5a.m. the next morning. Why couldn't the spirit leave the body without death occurring? I believe there is some debate among theologians as to when the soul inhabits the body of the fetus. We simply assume when the soul leaves, the body dies. It could be otherwise. I believe it was with Jane.

I woke once or twice during that night and noted Jane's breathing had not markedly changed. When I woke at 5a.m., the nurses were arranging her body. They said she just died. After they left I sat and held Jane's warm hand and said the rosary. Then I collected my things and left. Later that morning I went to the mortuary.

A lay minister from our church was there Wednesday afternoon to place ashes on the forehead of the Catholics on the unit. I received ashes and asked him to place them lightly on Jane which he did with the words, "Remember that thou art dust and unto dust thou shalt return." Jane was prepared for cremation the following morning.

There was another interesting coincidence that night on the nursing unit. The two staff members taking care of Jane were the two who had come to the apartment in the summer of 2010 when Jane was threatening to jump off the balcony.

3/7/12
How can the days seem so full when I feel so empty! They are filled with all sorts of things I feel pressure to get done as if they are important. Nothing is really important. I just act like it is.

I exercise shortly after 6a.m. I set the alarm but usually wake before it rings. I exercise longer than I could when Jane was napping in the afternoons. I shower and then prepare breakfast. Before eating I say the prayers we used to say as we stood together in the kitchen. It is one of the moments I feel closest to Jane. I hold my arms as if to embrace her and although I don't feel anything I know she fills them. I close the prayer as we always did, "We pray for courage, charity, compassion, patience, and our love."

I completed about thirty of the acknowledgement cards provided by the mortician. Yesterday morning I took five bags of Jane's clothing to the Christian Women's Charity. Then I went to Mass and had lunch with our friend Dennis.

I got rid of a number of things in the apartment. There were at least 500 paper doilies. They show up everywhere. I trashed about two dozens tissue boxes and about twenty of the cardboard cores from toilet paper rolls. Jane could not bear the thought of "trashing" them. I "disposed" of them. I put on a jacket I haven't worn in a while and found a little rock in the pocket. Jane, Jane what a sweet and innocent child of God you were.

Before leaving the apartment I usually tell Jane where I'm going and what I'm going to do. On return I expect to open the door without a key because she was always there when I came back. I usually tell her where I've been and what I did. All of this is an old habit. I have no desire to change it. She is still here with me. Of course she knows where I'm going and what I've done but I like to tell her about it anyway.

Her cinerarium and her eight-by-ten picture are on a beautiful antique trunk in front of our mantel. In her picture she is smiling the smile that charmed the world and filled our life with warmth and tenderness and beauty. It was taken shortly after we moved into Vantage House. Sometimes I sit nearby and say the rosary or just talk to her a bit and tell her how dear she was to me and how much I love her.

On the trunk I've added a few items that were hers, are hers. One is a piece of cement and rock which is actually a piece of the curb from the parking area at the Mall. A snow plow broke it off I'm sure. One day as we walked from Macy's back to the car Jane spotted it. Actually she saw it on the way in but I assured her no one would take it before we came out. It's a piece about eight inches long, five wide, and two on the higher end. It even has some of the red (do not park) paint on one end. It is so Jane. It was her treasure. Now it is mine. So it sits on the trunk by her picture. In front of it is a large perfectly shaped dried oak leaf. On the cement is a smaller dried leaf with a tinge of yellow and orange still present. On the cinerarium is one of her paper doilies (six inch diameter) with a piece of dried, beautifully tanned, beautifully shaped piece of bark, about two inches in size. Finally toward the front of the trunk there is a slender dried tree branch about six feet tall, slender at the bottom and spreading out about thirty inches at the top across the ceiling. Jane found it in front of our building well over two years ago and persuaded me to bring it home. It has been in its present position ever since.

While cleaning out things in my area of the studio I found the pair of white gloves Jane was wearing the first day I saw her. I have kept them through the years. I used to carry them in my briefcase when I went to the office. Now they help adorn the trunk.

In addition to all the above I placed the cards of sympathy and the Mass cards there. Yes, it is something of a shrine to this woman who enshrined me with her love and her goodness. It is a comfortable place to stand, to kneel, or to sit in a chair nearby and just be with her for a time.

It was nice to take this time and be away from "busy, busy" and think more clearly, more properly, more gratefully about this woman who not only filled my life with her own beauty but who filled me with God's beauty in trees and rocks and clouds and sunsets, who showed me the beauty of windows and doors and buildings and paintings, who brought me the beauty of life in all its fullness because she was here.

3/11/12

I went to the 9a.m. Mass this Sunday morning. It was for Jane. When her name was mentioned I couldn't hold back the tears. There were memories of the many times we attended that service. I don't think I was ever in that worship space without her. Memories of the times we were there when she was well. We were Eucharistic Ministers together then. Memories of more recent times when I held her arm to guide her up to Communion and then back to our place. The contrast struck me forcefully.

I'm not sure I realized how ill she was even though I lived with it every day. Now I can see more clearly how incapacitated she had become. How did she keep going! How could she face the day! Was she doing it so as not to fail me? Was it her determination to hold onto what little life she had? Was she keeping us going?

Was I deceiving myself that everything was all right? Was I too selfish, too self-centered to acknowledge her helplessness? She was really quite helpless. She had difficulty doing her make-up and her hair. She had difficulty choosing what to wear and getting it on properly. She had difficulty eating, picking up the food on her fork or spoon. She often spilled food on her clothing. She often spilled coffee on her robe during breakfast. She had difficulty brushing her teeth although she was very conscientious about doing so. That was probably a tribute to our son, Paul, who is our dentist. She had toileting problems which may certainly have contributed to the urinary tract infection that led to her death.

She was never aware of where we were going until we got there, even though I told her before we left our apartment. She recognized familiar places once we arrived. The unfamiliar was always strange and sometimes frightening. She never remembered where we had been once we got home. She never knew who people were or how we knew them. My attempts to identify "these strangers" were often futile.

Now I contrast this poor, helpless love of mine with the vibrant, enthusiastic, creative woman of our years prior to the onset of Alzheimer's. But I still found that earlier Jane in this increasingly infirm woman who became more dependent on me as the days turned to weeks, the weeks to months, and the months to years. Our presence to one another was not lessened by her increasing absence from life. The tender times of being together were not diminished by the harshness of her emotional storms. Our long conversations about her illness, future plans, death, and God, were never darkened by her lack of contact with the rest of our world. The warmth and pleasure of intimate intervals never lost what Alzheimer's could not take away.

I am shocked now when I confront the stark reality of her illness and how poorly she was doing. Her very presence, the tender times, the talking times, the intimate times did not conceal her illness but they made me overlook what was really happening. All our life I was overwhelmed with the depth and beauty of these features which consistently nourished our love. I could not believe her life was slipping away while our love continued to thrive. Now her life is gone; her love is not. Love has many forms, many disguises. Love does not die, not love like ours. I think of all the ways God has shown me love. I can't prove God's love; I just know it. I knew Jane's love; I know it still.

3/13/12
The following is a letter I wrote to the Director of Vantage House.

Dear Meriann,   March 12, 2012

During the past several years many Vantage House employees exhibited remarkable thoughtfulness and kindness to my recently deceased wife, Jane. They did a variety of things to help her be more secure, more comfortable, and more peaceful.

Employees from every department were involved in one way or another with her care either by some direct service to her or simply by a friendly greeting and a warm acknowledgement of her presence. I hope each of those employees fully realizes how meaningful and how reassuring it was for Jane to hear a cheerful hello, to see a pleasant smile, or to have the chance to stop and say a few words. Their responses made her dark days brighter and her stormy days less frightening. These Vantage House employees remained an important part of her shrinking world and brought some peace to her troubled times.

I will probably not have the opportunity to thank each of them personally, but I want each of them to know I will always be grateful for the gift of their caring. The memory of their kindness will always remain part of my world here.

As you know, you played an important part in all that transpired and I am grateful for your role in Jane's care. Please, let others know how grateful I am for their generous attention and gentle affection for this loving woman.

Sincerely,

Bob McAllister

I've been clearing out more things. Most of Jane's clothes are gone and I've been going through old letters she received and volumes of cards she bought to send the children and various other people. I'm sorting through our many books. Here and there I find little pieces of paper on which she wrote some thought she had. She did that all her life. Some of these are striking. "I go to a place where no one matters. I am there, but where . . . . indescribable . . . . no words could form a picture, no drawing a scene. I'm not even alone because I don't know myself, no words, just being there in full total fear. Only you would understand, only you would have the words that connect us, as always."

Other notes I found: "I hate this life. I hate where it's going. I wish I could die now! Of what am I afraid if I continue to live? Uncertainty? The change to death?" "Now I know, but do not 'understand' or 'remember.' Two very important points of almost everything. Not knowing of what I did . . . . what can I possibly act on, do, remember, or anything?" "Snow flakes. How strangely they fall? What causes that to happen? Why there? Why that direction? No answers ever needed. The thought of being there overcame every fear and worry, every other thought. I became wrapped in my warm soul and beating heart!" "I can find no peace in my heart and can't find my way back to it, or if it really still lives there." "Oh, Robbie. I love you so much. Let me hold you. I'm sorry I upset you. Please, forgive me." "I want to die now or as soon as possible. What I see ahead is like today, this evening. The present bonds are broken. I know not myself or my love, he is someone else!" Apparently she wrote this one at Mass. "My darling, you and I are within my heart and soul always, always. It allows breathing, peace. Actually I enter into a place of peace while still being part of God's Mass. What a gift!"

Finding these notes was like finding snapshots of recent years. Each one is a picture from her life and the radical fluctuations she experienced. She wrote bits and pieces of her pain filled story and she lived and studied every moment of it. If her keen observational ability made the beauty of falling snow fill her with warmth, it also increased the breadth and intensity of her fears and her sense of failure.

It is hard for me to read the sad and fear filled notes. Where was I? Why didn't she come and tell me these thoughts? The notes remind me of bad times. I know we had them. I have written about them in some detail. They were not our life. That was not who we were and not who we became. That was her illness. I knew that and could hold onto that knowledge. Jane could not hold onto it. When we sat and talked calmly and closely (that's a good expression for how we talked–closely), she could accept that the illness caused much of her behavior. Of course she never remembered. I think the worst part of her suffering was to believe she was a bad person and did things to hurt me and others. She wanted so much to be a good person. I think it was an element in her relationship with God. She wanted "to be true" to God the same way she was so completely true to me.

As I go over these things in my mind my overriding thought is, "Now she knows! Now she knows!" I cry when I write those words because that was the important thing I could never do for her. I could never convince her that deep down inside she was a good person, a good woman. My tears are for joy. Now she knows!

During the last years of Jane's life I recognized much of her world was separate from mine. I could not fully appreciate how strange, how different her world was. Her observations of events, her reactions to incidents, her response to others' behavior was often different than mine and different than what her response used to be. I tried to cross the distance that separated her world from mine. I tried to understand what her world was like for her. Although I never reached any clear grasp of its complexity and instability, I was comforted by my efforts and felt she was too.

Jane is now in a distant world and I know no meaningful way to span what lies between us. In the past I could devote myself to bridging the growing space between our worlds. I could do things. I could say things. I could feel the distance diminish and at times almost disappear. Now there is only mystery. I can pray and I do. I can talk to her and I do. I can love her and I do. But the air is empty of her words and her laughter. My eyes see the lovely, full smile of her picture and they see the branches she brought from the woods to add to the beauty of her decorating our small world. But they don't see her smile turn serious or playful. I touch the places she touched in our apartment. I feel the pillow she slept on, the dishes she washed, the clothes she wore. But I don't feel the hair I used to help her wash, the hand I used to hold when we walked, the lips I kissed one hundred times a day.

What do I do now? How do I live without Jane in my life? I want to believe she is still in my life. I want to believe she knows what I'm doing, that I miss her, that I love her, that she sees me, that she hears me. This spiritual world is a rather unsatisfactory world. It is terribly one sided. I continue on. I pray. I weep. I say everything is fine and I'm doing well. I go through the motions of living without the emotions of life. I'm enmeshed in the feelings of death.

There is no response from Jane. There is no response from God. How will I know if either one responds? I don't expect a voice or a vision. I don't need either one. What do I need? To wait and believe. God has never spoken to me but I strongly believe He has been very present in my life. I always believed Jane's presence in my life was a sign of God's love. It seems the only thing I can do to bridge the space between us now is to believe what my heart tells me and to forgo what my senses cry out for.

3/14/12

Lying in bed last night before I went to sleep it occurred to me I must prepare to end these notes. After all they began as notes about Jane's Alzheimer's. More correctly they began as an accounting of our struggle with the disease. And I thought the writing might help me maintain a clearer perspective as the complexity of Alzheimer's unfolded in the person of my beloved. Both of those goals were reasonably met.

Jane is gone. I will not say she died of Alzheimer's but had she not had the disease she would quite likely still be alive. None of that matters now. She is gone. And I live on without her.

It is not **our** life any more. It is **my** life. Alzheimer's is over for Jane and for Robbie. Why am I so reluctant to stop writing about it? Jane lives in these pages, painfully at times, fearfully and sadly at times. She also lives in them with spirit, determination, charm, wit, and warmth. To keep writing is to hold onto the latter but not without the stain of the former.

What I want most to do is just go on and on writing about her, telling different stories about her life, our life, telling about Jane before the illness came and began to creep mercilessly throughout the cells of her brain. She was so bright, so charming, so beautiful, so loving. She was the star of my life from the moment I first saw her. Others also knew her sparkle and her warmth and responded to it. I could go on page after page but it would all say the same thing in different ways, but the same thing. I might never stop writing about my love for her if I felt free to do so. But that was not the intent or the goal of these pages.

I went to Mass at the Shrine of Saint Anthony today. It's the place where we went last Christmas Day to see the crib. It was our only religious service for Christmas. It's where we went to Mass for a year or more after Jane was "done with our parish." It's where we went on warm fall days and sat by the replica of the Lourdes grotto. It's where she said to me one day last autumn, "After I'm gone, I will meet you here."

Mass was at noon. I got there a little after eleven. The day was unusually warm for early March. I sat on the bench where we always sat and talked. I talked to her and reminded her of what she said last October. I really didn't expect a response. But as I talked about it, the air stirred as it did in the room the night before she died. The breath of air was warm and gentle and seemed to encircle me. I am making more of it than I know it to be, but I had a feeling. In truth, there was a slight, unstable breeze and a warm sun.

As I looked at the statue of the Virgin Mary, white and glistening in her cove in the huge rock grotto, I couldn't help but smile. When we sat there together Jane hardly mentioned the statue. What attracted her was the intricate and complex construction of the grotto. And later as we walked a path looking at the beautiful bronze outdoor Stations of the Cross, Jane was captured by the blades of grass and various flowers and weeds that showed the bite of fall. While I saw and admired the obvious, Jane always found the mystery and beauty of what lay hidden in it or maybe along side of it.

I went by the Mall briefly today before going to Mass. There were a couple of people we used to wave to or say a brief hello. I somehow thought Jane would want them to know she is gone and that's why they don't see us anymore. If she was here and we were not going, she would want me to let them know "so they won't worry about us."

I plan to move to a one bedroom apartment soon. It is one floor up and has basically the same view we had from our dining room and living room. I will be able to take all the furniture she loved. The mirrors and pictures and statues and tree branches and jugs will suffer a selection process.

Laura will be down this coming Saturday and home on Sunday. She will take a number of things home with her, things we talked about when she was here for Jane's service. She and Paul and Kathie continue to be supportive and helpful.

I hope to be accepted to teach again in the Loyola University Pastoral Counseling Program. A grade school teacher we know would welcome my reading to some of the children in her school. I am considering going with a friend to work with Habitat for Humanity in home construction. All these things interest me and I have considerable enthusiasm for getting involved in one or more of them.

Paul wants me to go to Montana with him in August for the cowboy poetry contest. Bob and his wife come from Seattle, and my daughter, Fran, and her husband fly out from here. My nephew, Jim, has quite a reputation for writing cowboy poetry and he participates in the program. I am looking forward to being back in Montana and seeing the ranch again.

It is terrible to say but "I feel I have my life back." That sounds cruel, selfish. It sounds like Jane was a burden and I couldn't wait for her to be gone. Remember the line from the movie, Boys Town, when one boy is carrying another on his back, "He isn't heavy; he's my brother." Jane wasn't a burden, she was my sweetheart. Our life became narrow and limited. Jane accepted it willingly, knowing it gave her more emotional ease. It never felt like a sacrifice for me to live the way we did. Her smile, her presence, her love continued to enrich my life and fill my every want. There is no great joy in "having my life back" when it is empty.

It is "my life back" but it is not a life I wanted or a life that will ever be completely satisfying. I hope it will be of value to others in some way. It will have good times and bad times; it will have love from and for family and friends; it will have joy and sorrow. It will never have "times" with Jane, or love with Jane, or living joy and sorrow with Jane. It will never be the same. I am waiting to go home. That will be with Jane.

3/16/12

On the way to Mass today I felt I should mourn Jane more severely than I do. I used to think about her dying. I pictured I would go to Mass rarely and only on a Tuesday or Thursday, the days we usually went. I would not go to the dining room but would have my meals delivered for at least a few weeks. I would keep very much to myself. And I would be immeasurably and uncontrollably sad.

Why has my mourning not taken that course? For some time I have been praying to the Blessed Mother "to come to my aid in times of need and to comfort me in times of sorrow." I think my prayer life and my spiritual contacts have been of great help and comfort.

But there is something more. I have been mourning the loss of Jane for several years. I have been losing her a little more each day. It was not always noticeable. It was never really measureable. But now when I think of Jane I can't get back to the Jane of "the good old days." The Jane I remember is a Jane for whom life no longer came graciously or generously, a Jane who knew life was deteriorating and struggled gallantly but fruitlessly to restore what could no longer be.

Mourning Jane severely would be false. How can I mourn severely an event I do not completely regret? I mourn her loss in my life but I do not wish her back. I am grateful God took her in God's own good time. I could say it was an answer to my prayers. I did not pray for Jane to die but I prayed for her to be relieved of her fears and her despair. (I wasn't aware of the fine print either.) I prayed that when she died she would know me and she would not be frightened and would be at peace. My prayers were answered. I have moments of overwhelming sadness and a flood of tears but not one time have I wished her back.

I go to dinner, to Mass, and do other things because I think Jane would want me to do this. I know she wouldn't want me to sit around and weep for her or for myself. That was not her earthly character. She had spirit, courage, imagination, enthusiasm. I want to follow her in those graces as best I can.

3/23/12

I recently read through this complete section. A couple of items got my attention. On January 8th, "when I am with Jane, I am lonely for her." On January 30th, "I need to know now how it will end . . . How long, oh Lord, how long?" My mourning the loss of Jane began a long time ago. It was preparation for her ultimate loss.

Suddenly a biblical verse comes to mind: "Now is the acceptable time. Now is the day of salvation," St. Paul in 2 Corinthians. Perhaps my unconscious or perhaps Jane is suggesting this story should end now. It is the acceptable time. The Alzheimer's story is over. The love story will go on and that is the day of salvation.

To consider stopping seems momentous. This work became increasingly important to me during the past five years. It allowed me to put into words thoughts I could not speak, feelings I did not understand, and faith I could not fathom. It reported a journey into an unknown world filled with complexity and uncertainty with a companion who was braver than anyone I ever knew and with more love than I ever thought existed in one person.

There is no adequate way to end this story other than to use the prayer card that ended Jane's journey. When we went to a card store to buy a card for any occasion, Jane always chose a beautiful card with a short message. She always said, "I don't like cards that use a lot of words to say what can be better said in a few words."

It was so easy to choose Jane's prayer card from the hundreds that were available. On one side, a scene taken from God's world of nature: trees, clouds, sunshine. No words, just God's picture. On the other side:

In Memory of
Jane A. McAllister
January 24, 1930
February 23, 2012

Indian Prayer
Do not stand at my grave and
weep, I am not there. I do not
sleep. I am a thousand winds
that blow, I am the diamond
glint on snow. I am the
sunlight on ripened grain, I am
the gentle autumn rain.
When you wake in morning hush, I
am the swift uplifting rush Of
quiet birds in circling flight. I
am the soft starlight at night.
Do not stand at my grave and cry,
I am not there. I did not die.